the
hormone
z**o**ne

Navigate Metabolism Towards
Whole Health Transformation

Dr. John Alexander Robinson

The Hormone Zone: Navigate Metabolism Towards Whole Health Transformation

Published by:
Intermedia Publishing, Inc.
P.O. Box 2825
Peoria, Arizona 85380
www.intermediapub.com

ISBN 978-1-935906-88-9

DEDICATION

To those who believed in me, and to those who did not. A reminder that everyone you meet has a role to play in your development and that inspiration derives from your moral compass of truth and perspective.

This book is foremost dedicated to my faithful patients, trusting me with their most precious commodity. You all deserve my highest respect. The level of intimacy so graciously bestowed is constantly awe-inspiring for me and I thank you. You have all been and continue to be "patient" patients, and appreciative of my endeavors to improve my approach as your physician. I have learned the deepest of secrets from so many of you. This book is for you, by you, and to you.

To my daughter, who has inspired me to greater heights as a father with her mere presence and penetrating smile. To her goes a special kind of love emanating from some unknown distant place that lives so deeply and familiarly in my heart. To my mother, who has believed in me continually throughout my life. She is a rock of stability and a beacon of light. To my entire family and all my friends, who have supported me in my never-ending endeavors, providing a gentle compass reminder of where I came from and who I am.

And finally, let this book also stand as a small love note of appreciation to the one person I owe so much. She has been there for me through my entire development as a physician, providing a unique perspective of truth and a constant reminder of her faith in me. During the many hours I spent in my bubble pecking away at the keyboard for this book, she stood faithfully by, supporting me, encouraging me. Our connection has been, since the beginning, an almost ineffable desire. This love is often so inexplicable, so real, that it removes the very voice of the poet, and brings him, with a smile, to a calm sense of understanding and peace. She is the true love of my life. Humbly, I thank you.

Contents

Section 2

Chapter 4

Section 4   175

Completing the Metabolic Triad: Thyroid, Adrenals and Sex Hormones

Chapter 9   177

Adrenal Dysfunction: An Overview

Step 4: Balancing the Sex Hormones for an Optimized You

Step 5: Thyroid Hormone Treatment and Thyroid Gland Optimization:

Appendices

FOREWORD

Dr. John Alexander Robinson is undoubtedly one of the most hormone-knowledgeable physicians available today to patients and other physicians. As I read his book, *THE HORMONE ZONE: Navigate Metabolism Towards Whole Health Transformation*, I could not help but think of my face-to-face meeting with him at a conference four years ago where I had given a presentation. Most of us humans can sense extremely high intelligence and extraordinary knowledge when we meet it head on, and that was my experience with Dr. Robinson—despite his comparative youth. His youth is noteworthy in that, upon reading THE HORMONE ZONE, readers will take comfort in knowing that he has decades to provide wise clinical care and to write more exceptional books.

I remember my conversation with Dr. Robinson at that conference. I was impressed with the depth and breadth of his knowledge of metabolism and how hormones regulate it. I was not surprised, as most naturopathic medical physicians are well educated about metabolic disorders and their treatment. But Dr. Robinson's knowledge, obvious to me, went far deeper. As the contents of *THE HORMONE ZONE* tell me, his knowledge of hormones and health has grown even deeper, and it matches that of any other physician or researcher I know who is an expert in the field.

Dr. Robinson's descriptions of the various hormones, especially thyroid hormone, and their affects on our bodies and minds are crystal clear. With his clear prose, he explains how to use hormones and synergistic medicinal agents to enhance one's health, giving an abundance of treatment guidelines that will prove helpful to both patients and their physicians. *THE HORMONE ZONE* is comprehensive, covering each of the hormones our health depends on, and he has massively documented his full coverage from the scientific literature. One must admire the weight he bore on his shoulders, practicing clinically as he did, while assembling the complete coverage of hormones and health in his book.

Dr. Robinson eloquently explains that to acquire and maintain good health, we must cease to depend *exlusively* on conventional medical practice, while not abandoning it altogether. In the 1980s, the famed Robert S. Mendelsohn, MD turned away from that exclusive style of practice which he had taught at Loma Linda School of Medicine for some thirty years. He then called it "cut-burn-and-poison" medicine. Of course, conventional medicine has been a boon to mankind when we have used it thoughtfully and selectively. The mistake of those who advocate that style of medicine alone, as Robinson notes, is their overuse and over-dependence upon it. Dr. Robinson explains this in detail with the diplomacy of a nineteenth century British aristocrat. His clear and polite discourse is a refreshing tempering of tone. I say this as one of a cadre who opposed restriction to conventional medicine alone long enough ago that only with a harsh tone could we be heard. But Dr. Robinson explains the matter in terms palatable enough even for hardcore advocates of conventional medicine alone. And his words are persuasive as he explains how that approach limits personal responsibility and freedom and can deprive one of optimal health.

I strongly recommend *THE HORMONE ZONE* to physicians who have recently become interested in alternatives to conventional medicine alone. These physicians, often called "crossover doctors," will find Dr. Robinson's book a practical unabridged handbook, heavily scientifically documented, yet an easy-to-read segue into the integration of conventional and natural medicine.

All those seeking to improve their health—even those without a medical background—will benefit from Dr. Robinson's point-by-point guidance to integrating the best of both natural and conventional medicine. He adroitly expresses the philosophy of open-mindedly and flexibly using what works best from *any* health care discipline. His implicit rationale is that metabolic disorders can be sustained or relieved by physical, hormonal, nutritional, psychological, and spiritual phenomena, and he explains how one can properly address each of these.

Vade mecum is a Latin term that means "go with me." It refers to a book so valuable to the reader that he or she virtually always carries it around for easy and helpful reference. I predict that *THE HORMONE ZONE* will be the *vade mecum* of thousands of readers, myself included. I keep a few such books on my desk to refer to when I consult with patients and physicians. *THE HORMONE ZONE* is now among those reference books on my desk.

I trust that the value I feel in *THE HORMONE ZONE* and my admiration for Dr. John Alexander Robinson's extraordinary feat in writing the book is obvious. I strongly recommend that this exceptional book be in your library, close at hand for easy reference to scientifically-sound information on hormones and health. I trust also that you will find his unique style of prose as gripping as I have. Dr. Robinson and *THE HORMONE ZONE* have my most enthusiastic endorsement.

John C. Lowe, M.A., D.C.

Dr. John Alexander Robinson

PREFACE

"If I have seen farther than other men, it is by standing on the shoulders of giants."
—Sir Isaac Newton

This book has been a labor of love. It has been a compilation of experiences and research into the art of medicine and the complexities of the human condition. For me, this is the start of taking action on my passion for writing and sharing what I have learned. This book is for the curious patient who is willing to delve into their inner self, and for those looking for another piece to the puzzle of their status in health and in life. This book will help you explore your endocrine system, the world of hormones. I offer you a platform to learn about metabolic health and its "energy of change," the balanced complexities of nutrition, the effects of the mind on the body and many other things. But first things first....

I admit that I "stand on the shoulders of giants" while I, to invoke the spirit of poet Walt Whitman, "sound *my* barbaric yawp over the rooftops of the world" about *natural* things. But be neither fooled nor misguided about the perfection of the natural world, as the maxim has long been known…"nature unaided fails." This is not about controlling nature, but rather assisting it to come to boundless fruition. The natural world and physical phenomena desire the hand of human reason and choice to illuminate itself through the power of change, through the power of *metabole*. And we must ever diligently move towards perfecting the moment we find ourselves dubiously within, through research, reason and reflection. This book seeks to start that conversation towards betterment and change: for my patients, for my colleagues, for a world that may reach out to it, if only briefly.

In sharing my knowledge, personal perspective and experiences as a physician, it is "on the shoulders of giants" that have come before me, and those adepts who have shared a collective experience of medical knowledge with me. My professional relationship with Gino Tutera, M.D. has provided me with a wealth of knowledge and experience since I stepped, bright-eyed and green-eared, into the world of medicine. To him goes a very special level of gratitude and credit towards my understanding of endocrinology, particularly within the realm of sex hormones, gynecology and subcutaneous pellet hormone therapy, of which he has pioneered since 1992. We have shared countless experiences together about the subject in a very large practice with other talented and dedicated physicians, leading me to a deep sense of understanding, gratitude and pride. From this platform, and coupled with my training as a naturopathic physician, I have been able to develop my own personal and unique approach to endocrinology and hormone replacement therapy, in any delivery method, for my patients.

Without the blazing efforts and keen and meticulous mind of John C. Lowe, so many people would be suffering needlessly with thyroid conditions and fibromyalgia. From this world-class expert I have learned to look deeper into the rationality of medicine and am willing to act with painstaking precision when treating patients. His opus, *The Metabolic Treatment of Fibromyalgia*, provided a foundation of knowledge to properly utilize thyroid hormone treatment in my practice, knowing that what I was doing was supported by science and a rational perspective that is all to often devoid within the political landscape of medicine. Much of my work and expertise in the field of thyroidology is due to his diligent work. His passion for his craft and his patients knows no bounds.

Every naturopathic doctor knows his or her history, the lineage of physicians who helped inculcate the profession into a seamless paradigm of both past and present medical thought. Naturopathic medicine builds upon the generations before. The medical truths that are *re*-covered within the science and art of naturopathic medicine are, if observed correctly, timeless and consistent. Therefore, naturopathic medicine does not discard the old as dated and useless, but incorporates and conserves its collective truths about natural phenomena within the medical model, and thus uplifts any new medical perspectives towards improving the human condition. Any naturopathic physician you see comes equipped with the ability to tap into a very long lineage of medical insights. So, to all of them, from the past elders, to my teachers in medical school, from my effervescent classmates, to my current fellow colleagues, I am most deeply and humbly in debt.

*****

Disclaimer: *As with all information in this book, please seek the advice of a professionally licensed healthcare provider before making any changes. Medically prescribed medications must be treated with the utmost care and respect before stopping them. The advice contained within this book is not meant to consist of a diagnosis, but as a guide to be used by you and your healthcare provider so that you may work together to create your best overall health.*

Section 1
Defining Metabolic Health

Introduction

The words "metabolism" and "metabolic health" will be used often in the course of this book. Metabolism is the underlying process within all of your body cells, both physically and metaphysically, that drives the forces that allow you to realize health. The word "metabolism" comes from the Greek word *metabole* which

> The word "metabolism" comes from the Greek word *metabole* which means "to change."

means "to change." When I write of the concept of metabolic health throughout this book, I am referring to the process of creating a space for unbridled change to happen in all aspects of your being.

This book will provide you with some direction and guidance for your health goals in understanding how metabolism affects every aspect of your being. It is written for the patient as a handbook, guide and resource. It is also written for the healthcare provider as a guide, an alternative view and an additional perspective on a relevant medical topic that is open for debate and improvement.

We will see that metabolism, or the ability to offer change in the body, is affected by many elements, and metabolism in turn exerts its effects back on these elements. Some of these key elements are physical health including nutritional and structural components, mental health, emotional support and love, moral integrity and spiritual understanding. These key concepts are vital in order to keep human metabolism alive and well. My goal is to illuminate these key concepts to allow the reader to explore the layers of their own metabolic health to improve their well-being.

Often, metabolism is thought of only as the "ability to lose body fat" or "your sense of energy." These are two important physical aspects of metabolism, but only two of a multitude of processes within your body. I will show that when metabolism is negatively affected and out of balance, every cell in the body will be affected, and this leads to a multitude of symptoms and signs. I will explain how altered metabolism affects thinking and emotions, physical well being, and even spiritual endeavors. You will see how the endocrine system and its vast array of hormones affects metabolism, including a focus on thyroid health. This is a journey about health and change.

What are the Common Diseases of Altered Metabolism?
- Hypothyroidism (low thyroid function)
- Hyperthyroidism (high thyroid function)
- Weight Gain
- Obesity
- Insulin Resistance
- Diabetes
- Menopause
- Andropause
- Fibromyalgia
- Chronic Fatigue Syndrome
- Adrenal Insufficiency/Adrenal Fatigue
- Depression

This book explores altered metabolism with specific attention to diseases of the thyroid and how to overcome them as comprehensively as possible. However, other related metabolic conditions are discussed. The details of the conditions will be explained along with conventional and alternative medical solutions to overcoming conditions related to altered metabolism.

How Do I Use This Book?

This book is written mostly for the patient with a consideration that a healthcare provider will read it and reference it. As the patient, you need to explore every aspect of this book, all the suggestions, all the nuances of the **Metabolic Health Protocol** described in the last section of the book, and then…explore further. There is nothing complete about this or any other book. Continue to explore.

The book is designed for the patient to use as a checklist of conditions, strategies, and possibilities to improve your health. The focus of the book is largely concerned with metabolism, hormonal health and endocrinology, and particularly thyroid disease and its treatment. But the ultimate goal of this book is to guide people towards improved health. Multiple examples of this are presented. Below is an overview:

- **Section 1** reviews some basic concepts about health from an integrated and holistic perspective, the alternative medical art and science of naturopathy and a basic review and explanation of the endocrine system.

- **Section 2** explores thyroid disease, explains conventional diagnosis and treatment, reexamines the utilization of natural thyroid hormone medications and demonstrates how to support thyroid health holistically.

- **Section 3** provides an overview of both menopause and andropause and their hormonal abnormalities. Additionally, the poorly understood and unrecognized condition of adrenal fatigue will be explained by expert and Yale trained naturopathic physician Cristina Romero-Bosch, NMD.

- **Section 4** tackles the very complex and confusing concept of diet, exercise and weight loss with practical and effective solutions.

- **Section 5** brings it all together by offering an in-depth Seven Step Metabolic Health Protocol that takes the reader through a multitude of possibilities to improve their health.

- The Appendices offer a whole host of references and resources.

Be sure to utilize the book continually, reference it often and bring the concepts to your healthcare provider to assist in your health concerns.

Patients today must navigate a lot of change that is happening in the world of medical treatment. There is more information available to patients today than ever before. Many doctors are aware that patients are researching their symptoms by using the Internet or books and they will be open to your questions. Some doctors may not want to be second-guessed.

When feeling ill spurs you to go to the Internet to learn more about what you are feeling, let your doctor know what pieces of information resonated with your particular situation. Then let the doctor use his or her best judgment and knowledge to test your assumptions. Establish that both of you are trying to work toward the best solution for your particular situation. When you both are able to reach this ability to work together, you will have established an ideal doctor-patient relationship. However, sometimes it is difficult to establish this relationship when your ideas about where you want to go with your health completely contrasts with your doctor, particularly in the case of alternative health.

My goal is to lay out suggestions and ideas about the philosophy of healing. But my true desire is for readers to find out what the process of healing, in its true and complete definition, means for them. Let me start with some basic definitions.

Chapter 1
What is Health?

Patients come to me with questions about how they are feeling, their symptoms. They want answers and sometimes they assume that the remedy is simply a certain pill, natural or otherwise, a hormone adjustment or other such isolated item. What I have noticed is that patients are not really telling me that they want an herb or a hormone or a pill. What they really want is the wellness and peace that those things have the potential to represent.

A good analogy of this is money. If you said you wanted money, you do not really want little green pieces of soft paper with dead presidents' faces on it. You want what that money has the potential to represent, such as freedom, power, peace for your family or any of the other myriad things it could represent.

This book is an attempt to present a perspective about health that attempts to demonstrate a system of organization regarding change that can guide you to the wellness and peace you really desire. Yes, it will involve instruction about natural remedies, hormone therapy, thyroid health, nutritional advice and many other things. But it will integrate these isolated items into a system that helps guide you towards a true lifestyle change, which helps to provide you with what you really desire.

Many people view health as it relates to the proper function of their body, without pain or symptoms of any type. This ideal is a singular piece to the overall complex entity that is full human health. As human beings, we possess an integrated system that includes an enormous complexity of potentials.

These potentials include four major health categories:

- 𝕫 Physical: Our body in space and nature.
- 𝕫 Mental: Our intellect and reason.
- 𝕫 Emotional: Our ego and sense of morality and integrity for self and towards others.
- 𝕫 Spiritual: Our essential selves.

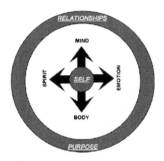

For full health to be realized, all aspects of our being must be nourished and cultivated in order to find the health that we are seeking.

Each of the major health categories is interrelated. One is dependent on the other. Mastery of the physical body allows us to better understand our spiritual nature. If we do not cultivate an understanding of our spiritual nature, then physical symptoms have difficulty in leaving. This holistic approach to the definition of health brings us into a position that permits the realization of the full potential of health to be realized. Ultimately, this holistic view of health will better provide a patient with the ability to create a space where symptoms and pain have difficulty in residing.

> **For full health to be realized, all aspects of our being must be nourished and cultivated in order to find the health that we are seeking.**

Each of these four major health categories contains their own metabolism, their own ability to change, and their own energy process that needs to be properly charged to make the entire human metabolism balanced.

If your goal is complete health, then at some point and on some level, you will need to delve into all the aspects of your health: physical, mental, emotional, and spiritual. Health is a journey of self-realization and a process of transmutation of negative concepts into positive potentials.

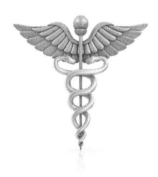

To Heal, To Cure

Two words exist that relate to medicine and its actual pragmatic utility: cure and heal. The words appear to be the same, but there are distinct differences between the two. To cure by definition is to "provide a complete and *permanent* remedy or solution to a *defined* state of being." To heal means, "To *cause* an undesirable condition to be overcome, *restoring* health." The first definition depicts health as an entity; in the second definition health is described as a process. I believe that health is an ongoing process, something that changes constantly, something that you must restore. Health ebbs and flows as a tide, rhythmically. The moment we try to grasp it and define it at a particular moment, it changes, even if only subtly.

We must be prepared to change with our health from moment to moment and remain steadfast on the journey. Disease, therefore, is more of a process than a physical permanent entity. Health is all too often viewed as a static unchanging entity that we are grasping to hold onto. The logical extension of that myth is the view that *disease* is also a static permanent entity that must be excised by surgery or suppressed by drugs. This is called "cure." But this cure does not allow, in most cases, the rest of the system to "change within a process," or to "heal," actively, consistently and constantly to restore balance. To *restore* balance implies constantly moving and changing position to maintain the system. To "restore" also implies replenishing stores constantly as they are utilized. It never ends. Therefore your quest for health never ends; it is a constant journey. Healing is a process that does not fight nature, but honors the physical and quantum laws that dictate it.

If health is a process, then disease also is a process. As we attempt to get well and restore balance to our life, we must honor the process, and give the disease the time and patience any process deserves. In our fast paced culture, we have the expectation of "instantaneous cure" versus "cultivated healing." The social culture of America of instant gratification melds with our ideas of philosophy and science within our medical culture. This is a key reason why the pharmaceutical drug industry is so inculcated within our social consciousness; an instant gratification for a disease "entity" that must be immediately and wholly eradicated and "cured" with a simple pill. The expectation of instantaneous cure comes forth from our instant gratification social norm. Patients fear the time it takes to actually get well and view their health as a process. What they also often fear is the mirror the process inevitably places in front of them, forcing an examination of lifestyle choices, both past and present, and psychological and emotional beliefs and patterns that keep them

> Patients fear the time it takes to actually get well and view their health as a process. What they also often fear is the mirror the process inevitably places in front of them, forcing an examination of lifestyle choices, both past and present, and psychological and emotional beliefs and patterns that keep them in the same state. The fear is of the change. "Resistance to the change" is the definition of pain itself.

in the same state. The fear is of the change. "Resistance to the change" is the definition of pain itself.

This book is about providing instruction and guidance for a process to help heal a common condition so many people face: altered metabolism. This new and holistic paradigm of "disease as process" requires a shift from the old paradigm of avoidance of engagement in every aspect of our health, including the physical, mental, emotional, moral and spiritual elements it contains. If complete health is truly your goal, then take the first step on the journey of health, hold on tight and enjoy the ride. The deeper you delve and the longer you travel the more interesting and rewarding your journey. Seek out experts who listen, experts who see health as a process, experts who honor you as an individual. You will know these experts because they will be looking past their own opinions into the eyes of the patient sitting before them.

A Process of Healing: Begin at the Beginning
The First Step—Become Self-reliant

To do this, you must know yourself. If you do not yet know yourself, have courage towards self-discovery. Plato said we must govern ourselves in finding our own personal autonomy. We must govern our own thoughts and desires, our

> We should not look for answers for ourselves when trying to heal, but answers about ourselves that will lead us to unprecedented understandings and healing.

own beliefs and realizations of truth. But we must know ourselves in order to accomplish this. The process of knowing yourself often comes through a spiritual practice that teaches you to let go of your ego enough to see the true you that remains.

When we are self-reliant, we do not blame others. That which comes from the outside of ourselves is not as much the problem as the things that come from inside ourselves. Blame always hinders the process of healing. We should not blame ourselves; it only leads to festering of our wounds. We often look to blame others for our state of being, versus taking responsibility for our actions. Responsibility does not automatically mean blame; it implies an honoring of the moment and the circumstance in which you find yourself. So take up the responsibility of self-healing whenever you can. Too often, people look for a panacea to solve problems or an outside entity to rectify the existence of the disease entity within us. Medicine should not hinder our ability to think about our own responsibility and integrity. The concept of taking a pill that masks symptoms (and therefore understanding) often does exactly this. We should not look for answers for ourselves when trying to heal, but answers about ourselves that will lead us to unprecedented understandings and healing.

> **Look forward to being something completely new, not getting back to what you were before. Be willing to change your personal mythology, or the definition of yourself, by letting go of old patterns and hindering beliefs.**

> **Self-discipline refers to a process of knowing yourself, knowing what you truly desire, and then using reason to maintain focus on that true desire over other lesser desires that get in the way of the true goal.**

Perhaps this is already happening for you now. By reading this book, you have already made a conscious effort towards taking responsibility for your health. Continue down the path of self-exploration, educating yourself as much as you can about your health, seeking out the healthcare providers who are willing to assist you. This is the first step towards renewed health. It is the first step towards creating the "change" that you are seeking.

The Second Step—Be Willing to Change

Seek to change your ways—your patterns—and amplify the process forward towards what you want. Remember that the very definition of metabolism refers us back to the idea of *change*. Look forward to being something completely new, not getting back to what you were before. Be willing to change your personal mythology, or the definition of yourself, by letting go of old patterns and hindering beliefs. Sometimes, you must liberate yourself from the very things that you had assumed were good for you. Do not fear this process; your heart will tell you the difference between what is or is not good. And when you go through the process of letting go of everything, you can always pick up the necessary elements that help you move onward again.

The Third Step—Become Self-disciplined

Once you have accepted change, and sought to change old harmful patterns, then you must seek to discipline your actions throughout the day. Self-discipline refers to a process of knowing yourself, knowing what you truly desire, and then using reason to maintain focus on that true desire over other lesser desires that get in the way of the true goal.

> Nature has particular rules that must be followed. You cannot continue to break the rules and expect to obtain the healing and understanding that you are seeking.

So, take time to truly define what you want, what you desire. The next chapter will specifically discuss how to sit down and take the time to write out what you truly desire. You may find that these desires are about your health or about other personal aspects of your mind, soul, and long forgotten desires. And then, you must know it to be so in your heart with no doubt, and will it to be so with your entire being.

The Fourth Step—Have Personal Integrity

People often want to do whatever they please. I am not a proponent of telling someone to not do what they want to do. I believe that people should always seek out how to obtain their own personal desires and be free to express themselves. However, there is always a natural and inevitable consequence to any choice you make. And sometimes the things you seek and the choices you make are not what you truly desire. This is why knowing yourself is so important because you can focus on the things that you truly want. Remember, people can make any choice they want, even if detrimental, but they must be *responsible* for that choice.

> In order to discover this purpose, you must realize there is something bigger than yourself and then what is your personal, unique role in it all. Nature does not create anything solely for its individual needs, but always within the context of the larger system of nature.

Nature has particular rules that must be followed. You cannot continue to break the rules and expect to obtain the healing and understanding that you are seeking. Nurturing your own personal integrity will help you to follow the natural laws. To heal, you must understand the benefits and healing quality of your own personal integrity and your understanding of what you truly desire. Greater integrities, greater sincerities with lack of ulterior motive, will lead you to health.

The Fifth Step—Find a Purpose

To be healthy, you must find your purpose. Another term for this is providence, which implies that everyone has a singular purpose that will fulfill their own desires and help others along the way. Very often, patients come to me very unhappy and ill after spending many years in situations that are unfulfilling, whether it is an unsatisfying job or an unhappy relationship. Their current unhappiness really has a lot to do with an unrealized purpose, something that they have wanted to do or become but have not figured it out yet or were too fearful to make the leap towards fulfilling it. In order to discover this purpose, you must realize there is something bigger than yourself and then what is your personal, unique role in it all. Nature does not create anything solely for its individual needs, but always within the context of the larger system of nature. So, attempt to find out how you fit into it all.

The other steps towards healing will all be easier to understand, attempt and to achieve in the context of knowing your own purpose. But if you do not yet truly know your purpose, then simply moving towards discovering it will sustain you. If you strive towards truth, you will be sustained by truth.

How to find your Purpose:

- Understand that *you are not alone* and that there is something bigger than yourself.
- Release your *fear of fear*. Learn to live and function in the midst of your fear. Articulate it, own it, and know it is ever-present but that it is also something which can be overcome. When you overcome your fear, you will experience a feeling of relief.
- Always *push your own limits* on a physical, mental, emotional and spiritual level. Live your life on the very edge of your own limits, pushing just beyond, testing the current definition of your own boundaries. This is where growth abides and it is how health can be achieved.
- Once a purpose reveals itself, grab it and go for it. It does not have to be your exact purpose, but it will get you started and you will learn how to then continue to strive towards your ultimate purpose.
- *Discipline your whole life* around fulfilling this purpose.

Finally, *learn to laugh...*

Learn to laugh at all things, even the most horrible things. Laughter does not imply being unpresent to the seriousness of a situation, it implies an understanding that all things have a divine plan and that in the end we will be fine. Laughter at all things means we have let go of our ego and see past ourselves to something bigger. I do not mean to trivialize anyone's pain, but laughter will heal the weary soul.

Summary:

- Be sure to continually go through each of these items often while on your health journey.
- Become self-reliant. Ask, "Am I self-reliant?"
- Be willing to change. Ask, "Am I willing to change?"
- Become self-disciplined. Ask, "Am I self-disciplined?"
- Have personal integrity. Ask, "Have I found my personal integrity?"
- Find a purpose. Ask, "What is my purpose?"
- Learn to laugh.

On Healing and the Naturopathic Philosophical Paradigm: Integration

Medicine and health is a process of integration of all aspects of our being into one cohesive system that helps us to realize more about ourselves.

—John A. Robinson, NMD

Naturopathic medicine, as a distinct medical system, attempts to integrate philosophy, science, spirituality and art into a cohesive perspective and narrative regarding the human condition. The integrative approach offered by naturopathic medicine attempts to provide a healing model of cohesiveness of all internal disciplines, all internal reflections of the human condition and all outward manifestations of being. This model can help to stand as a shining example of how a person can integrate their own health.

This integration conjoins the aspects of our humanness; that is, the pure inspiration of the spirit begetting the pattern of the soul, the soul giving rise to the expression of thought and mind, the mind whispering the secrets of the human body, the human body circulating back to the source of spirit. This is a scientific expression of human integration that, when understood and incorporated, helps provide the model for realizing true health. A person that is integrated in this respect both within and without will be ready to handle most problems related to health.

Remember that the answers are within you. At times we need reminders from those things and people around us, and if I can ever be that humble guide for you, then I stand at the ready. But any empowerment you receive from without is always a reminder of a truth, and *health*, that you *already possess* from within.

To Your Health…

Chapter 2
Defining What You Want:
The Health Affirmation Statement

If you have decided to walk on a path towards finding health and balance, you must set out with the actual map and the true picture of what it will be like when you arrive. Getting there is what *you* create. Where you arrive is up to you and the decisions you make. Creating a statement of intent is the preamble to your personal constitution of your life. You can create a Health Affirmation Statement. It is designed to bring your intention to the forefront of your conscious awareness and create goals that your mind and body will seek to accomplish, if it is done and utilized correctly. This will occur on a subconscious level also.

Why should I do this?

Writing out your goals and where you want to be in terms of your health provides practical understanding about any difficulties you are having with illness. It aligns you with the picture of your goal as you see it and directs you to the means to achieve it. Goal setting is a common practice in projects like business, athletics, architecture and construction so why shouldn't it be used extensively in medicine and health for and by an individual? Know what you want, write it down, change it to fit the situation, then implement the plan. Although, a health plan is not as straightforward as a blueprint for a house, because you are a complex human being.

Sometimes patients do not even know what a list of health concerns should look like. Or they know the list of concerns but do not know where to start to address those concerns. This process helps you articulate what you want for yourself, and then communicate it to your healthcare provider. You must ask and inform your healthcare provider of what you want in terms of your health. When new perspectives and technical information are gained through this open communication, you can alter your health affirmation statements to fit the new situation.

You should take the time to write out exactly *what* you want yourself to be in terms of your mental, emotional, physical and spiritual health. A short paragraph will suffice, but it must contain specific details about *exactly* what it means to you.

Here are important points to keep in mind while you create the statement:

- The more detail the better.
- Keep your statements in positive terms, avoiding terms such as "no," "not," "won't," etc.
- Always keep your wording and phrasing in the present tense. Avoid the future tense.
- Use power words and phrases: "I AM…," "I WILL IT…," "I BELIEVE…," "I KNOW…," "I LOVE…."
- Note: The psychological and physical power of the statement "I am" cannot be overstated. Always pay attention when utilizing this statement. Your entire being will incorporate whatever you attach to it.
- See the chapter on Endocrine Basics in this section of the book. In that chapter, there is information regarding mental, emotional and even spiritual perspectives as they relate to your *endocrine system* and your *hormonal health*. You may choose to incorporate some of these concepts into your Health Affirmation Statement.
- In your Health Affirmation Statement consider all the different aspects of your being:

PHYSICAL: What do I want my health to look like? How will I look? Add colors to the description such as a healthy skin glow, muscle definition, the way your posture will be, the way you will move, etc. Will you be free from pain? Be specific.

MENTAL: What state of mind do I want my health to show up as? Am I focused towards my goal of being in a state of balance and health? Will my thoughts be centered and focused? Will my thinking be clear and poised? Will I create happiness and peace? Will my intellect be keen and aware?

EMOTIONAL: What do my healthy emotions feel like? How will I feel? What sensations would I like to have on a consistent basis? What does that look like, feel like? Are there any smells that are there or not there? How will I be breathing? Deep and centered? Steady and focused?

SPIRITUAL: What is my relationship with Spirit or God or The Other or The Source? Is my goal of health in line with my inner beliefs? Do I see the peace that I want and desire? What does it look and feel like?

APPLY ACTION: What specific things must I do in order to achieve the health that I desire? What actions must I take consistently to be in the state of health I desire? Do I know that I deserve to help myself in order to help others around me?

USE IT DAILY: Once you have created your detailed Health Affirmation Statement, you must utilize it, meditate on it, pray over it, repeat it daily in the morning upon rising and before you go to bed. Commit it to memory over time. Change the statement to meet your personal changing needs.

And along your health journey you may decide to add more things to your Health Affirmation Statement, changing your map slightly to fit your current needs. Remember that your health and your perspectives towards your health are constantly changing. Just keep moving towards what you truly desire. In the next chapter, you will be given another layer of understanding regarding positive affirmations as they relate specifically to the endocrine system that can be added to this first phase.

Here is an example of a Health Affirmation Statement written by a patient:

Health Affirmation Statement

By

Jane Smith

PHYSICAL: *I want my health to look like I radiate positive energy. By radiating positive energy, I will look as if I am bathed in a glow that will be noticed by others. I will view the world through eyes that behold my own inner strength, and because of that, my eyes will appear clear and sincere. My skin will be free of blemishes, feel smooth and properly hydrated. My movements will be graceful but strong, and I will feel no pain in any area of my body.*

MENTAL: *To be in a state of constant good health, I will wake up feeling strong and refreshed. I will move through my day being conscious of my breath if I feel anxiety and I will take time to calm down. When I put on my clothes, I will pay attention to every area of my body and make a point to be grateful for the lack of pain. If I encounter pain, I will focus on my breath for as long as it takes me to feel centered and then I will think healing thoughts to myself. As I feed myself I will pay attention to what and how much fuel I put into my body, always being grateful for proper nourishment. I will sleep well each night by reminding myself that getting rest is for my greater good.*

EMOTIONAL: *Because I know my emotions play a big part in the way I experience life, I want to respect them and allow them to guide me in all my interactions with others. Above all, I value honesty with myself and with others. If anger arises, I will commit to understanding the source and instead of holding it in, I will express it appropriately with an eye toward an adequate solution. When sadness occurs, I will express it to myself first and then seek comfort from others. I will take time each day to engage in about fifteen minutes of meditation where I close out the world and focus only on my own peace of mind through the practice of attentive breathing. I will develop the capacity to hold faith and trust that the Universe desires my greater good. I will take time to use discernment when I face choices that may affect the way I see myself. I will ask others to respect me by allowing me time to think before making a decision. I want to feel trusted, and I expect trust from others. To enhance my personal environment, I will take time to light a scented candle during moments when I am focused on tasks like paying bills, meditating or cooking.*

SPIRITUAL: Because I believe in an entity that is far greater than myself and all of humanity, my heart is full of reverence for both the seen and the unseen. Out of this reverence comes a sense of being loved, and being able to love. From this love, I am able to trust that a path of learning is set for me that I may interact with by using my own free will. In difficult times, I will be conscious of what I am supposed to be learning. In good

times I will appreciate what has been given to me as a gift and I will also see a lesson in receiving it. In all of the learning, I will have a greater understanding of the lives of others and will be able to be a loving witness to them, bearing them no judgment, offering help through the power of thought and prayer and giving them only as much support as necessary for them to learn their lesson.

APPLY ACTION: My actions will be as follows: daily exercise (a thirty minute walk minimum, some free weights and calisthenics as time permits); daily meditation (fifteen minutes); protein for breakfast and small meals throughout the day; daily journaling; a goal of seven hours of sleep each night; scheduling routine checkups in order to allow assessment by a medical professional who will be my partner in maintaining my health.

Chapter 3
The Endocrine System Basics: A Naturopathic Perspective

Note: This chapter has two sections. The first section is devoted to reviewing and explaining the different hormones and their function. Be sure to not get bogged down in the details of this section, but rather use it as a reference if you have questions. Of course, there are always very enthusiastic readers who want all of the detail, so there is a lot of it here. The second section provides details about your endocrine system and hormones that is important to achieving success. I recommend reading this section with attention to the details, but have some fun with it like you would if you were putting together a jigsaw puzzle.

The endocrine system is one of the most elaborate and intricate systems in the human body. Its multiple hormones relay an interplay of messages and signals to every cell in the body, all in a poetically orchestrated fashion that functions to do things as complex and beautiful as keeping us breathing to helping us pass on our genetic code to our children. The endocrine system is in constant flux and change, and its hormones and related glands allow this change to occur on a moment-to-moment basis and beyond. Your metabolic health is vitally dependent upon the proper function of the endocrine system. This chapter will define the basics of the endocrine system. Additionally, a brief review of some of the overall holistic viewpoints of the endocrine system will be provided to explain a more global view of this system and how it affects humans from a physical, mental, emotional and even spiritual perspective.

Your Key Endocrine Organs

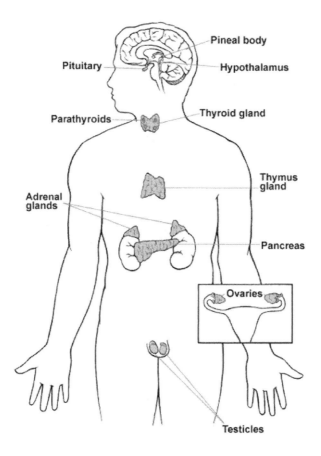

As you can see, several major endocrine organs exist in the body, centrally positioned along the midline. Each gland is responsible for secreting its own various hormones directly into the bloodstream where they travel to their target tissues. Most of the endocrine organs also have a corresponding and associated anatomical nerve bundle called a plexus. Your sensory perception of the environment around you is created by your nerves and your hormones.

In general, the endocrine system works through a series of steps:
- An endocrine organ such as the thyroid **senses a change** in the body such as lowered cellular energy.
- Responding to that change the thyroid **secretes a hormone**.

> ❧ Via the bloodstream, the **hormone arrives** at tissue or organ cells.
> ❧ By a lock and key mechanism the provided stimulus **creates a necessary change**.
> ❧ **Balance**, or homeostasis, is maintained.

Let's explore these organs and their associated hormones. We will begin with one of the most unlikely endocrine tissues, the digestive tract, and another recently redefined endocrine tissue, body fat. Then we will explore the endocrine organs, such as the gonads and adrenals up through the pineal gland. This section describes the normal function of these organs and hormones and can be used as a reference in the future as you proceed to the other sections of the book. Sections 3 and 4 will focus on the actual diseases of these organs and their associated hormones.

Digestive Tract

The digestive tract actually secretes hormones that are generally responsible for digestion and weight control. These hormones are secreted based on food consumption rates and even types of food.

Cholecystokinin is a hormone secreted from the intestinal tract when predominantly protein and fat rich foods have been eaten. Cholescystokinin causes a sensation of satiation or fullness. This hormone opposes another hormone called ghrelin, which is known to increase appetite.

Glucagon-like peptide is another gut hormone that is secreted by the digestive tract during the process of digestion. Some of the basic functions of this hormone include increasing insulin secretion from the pancreas which helps to clear the glucose (sugar) from the blood, increasing beta cell mass (pancreatic cells that produce insulin), inhibiting acid secretion and stomach emptying, and decreasing food intake by increasing satiety or fullness.

Peptide YY is a hormone that is secreted from the stomach in response to food ingestion. Peptide YY has been shown to blunt ghrelin secretions, therefore lowering appetite and reducing food intake. Peptide YY works by slowing gastric emptying thereby increasing the efficiency of digestion and nutrient absorption after meals.[1] The strategy of eating smaller meals keeps this hormone stimulated and consequently keeps the appetite down. Obese people produce less of this hormone.

Adipose (fat) tissue has more recently been reclassified as an endocrine organ. For years, doctors and scientists simply observed fat tissue as an inert substance with little metabolic activity. This is no longer true.

Resistin is a pro-inflammatory hormone produced by fat tissue and it will increase when inflammation is present in the body. Resistin is secreted by fat tissue as an inflammatory cytokine in response to a perceived immunological threat. Increased amounts of resistin are linked to insulin resistance and type II diabetes. As fat tissue goes up, resistin levels go up, and as fat tissue declines, resistin follows. Central obesity or fat that accumulates around the middle of the abdomen is related to both type II diabetes/insulin resistance and increased resistin levels.

Ghrelin and Leptin

Both ghrelin and leptin have emerged recently as a very popular hormone associated with appetite and weight control. They work as counterparts, with ghrelin stimulating appetite and leptin stimulating satiety or the sensation of feeling full and satisfied. Let's explain ghrelin in detail first. Ghrelin is largely secreted by the stomach and stimulates hunger centers in the hypothalamus of the brain telling you to eat more and increasing the deposition of fat. Interestingly, this hormone is also associated with the pleasure and reward centers of the brain, which increases desire to eat. When you are finished eating, levels decrease. It even encourages addictive behaviors. Ghrelin also displays strong growth hormone releasing activity through the binding to and activation of growth hormone receptor type 1a.[2] Paradoxically, in obese individuals, ghrelin levels are lower, and the opposite is true of thinner people. This is an attempt made by the body to lessen food intake in obesity by limiting ghrelin. There is also a link with obesity and shorter sleep durations, as ghrelin levels are higher when sleep is short and deprived.

Leptin has its source in adipose tissue, but the ovaries, skeletal muscle, stomach, breast tissue, bone marrow, pituitary and liver all produce small quantities. This hormone controls appetite by sending signals back to the brain inducing satiety, or fullness. If you are starving, then leptin increases to stimulate your appetite at the brain level.[3] Therefore, the less we eat, the more we signal to the brain to increase the appetite. This could be why many starvation type diets have a rebound effect on eating and weight control.

Here are some of the other known functions of leptin:

* Leptin is also responsible for proper metabolism of stored sugar or glucose, called glycogen, within the liver.
* Hypothalamic regulation or indirect association with regulation of body temperature, heart rate, hunger sensations, the fight or flight stress response, fat burning or storage, reproductive behavior, bone growth and blood glucose (sugar).
* Pro-inflammatory hormone which relates leptin back to the inflammatory state of diabetes and other chronic diseases such as heart disease.
* Leptin determines how much fat you have, but also where that fat is deposited. When you are leptin resistant, you put that fat mostly in your belly (your viscera), causing the so-called apple shape that is linked to disease. Some of that fat permeates the liver, impeding the liver's ability to listen to insulin and further hastening diabetes. One counterpart to leptin is ghrelin, the hormone produced largely by the stomach and the brain, responsible for increasing appetite.

It also important to note that obese people are resistant to leptin, just as they can be resistant to insulin. Insulin is another counterpart to leptin and they both are associated with blood sugar handling problems such as metabolic syndrome and diabetes, which are both insulin and leptin resistant conditions. The easiest way to regulate insulin and leptin is to decrease carbohydrate and sugar intake and to increase quality sleep.[4]

Ovaries

Females have two ovaries, one on each side of the body, which are responsible for reproduction. The ovaries house a finite amount of ova or eggs which, when combined and fertilized by male sperm produce a fetus.

The ovaries produce estrogen. There are three main types of estrogen:

- ❧ E1 or Estrone (-one refers to "one"). This is a relatively weak estrogen and a breakdown product of estradiol. Estrone in high levels is related back to breast cancer and is in higher levels after menopause.
- ❧ E2 or Estradiol (-di refers to "two"). This is the main potent form of estrogen that characterizes most of the benefits known about estrogen in general.
- ❧ E3 or Estriol (-tri refers to "three"). This is the weakest form of estrogen and is also a breakdown product of estradiol. This form of estrogen has very little physiological effect and benefit in people.

Estradiol (E2) has a direct affect on the function and development of the reproductive system, the nervous system, the cardiovascular system and the skeletal system. The main functions of estradiol (E2) are many:

- ❧ Estradiol improves vaginal lubrication and prevents atrophy (shrinking).
- ❧ Estradiol keeps the urinary tract lubricated and healthy, preventing infection and urinary incontinence (leakage).
- ❧ Estradiol can directly increase libido (sexual desire), interest and responsiveness.
- ❧ Estradiol improves blood glucose (sugar) metabolism by increasing sugar uptake in muscle cells and therefore decreases the risk of developing high insulin levels and insulin resistance.
- ❧ Estradiol influences and improves neurochemical balance in the brain helping with depression, anxiety, memory and focus. Estrogen particularly increases serotonin production[5] by both making more of it[6] and retaining it by selectively inhibiting its re-uptake,[7] much like the medications Prozac® and Wellbutrin®.

- Estradiol helps maintain the size and normal density of breast tissue and serves as a powerful antioxidant for breast tissue.
- Skin thickness, collagen, water content, skin softness and blood flow are all enhanced by estradiol.
- Bone formation is greatly influenced by estradiol. The activity of bone clearing osteoclast cells are kept in check while bone building osteoblast cells are influenced and stimulated.
- Estradiol has been shown to lower total cholesterol levels and LDL (bad cholesterol) levels while increasing HDL (good cholesterol) levels. Estradiol also causes a reduction in the level of lipoprotein (a), which results in a significantly reduced risk of developing heart disease.[8]
- Estradiol, in the presence of balanced testosterone, can help to *decrease* body fat.

Progesterone is another important ovarian hormone. Progesterone causes the endometrium or uterine lining to prepare to receive and nourish an implanted fertilized egg. If implantation does not occur, estrogen and progesterone levels drop during the second half of the menstrual cycle and the endometrium breaks down leading to menstruation. If implantation and pregnancy occurs, progesterone is produced in larger amounts in the placenta and it remains elevated throughout a pregnancy.

One more product of the ovaries, testosterone is typically thought of as a male hormone; however, testosterone is extremely important for a woman's health. Among its many benefits and functions are enhancing memory and focus, assisting in recall of information, regulating moods and improving anxiety, helping with drive, stimulating the metabolism, boosting energy, assisting in bone growth, helping with weight loss, enhancing the function of insulin and therefore lowering the risk for diabetes, benefiting the structures of the vulva thus helping with incontinence (urine leakage) and enhancing vaginal secretion, and finally, stimulating the libido or psychological drive to have sex.

Although it is produced in a small amount by the ovaries, DHEA is considered an androgen, just like testosterone, but has an overall weaker effect to the system. See the section below under "Adrenals" for more detail.

Testicles

The two testicles produce a variety of hormones, but testosterone is one of the most potent and abundant. Testosterone has many functions. It is responsible for the secondary sex characteristics in men such as increased muscle mass and strength, facial hair growth and development of the larynx (Adam's apple) and voice deepening.

Testosterone is typically thought of as a male hormone; however, testosterone is extremely important for a woman's health.

The main physiological effects of testosterone are that it:
- Lowers insulin resistance and decreases the risk for type diabetes.
- Improves bone formation and decreases the risk for osteoporosis.
- Improves cardiovascular function and improves blood lipid (cholesterol) levels.
- Enhances short-term memory recall and improves mood stability.

Kidneys

Erythropoietin, a peptide hormone, is extremely vital in red blood cell production. It has multiple actions including controlling blood pressure, stimulating the production of new blood vessels and controlling the proliferation of smooth muscle fibers.

Renin is more of an enzyme than a hormone and it has the important function of maintaining blood pressure. Renin works intimately with aldosterone, another adrenal hormone in balancing the blood pressure through sodium regulation.

Adrenals

There are two adrenal glands in your body, each atop a kidney. The adrenals are about the size of a grape and their function is absolutely necessary for life and overall health. These glands are involved in the fight-or-flight stress response which allows the body to properly regulate and cope with any perceived threat to the system.

The adrenals are composed of two layers: the outer portion, called the adrenal cortex, and the inner portion called the adrenal medulla. The adrenal cortex secretes aldosterone, cortisol and the sex steroids androstenediol and androstenedione, DHEA (dihydroepiandrosterone), estrogen and testosterone. The adrenal medulla secretes epinephrine, norepinephrine and dopamine.

> **The adrenal glands also contribute to the overall content of testosterone and estrogen in the blood for both men and women. When the adrenals are functioning suboptimally, then a larger pressure exists on the ovaries or testicles to produce them.**

The Hormones of the Adrenal Cortex

Aldosterone regulates salt and water balance by retaining salt and water and excreting potassium. This is an important hormone for maintaining proper blood pressure.

Cortisol is one of the most important adrenal hormones in the body and has a multitude of effects and functions. Cortisol production undergoes a diurnal or cyclical variation, with the highest levels produced in the early morning and the lowest around midnight, or three to five hours after the onset of sleep. Functions of cortisol include:

- It is one of the most powerful anti-inflammatory substances known. It reduces histamine secretion which is related to the inflammatory responses.
- It is also vital for maintaining your blood sugar levels by counteracting insulin by increasing gluconeogenesis or the creation of sugar from the breakdown of fats and proteins. This is important in preventing insulin resistance that leads to diabetes.

❧ Cortisol also functions similarly to aldosterone as it helps to control salt (sodium) and water balance, and therefore blood pressure.

❧ It is also involved in overall muscle strength and even memory.

❧ Additionally, cortisol stimulates gastric acid secretion and as a result, improves digestion.

❧ And cortisol is responsible for enhancing copper availability for enzymatic reactions for the immune response.

DHEA is a potent sex steroid that has many functions in the body. Most of the available DHEA in the body is produced by the adrenal glands with some of it being produced in either the ovaries in women or the testicles in men. It is important to note that most of the DHEA in the body will convert into testosterone. Therefore, most of the physiological benefits known for DHEA are very similar to testosterone. Some of the basic functions of DHEA are:

❧ Possesses basic androgenic and anabolic effects, allowing tissue to repair and grow.

❧ It converts readily into testosterone.

❧ Balances excess cortisol levels.

❧ Stimulates bone growth.

❧ Improves lipid profiles by lowering total cholesterol and LDL levels.

❧ Increases muscle mass and lowers body fat.

❧ Stimulates T-cell proliferation and interleukin-II synthesis, therefore improving immunity.

❧ Improves short-term memory.

❧ Improves conversion of T4 to active T3 in the thyroid gland.

The "prohormones" androstenedione and androstenediol have less physiological potency than the other sex steroids testosterone and estrogen. The term prohormone implies that most of this hormone will be converted into a more activated form.

Let's get back to testosterone and estrogen. The adrenal glands also contribute to the overall content of testosterone and estrogen in the blood for both men and women. When the adrenals are functioning suboptimally, then a larger pressure exists on the ovaries or testicles to produce them.

The hormones of the adrenal medulla include: epinephrine and norepinephrine (adrenaline). The outer portion of the adrenals, called the adrenal medulla, produces these very potent hormones, more commonly referred to as adrenaline. They are directly responsible for the fight-or-flight stress response. Many other tissues, including the brain, produce these hormones. During stress, these hormones increase the supply of oxygen and glucose to the brain and muscles. Adrenaline increases heart rate, dilates the pupils, constricts arterioles in the skin and gastrointestinal tract while dilating arterioles in skeletal muscles, elevates the blood sugar and breaks down fats, all to prepare the body during extreme stress.

Dopamine. Although dopamine is an adrenal hormone and listed here in this section, it is also a very common neurotransmitter in the brain. Dopamine has roles in behavior and cognition, voluntary movement and reward. It is involved in attraction, passion and desire. It is the major hormone for inhibition of prolactin which is involved in lactation. It is also involved in sleep, mood, attention and learning.

Pancreas

The pancreas has two portions, an endocrine portion that secretes hormones into the blood, and an exocrine portion that secretes hormones directly into the small intestine in response to digestive enzymes and activity. The hormones of the pancreas are insulin, glucagon, somatostatin and pancreatic polypeptide. Because the key hormones are insulin and glucagon, they are my focus here.

Insulin responds to the presence of carbohydrates, proteins and fats when ingested. It assists cells in the absorption of glucose or sugar in muscle and fat tissue, increases protein creation for body repair and maintenance and improves the function of other metabolic enzymes in the body. But insulin has other functions. It increases:

❧ Glycogen synthesis or the "storage form" of energy in the liver and muscle.

- Fatty acid synthesis. This is a very important concept as it relates to weight management. Insulin forces fat cells to take in blood fats or lipids which convert to triglycerides and are stored in fat cells making them larger. When insulin is not present, fat cells liberate their triglycerides freely.

- The secretion of hydrochloric acid by parietal cells in the stomach. And why is this important?

Glucagon is the counterpart to insulin, largely acting in an opposite way to balance the actions of insulin. When blood sugar is too low, glucagon is secreted instructing the liver to release glycogen that is the storage form of glucose or sugar. This increases blood sugar levels back to normal. Interestingly, glucagon then signals the release of more insulin that is to regulate the newly secreted blood sugar. Much of this blood sugar, if not used appropriately, will be stored as fat. This is another reason why keeping the blood sugar balanced is important to prevent the starvation effects of skipping meals and restricting food when trying to lose weight. Hormonally, the body wants constant sources of the right kinds of foods.

Thymus

The thymus is a relatively small organ located in front of the heart and behind the sternum. It is a part of the immune system and makes the all-important T cells that fight foreign invaders in the body. Thymus hormones, called thymosins, stimulate the development and differentiation of T lymphocytes. T lymphocytes play a role in regulating the immune system by stimulating multiple types of immune cells, including protective antibodies. There has been some suggestion that the use of thymic extracts can boost the immune system helping with various diseases including cancer.[9, 10] These extracts have been used in homeopathy for over 200 years and new studies of its various uses are being published.

Thyroid

The role of thyroid hormone is immense and pervasive within the body. The subject is thoroughly examined in later chapters. For consistency, a brief explanation of the main thyroid hormones are provided here.

Thyroid Hormone

The follicular cells of the thyroid gland produce the main hormones thyroxine (T4) and triiodothyronine (T3). These are the key hormones of metabolism and are responsible for a multitude of functions of both development and cellular maintenance. Be sure to see the additional chapters that are devoted to thyroid hormone physiology.

Calcitonin

This hormone is produced in a different part of the thyroid gland known as the parafollicular cells and acts to reduce blood calcium, opposing the effects of parathyroid hormone. Its importance in humans has not been as well established as its importance in other animals, but there are specific actions known, such as protecting against calcium loss during stressful events such as pregnancy and lactation, regulating blood levels of calcium through vitamin D regulation, and it may even be involved in appetite control.

Parathyroid Glands

You have four distinct parathyroid glands located just behind the thyroid gland, two on each lobe of the thyroid. The sole purpose of these glands is to produce parathyroid hormone (PTH).

This hormone is responsible for increasing calcium levels in the blood, which is opposite to the effects of the thyroid hormone calcitonin. Calcium is needed, in very specific amounts, to regulate the vital actions of muscle contractions and nerve impulses for your entire body. Without proper calcium regulation, you would soon die. Parathyroid hormone acts specifically on bone to release calcium stores. In the kidney, PTH will prevent calcium from being excreted, and in the intestine, PTH will activate vitamin D which improves calcium regulation.

The role of PTH on vitamin D regulation cannot be overstated. Vitamin D is important for bone health and it provides a multitude of other health benefits that will be addressed in section five of this book.

Pineal Gland

The pineal gland is one of the most mysterious of all endocrine tissues. Relatively little is known of its function. In Latin, it is termed the *epiphysis cerebri* or the third eye. This structure has been studied for centuries. René Descartes wrote that the pineal gland was "the seat of the soul." It is a small, pea-sized organ located in the center of the brain, just above the pituitary gland. It secretes melatonin.

Melatonin is partly responsible for regulating sleep and the circadian rhythms that set our internal clocks knowing when to sleep and wake. This hormone can be used for improving sleep if it is administered correctly. Melatonin is also involved in reproduction, retinal and eye physiology, the cardiovascular system, immunity, cholesterol and blood sugar (glucose) metabolism, and it acts as a powerful antioxidant free-radical scavenger. Melatonin also functions in cancer control.

Pituitary

The pituitary gland is located in the center of the brain and has been coined the "master gland" due to the multitude of stimulating and regulating hormones it produces. The pituitary has two lobes, both anterior and posterior, which are discussed here. The hormones produced by the pituitary tend to be hormonal messages that are actually targeting an endocrine gland to secrete its hormone product. In other words, their physiological effects are focused to the main glands they target.

Antidiuretic hormone (vasopressin or ADH) causes the kidneys to retain water and control blood pressure with the help of aldosterone.

Adrenocorticotropic hormone (ACTH) is a chemical messenger that controls the secretion of hormones from the adrenal glands.

Luteinizing hormone (LH) and follicle stimulating hormone (FSH) are messengers that stimulate the testicles for the production of sperm and semen in men, and in women stimulate the ovaries for egg maturation and menstruation. FSH is specifically related to menopause in women. FSH will go considerably high, indicating the presence or onset of menopause.

Thyroid stimulating hormone (TSH) is the chemical messenger from the anterior pituitary that is responsible for stimulating the thyroid to produce thyroid hormone. More will come on this hormone later.

Human Growth Hormone (hGH) is a very potent hormone related to proper development and growth in children stimulating the division and multiplication of bone and cartilage cells. Growth hormone also stimulates insulin-like growth factor 1 (IGF-1), a hormone that has growth-stimulating effects on many body tissues, including bone tissue. Typically, an adult will produce about 350 micrograms of human growth hormone per minute. Hypothyroid (low thyroid) patients have considerably lower production rates at about 160 micrograms per minute.[11]

There are many other functions associated with hGH including:
- Promotes fat loss.
- Improves protein synthesis and therefore increases muscle mass and function.
- Stimulates the growth and development of internal organs.
- Maintains the function of specialized cells in the pancreas known as islets.
- Stimulates immunity.

The use of hGH for anti-aging outside of standard reasons, such as children who are not growing, remains controversial.

Prolactin is secreted by the anterior pituitary gland. However, other tissues including the breasts, parts of the central nervous system, the brain and the immune system secrete this important hormone. Prolactin normally elevates after orgasm and is therefore associated with sexual gratification. However, when levels are too high, it can be associated with lowered libido or sexual desire and lowered sexual function, such as impotence and erectile dysfunction.[12]

Reasons for an elevated prolactin level include:

- A possible prolactinoma which is a prolactin-secreting tumor normally on the pituitary gland itself. A CT scan would be necessary to properly follow up and diagnose.
- Prescription medications such as the dopamine suppressing drugs trifluoperazine (Stelazine), haloperidol (Haldol), risperidone (Risperdal), and molindone (Moban), the GERD medication metoclopramide (Reglan), and to a lesser extent the high blood pressure medications verapamil, alpha–methyldopa (Aldochlor, Aldoril), and reserpine (Serpalan, Serpasil).
- It is interesting to note that thyrotropin-releasing hormone (TRH) stimulates prolactin release. TRH is responsible for stimulating the release of thyroid stimulating hormone (TSH), which in turn stimulates that thyroid gland to produce thyroid hormone. If the thyroid is not functioning optimally, TRH will increase to stimulate the release of TSH. This could also increase the release of prolactin. It is not uncommon for hypothyroid (low thyroid function) patients to have elevated prolactin levels.

A Naturopathic and Energetic Endocrine Perspective

Integration and holism is the philosophical paradigm upon which my training exists. Holism is also, in my opinion, the proper way to view the body, with its physical, mental, emotional and spiritual aspects melded into a singular, integrated perspective. Therefore, the naturopathic medical focus on the endocrine system finds itself organized and orchestrated into a large integrated entity that includes the natural science of the physical, mental, emotional and spiritual aspects it possesses.

The endocrine system from this viewpoint is the keystone to your metabolic health. This naturopathic perspective has several key points:

- Each hormone interplays with all other hormones.

- Each organ in your body can be technically viewed as an endocrine organ since all tissues in the body react to and with hormonal signals.
- If there is an imbalance within the endocrine system, the science and art of naturopathy asks key questions:
  - *Tolle causam* (treat the cause): What is the underlying *cause* of the hormonal imbalance, such as a nutritional deficiency?
  - *Tolle totum* (treat the entire person): How can the *entire individual* be treated in this situation, even if it is "hormonal?"
  - *Vis medicatrix naturae* (the healing power of nature): How can the healing power of nature, or the healing power that the human system possesses, be incorporated to help balance the endocrine system in a safe, natural and gentle fashion?
- As we are integrated beings, what are the mental, emotional and even spiritual difficulties that are playing into the hormonal imbalance?

The Physical Balancing of the Endocrine System for Metabolic Health

This entire book is devoted to optimizing the metabolism as it relates to your endocrine health with a particular focus on thyroid health. Some of the direct ways to affect the hormonal balance of the endocrine system are:

- Proper diet that allows for enhanced function of all of the endocrine organs and their associated hormones:
  - Improved digestive health enhances endocrine hormonal health through assimilation through the liver and excretion.
  - Dietary supplementation and herbal enhancement to promote hormonal health.
- Proper exercise promotes the hormonal profile of energy and weight management.
- Lifestyle choices such as good sleep hygiene and meditation enhance the production of hormones when you need them.

❧ Direct replacement of hormones utilizing safe, natural and effective bioidentical hormones including sex hormones, adrenal hormones and particularly thyroid hormones.

Finally, repeated attempts at clarifying the need to incorporate the physical, mental, emotional and spiritual aspects of your being to improve your endocrine health are emphasized. The remaining parts of this chapter help to illustrate this point by demonstrating the deeper internal relationships of your endocrine system and your entire being.

Emotions, Spirituality, and the Endocrine System

Your body responds to emotions—any emotion. Upon the perception of an emotion, whether it is joy, happiness, desire, fear, or anger, distinct and unique neurochemical and hormonal responses activate and guide your body and perceptions in a particular direction either enhancing or redirecting the emotion. For example, when you feel the emotion of desire, particular neurochemicals such as endorphins, dopamine (a brain neurochemical hormone of intense animalistic desire), testosterone, and others are released, which express this state. If your emotions are geared towards positive things, your body will create the necessary physical manifestations of that in the form of neurochemicals and hormones.

Your emotions also have a direct link to spirituality and spiritual choices. Some of these choices empower and some can hinder your growth and health. So, the endocrine system becomes the conduit of how a spiritual choice, good or bad, presents itself in our bodies. If you make a spiritual choice to give power to a particular fear, for example, the fear you continue to allow yourself to feel will chronically increase the stress hormone response in your body and possibly result in ill health.

Real knowledge of your body and its related emotions is found within the endocrine system and its hormones. As you explore your true purpose and your true desires from a physical, mental, emotional and spiritual level, for yourself and your personal relationships, you will have the ability to possess more balance and health. There is a lot of work involved, including giving yourself several personal interviews over the course of your life and then providing yourself honest answers.

The Science and Art of the Endocrine Relationship to the Chakras

There exists an ancient understanding of particular energy systems in the body known as chakras. The following table demonstrates the spatial relationship between the endocrine organs and the charkas. Chakras relate to the culture of India but their concepts are found in all ancient cultures and religions of the world, in one way or another. There is also a medical and scientific relationship to these energies that hold the potential to reveal additional layers of clarity to the understanding of the endocrine system and overall health.

The following chart is an overview of some the main correspondences of the chakras and their relationship to the endocrine system and other physical, mental, emotional and spiritual aspects. I have kept the chart specific to these concepts and resisted the need to elaborate any further. The study of the chakras is complex and is left outside the scope of this book. However, I encourage anyone, if this information resonates, to further explore.

You will see that there is a frank anatomical relationship of the nervous system and the endocrine system to the chakras. The chakras are not simply perceived—belief that they exist is endorsed by their direct physical manifestation and correlation to the human operating system. In addition to defining physical insight, the chakras encompass the intellectual and emotional aspects of human psychology. The spiritual aspects depicted by the chakra system are varying expressions of who we are and who we aim to be, but the chakra definitions are by no means exhaustive and complete. The term "spiritual" here and throughout this book refers only to the connection each of us has (or strives to have) with a source of being outside ourselves, and our inner connection with that source. Even though the word "spiritual" is typically related to a belief and understanding of a supreme being, it does not need to have that connotation. I leave it up to the individual to define this important aspect of humanity for themselves while attempting to achieve their ideal health.

The practical use of this information for your metabolic health is to recognize any of the physical, mental, emotional or spiritual aspects presented here in an attempt to work on, admit, clarify, intensify and open up in order to approach any possible endocrine system imbalances and improve your overall metabolic health needs.

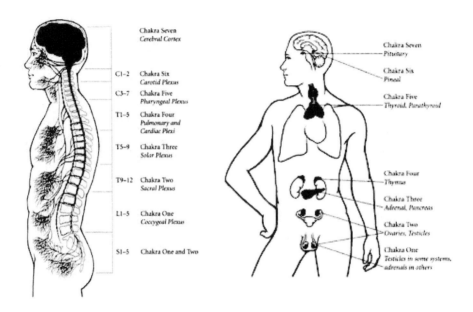

How to Use the Chakras for Hormonal Health

Go through each aspect carefully and admit to yourself what you may need to work on, but also focus on the inevitable strengths that you possess and learn to further cultivate them. If you have any particular issue with a negative emotion, use the positive affirmation that is its counterpart. Add this affirmation to the Health Affirmation Statement exercise that was done in the previous chapter, which will produce an even more specific declaration for you. Read and repeat this new set of goals and affirmations aloud daily or whenever you feel the related negative emotions.

After you review the concepts in the chart, I also encourage you to write in a journal about the specific mental, emotional and spiritual aspects on any chakra or endocrine organ that is imbalanced to understand what it personally means to you. Remember, these exercises include the physical aspects also. The more you delve into all four aspects of your being, the more complete your attainment of health will be.

CHAKRA	PHYSICAL		MENTAL		EMOTIONAL		SPIRITUAL
	Plexus (Anatomical Nerve Bundle) and Spinal Vertebra	Endocrine Organ	Psychological Function	Mode of Intelligence	Positive	Negative	Purpose/ Affirmation
Root	Coccygeal Plexus and 1st Sacral Vertebra	Adrenals	Survival, Primal Sexuality, Courage, Impulsiveness	Administrative Intelligence; clear thought, speech and action helps to govern the world	The right to be here, "dominion"	Fear, "slavery"	I am, Will to Be Affirmations: I am safe and secure at all times while expanding my awareness and enjoyment of life. I am responsible for the quality of my life.
Sacral	Prostatic Ganglion and Sacral Plexus and 1st Lumbar Vertebra	Ovaries Testicles	Feelings, Intimacy, Procreation, Sensuality, Sociability, Freedom	Exciting Intelligence: Breaking down old ways of thought and action and impels you to seek out new forms of expression.	The right to feel, "fertility"	Guilt, "sterility"	I feel, Will to Feel Affirmations: I unconditionally love and approve of myself at all times. I release my negative attitudes which block my experience of pleasure. I am in control of my own sexuality.

CHAKRA	PHYSICAL		MENTAL		EMOTIONAL		SPIRITUAL
Solar Plexus	Solar Plexus and 8th Thoracic Vertebra	Pancreas (Digestion)	Will, Knowledge, Mental Clarity, Humor, Optimism, Self-Control	Conciliation Intelligence: The longing desire of earnest quest of the true nature of things—going home	The right to act, "grace"	Shame, "sin"	I do, Will Power Affirmations: I love and respect myself at all times. There are no failures; I learn from everything I do; I love life and trust love; I release judgment and let my life flow.
Heart	Cardiac and Pulmonary Plexuses and 1st, 2nd, 3rd Thoracic Vertebra	Thymus (Immunity)	Relationships Love, Compassion, Forgiveness, Harmony, Growth	Collective Intelligence: Combining all forms of knowledge and experience into one cohesive stream.	The right to love and be loved, "wealth"	Sorrow, "poverty"	I love, Will to Love Affirmations: I am willing to love everything about myself. I forgive myself and those who need forgiving for not being what I wanted them to be. Love is the purpose of my life.
Throat	Pharyngeal Plexus and 3rd Cervical Vertebra	Thyroid Parathyroids, Medulla Oblongata	Communication, Wisdom, Speech, Trust, Creative Expression, Planning	Luminous Intelligence: Relating to the intelligence of the subconscious mind which gives force to our creative ideas and particularly wisdom.	The right to speak and hear truth, "wisdom"	Lies, "folly"	I speak, Will to Create Affirmations: I am able to harness my will power to control addictive influences in my life and put my negative habits to one side and openly develop my creativity. I release the fear and doubts which block the way to my creative expression. I substitute love, joy, and creative expression for old patterns of addiction and abuse.

CHAKRA	PHYSICAL		MENTAL		EMOTIONAL		SPIRITUAL
3rd Eye	Carotid Plexus and 1st Cervical Vertebra	Pituitary Hypothalamus Both hemispheres of the brain	Intuition, Invention, Self Realization, Understanding, Fearlessness	Uniting Intelligence: bringing together the personal ego with the universal ego	The right to see, "peace"	Illusion, "strife"	I see, Will to Serve through Wisdom Affirmations: I open myself to my intuition and deepest knowing. I acknowledge I am the source in creating my life the way I would like it to be. I create clarity and unlimited vision for myself about my life, and I trust whatever comes to me is for my greatest joy and highest good.
Crown	Cerebral Cortex	Pineal Gland, Upper portion of the brain	Knowingness, Wisdom, Inspiration, Higher Self, Meditation/ Prayer, Self Sacrificing	Transparency Intelligence: Seeing through the illusions of bondage and death	The right to know, "life"	Attach-ment, "death"	I understand, Will to Do Affirmations: I am open and receptive with understanding to all life knowing love makes me free. I am always willing to take the next step in my life to go beyond my limitations to express and experience greater joy. I go beyond limiting beliefs and accept myself totally.

This chart was adapted from various sources including the work of the Western Mystery Schools, also *The Book of Chakras*, by Ambika Wauters, The Brofman Institute for the Advancement of Healing, and www. chakraenergy.com.

Section 2
Keystones to Your Metabolic Health Foundation

Introduction

The following two chapters focus on two important factors in your metabolic health, diet and exercise. Proclaiming the benefits of "diet and exercise" has been done so many times now that I have found most patients simply glaze over when it is mentioned.

When I say "diet and exercise" people have a less than excited reaction for several reasons:

- Many patients have no idea how to maintain a proper diet and to effectively exercise, so they give up out of lack of understanding.
- All too often, patients have followed various fad programs that have led to minimal or no results.
- Diet and exercise always seem to be perceived as something that is "extra" to our daily regimen of living, and therefore something that is not a lifestyle necessity.
- The conventional approach to medicine has created the attitude that diet and exercise are simply a secondary afterthought to the primary motivator of health correction like the instant gratification of the prescription drug. In other words, our healthcare system does not promote a culture of true importance and medical effectiveness to diet and exercise for our health.

This section will offer strategies towards a healthy and effective way to exercise and eat. It is by no means exhaustive in its scope, but I provide what I have found to be the most broad-based, scientific and practical approach to diet and exercise to improve overall health, decrease joint trauma, enhance metabolism and improve weight management goals in the long term.

Chapter 4
The Metabolic Diet for Weight Management and Beyond

The Physiology of Fat Loss

Do you really want to know the secret to weight loss? It is simple and you have probably heard about it before in some direct or round about way. But, to sum up a complicated concept in one simple statement, it is: "Avoid grain-based carbohydrates."

That's it. When looking at weight loss from a strict food perspective, then this statement works. This concept has been touted since the late 1800s, it was studied extensively in the 1930s and 1940s and was revitalized in the popular Atkins, Zone and South Beach diets. In short, if adopted as a lifestyle versus a temporary diet to lose weight, eliminating grain-based carbohydrates regulates weight. But, there's more to the story.

> Does calorie counting and calorie restriction work? Over the past thirty years fat consumption has decreased by 11 percent while total calorie consumption has decreased by 4 percent. That's correct, Americans are actually eating fewer calories and they are getting fatter!

Since this book and its approach focuses on the inevitable interrelationship of your mental, emotional and spiritual approach to health, simply "avoiding grain-based carbohydrates" will not cover the fully integrated approach to weight loss. You will find more information on the complete comprehensive approach to food and nutrition in "Step One of the Metabolic Health Protocol." Here we will focus on the actual physiological nuts and bolts of weight loss, so hold on for the ride.

Let's explore how the physiology of weight loss actually works and why eliminating most grain-based carbohydrates can significantly turn on your metabolic furnace and help you to shed unnecessary fat.

Does calorie counting and calorie restriction work? Over the past thirty years fat consumption has decreased by 11 percent while total calorie consumption has decreased by 4 percent.[13] That's correct, Americans are actually eating fewer calories and they are getting fatter! Why? Because all of the good fats have been replaced with more carbohydrates. Remember, one gram of fat has over double the amount of calories than one gram of carbohydrate. So, we have netted less calories but have inevitably increased the amount of grain-based and processed carbohydrates.

This enigma relates to the concept of "calories in, calories out." If you eat less then your body is utilizing and burning, then you will automatically lose weight. One of the key paradoxes offered by Gary Taubes, a prominent scientist and author of the book *Good Calories, Bad Calories*, explains that calorie counting for weight loss or weight maintenance does not work. Here is an excellent example of this concept: If a person eats an average of 2,700 calories per day over a ten year period, this would equate to one million calories or about twelve tons of food. In order to maintain your weight within five pounds, you would have to have eaten your daily calories within a 0.1 percent accuracy. This means that if you eat even slightly outside of that range, then you would gain weight... considerable weight. And even the most prudent dieter cannot possibly keep up that level of accuracy over an entire decade. So, how is it that everyone is not either completely obese or completely anorexic?

Typically, most weight loss programs are predicated on the belief that fat cells are sitting around, inactive and minding their own business. Then along come too many calories and they are forced into the fat cell, making the *cell* larger and *you* fatter. In physiology, adipose cells (fat cells) have been assumed to be inactive, inert and passive. But there has been a long history of physiological study that has shown that fat cells are very active. Recently, endocrinology has placed new emphasis on the physiology of fat tissue and has discovered fat secreting hormones such as grehlin and adiponectin. **Fat tissue is therefore hormonally active and possesses a dynamic physiology.** This perspective lends to a different theory on weight loss, one of a hormonal and cell signaling interplay with fat tissue. If we can understand and influence the hormonal signals of fat tissue, then we can influence and experience desired fat loss. So, you have to create the proper hormonal environment.

The Hormonal Influence of Fat Loss and The Paleolithic Diet: A Metabolic Furnace

A quick summary is listed here of the metabolic enhancement of a high protein, moderate fat and very low grain-based carbohydrate diet:

- Protein increases your metabolism more than carbohydrate or fat. Simply, protein takes more energy by your body to digest. The resulting effect is an increase in thermic or heat energy. Protein has a thermic effect of 25 percent, meaning you only get seventy-five grams of effective energy from one hundred grams of protein eaten. Carbohydrate has a thermic effect of 15 percent, meaning 85 percent is digested and utilized and fat has a 0 percent thermic effect, as all of the energy is used by the body.
- Your body will be more conditioned to burning fat for energy when you stop relying on sugar, starches or complex carbohydrates for energy. The low levels of insulin in your blood opens up for the fat burning process and you will feel more energized.
- Fat and adequate protein will prevent loss of lean body mass. Maintaining muscle and/or gaining muscle will keep your metabolism up.

I believe that patients would like their fat cells to go away or truly go to sleep, never to be around again. But it is time for fat cells to wake up! We don't want them sleeping, we don't want them dormant, we want them active! With fat cells mobilized and activated, sending signals and messages to wake up, fat will start to liberate its contents. The diet lifestyle and other hormonal factors explained in this book provide powerful influences towards your goals of fat loss and metabolic health.

Carbohydrates Make Alpha Glycerol Phosphate (AGP)

When you ingest sugar in all its forms it will be metabolically broken down into a product called alpha glycerol phosphate (AGP). AGP is the actual backbone to triglycerides or the fatty acid molecule that is stored in fat cells making people fat. If you do not have adequate AGP being formed from sugar intake, then the body must utilize its stores within fat cells by pulling out the triglycerides with their AGP backbone. This translates into fat loss. So, keeping carbohydrate intake low keeps AGP low, which tells fat cells to dump their triglyceride (fatty acid) contents, leading to overall fat loss.

But there is more to the story…

Insulin is the fat storage hormone. Let me start off by clarifying that insulin is not a direct enemy. It is needed to keep us functioning properly on many levels. However, in excess amounts over time it continues to signal our fat cells to store fat, or worse, it tells our fat cells to not liberate their contents of fatty acids. The goal is to limit the amount of insulin secreted in order to optimize fat loss.

There are a couple of ways to keep insulin low in your body to optimize weight loss:

- Prevent it from being secreted in large amounts in the first place. This means avoiding grain-based carbohydrates as much as possible. Keep in mind that insulin responds to the amount of carbohydrates, NOT the amount of calories.[14] If calories are still relatively adequate or high but devoid of most carbohydrate, then insulin will be minimally secreted. Also, despite what we have been told for years, dietary fat cannot enter adipose cells (fat cells) unless *carbohydrate* and its resultant AGP helps to shuttle it in.

❧ Inhibit the release of insulin through other pathways. This idea refers to increasing catecholamine hormones such as epinephrine, norepinephrine and dopamine through exercise and certain dietary supplements (see Step 3 of the Metabolic Health Protocol). These hormones activate the breakdown of the triglyceride fatty acid molecules in your fat cells by activating hormone sensitive lipase. Lipase is necessary to prevent the triglyceride from going back into the fat cell once liberated by the low carbohydrate diet.

Stress and Weight Management: The Cortisol Factor

Cortisol is the stress hormone. It is responsible for a multitude of functions including inflammation regulation, immunity, blood sugar control and mobilization of energy when under a stress response. Cortisol keeps you alive. However, when you are under consistent stress, cortisol levels can remain elevated in direct correlation with abdominal and visceral (organ) fat accumulation, or belly fat.[15] The constant stress and high cortisol levels also leads to a chronic inflammatory state that further lessens the ability to lose weight. Stress and inflammation lead to an accumulation of fat.

The Lectin Connection

Lectins are protein complexes found in all foods, but in varying amounts depending on the food. Lectins are difficult to digest and pass undigested through the hydrochloric acid conditions of the stomach. They then can damage the lining of the intestines and pass directly into general circulation. Various tissues are sensitive to lectins including endocrine tissues such as the pancreas, adrenals and thyroid. Lectins have been associated with a multitude of diseases including arthritis, heart disease, allergies, high blood

> The potential problem with lectins is the pro-inflammatory state they create. Remember, when our bodies are inflamed, we have great difficulty losing weight.

pressure, fibromyalgia, chronic fatigue, thyroid disease and hormonal imbalances including elevated cortisol levels. The potential problem with lectins is the pro-inflammatory state they create. Remember, when our bodies are inflamed, we have great difficulty losing weight.

The most common lectin-containing foods are grain-based carbohydrates, particularly gluten-containing foods such as wheat and wheat germ. Also, quinoa, rice, buckwheat, oats, rye, barley, millet, corn, legumes including all dried beans and soy and peanuts, and members of the nightshade family such as potatoes, tomatoes, eggplants and peppers.

Any pasteurized dairy product also contains lectins because it has been heated which decreases secretory IgA, an immunoglobin that binds to lectins rendering them harmless to the body. Raw, unpasteurized milk contains significant secretory IgA levels that can bind to the lectins naturally found in milk. The second section of this chapter discusses the benefits of raw milk in more detail.

Lectins have been recently suggested to be associated with interfering with an important fat hormone called leptin, leading to what is called "leptin resistance."[16] Leptin is a hormone that signals the brain to feel satisfied or satiated. Without it, we would just keep eating. Leptin also affects the growth of blood vessels and bone, the immune system, glucose and fat metabolism and the reproductive system. If you give leptin experimentally to rodents, it promotes weight loss. However, giving leptin to obese humans does not promote significant weight loss. And interestingly, most obese people have high levels of leptin, not low levels as you might expect. This suggests that "leptin resistance" may be a significant cause of human obesity.[17, 18] Lectins from grain-based carbohydrates may be interfering with the actual receptor on the cell surface that allows leptin to stimulate the cell and improve satisfaction from eating.

Leptin resistance is also associated with increased inflammation and elevated blood levels of CRP or C-reactive protein, an inflammatory marker.[19] Leptin resistance also seems to be associated with the very potent pro-inflammatory lectins. So, it seems that eliminating lectins and lowering overall inflammation in the body would be extremely key to controlling the important fat-regulating hormones. And the first dietary step towards this end would be to eliminate or at least greatly reduce, grain-based, lectin-containing, pro-inflammatory carbohydrates.

A Word on Fad Diets and HCG
(Human Chorionic Gonadotropin)

This chapter and Step 2 of the Metabolic Protocol explores and introduces a nutritional lifestyle that is more sustainable over time, versus a limited, brief diet process that is not realistic or sustainable over time.

We have seen and heard of the fad diets because they grow like weeds in the public nutritional landscape, offering levels of hope of weight loss that sometimes do and sometimes do not work. Radical cleansing diets such as the "Master Cleanse" employed by people who have never cleansed in their lives that can do more harm than good. We have heard of the typical yo-yo dieting process, and many have experienced it first hand, but we still look for the easy, temporary solution that never really teaches us how to live and eat.

One of the not-so-new diet fads is the HCG Diet. It was first introduced officially in *Lancet* by Dr. A. Simeons in 1954 [20] and quickly fell out of popularity. But the relatively recent abundant acceptance of hormone therapy coupled with the obesity epidemic in America, the HCG hormone has made a new emergence for weight loss. HCG is a hormone abundant during pregnancy and is measured in pregnancy tests as its levels elevate early on after fertilization. HCG also mimics a pituitary hormone known as leutinizing hormone (LH), and in fact is a powerful stimulant of many endocrine tissues including the ovaries and testicles. I have seen spikes in hormone levels while patients are taking HCG, but of course, this stimulation to the endocrine system is temporary and transient and varies from individual to individual. There are some variations on the way the diet is offered, depending on the practitioner. The diet often employs either injectable or sublingual HCG administered weekly or biweekly in varying doses from 250 IU per injection up to 500 IU per injection. The HCG is harvested from pregnant women's urine who have consented to its use for infertility. The HCG is coupled with a calorie-deprived diet ranging from the more traditional 500 to 800 calories per day to more recent variations of up to 1,200 calories per day. Exercise is sometimes, but not always encouraged. Claims are made of rapid weight loss and actual redistribution of fat from one area to another.

> In general, I do not believe that the HCG diet is the best solution for weight loss. Even though it is obvious that people in fact do lose weight on the diet, and I have seen this in many of my patients, the actual HCG hormone component does not seem to be overly important in this weight loss.

In general, I do not believe that the HCG diet is the best solution for weight loss. Even though it is obvious that people in fact do lose weight on the diet, and I have seen this in many of my patients, the actual HCG hormone component does not seem to be overly important in this weight loss. Two key double-blind placebo controlled studies from 1977 [21] and 1990 [22] showed no difference between groups using the calorie-deprived diet without the HCG component versus the group following the same diet and using the HCG. In other words, if you starve someone, very often they will lose weight, but even more often they will gain it back. This type of diet is not conducive to teaching someone how to manage their relationship with food. Of course, certain practitioners will be better than others in their educational approach to maintenance, but once you dangle the carrot of easy, quick weight loss, then this will be the path that the patient will likely want to continue to take.

There are far more studies that demonstrate HCG does not work. The American Society of Bariatric Physicians clearly states this in their official position statement on the HCG diet.[23] A 1995 meta-analysis of all the published articles on the use of HCG in weight loss concluded "there is no scientific evidence that HCG is effective in the treatment of obesity;

it does not bring about weight-loss or fat-redistribution, nor does it reduce hunger or induce a feeling of well-being."[24]

Additionally, HCG is not FDA approved for the specific use of weight loss but for use in infertility. There are many medications that are effectively and safely used "off label," meaning not the original FDA approved usage. I bring this point up as salient to the medical-legal aspect of medicine, and as a reasonable warning to practitioners utilizing this therapy. So it is very clear, the literature does NOT contain any negative effects of the use of HCG injections per se.

There is also some question as the safety of calorie deprivation during an HCG diet protocol course. Many unhealthy people cannot handle a serious reduction in calories utilized in the HCG diet protocol. As a naturopath, I believe that careful cleansing and brief food and calorie restriction is a cornerstone of health and therapy for patients. However, the cleansing diet and protocol is usually more controlled and finite in comparison to the longer-term calorie restriction of the HCG diet that lasts a month or more. Over time, many of the patients, particularly if they are left to their own devices, will gain the weight back. But, even if monitored, they will still often gain the weight back. The body always desires balance, and if weight loss is too rapid, then the body will make the pendulum swing further to the other side, and weight gain follows.

In summary:

- Fad diets and calorie deprivation diets do not teach the body to gradually lose weight nor tend to teach and promote a healthy relationship to food.
- If you starve a patient, they will often lose weight, but not necessarily, as it depends on what they eat.
- The hormone HCG does not *necessarily* cause weight loss or fat redistribution and most studies support this.
- Empirical and experiential evidence exists that the HCG diet works but it is suggested that this is due mostly to the calorie-deprivation and placebo effect of using the hormone.

- ❦ HCG stimulates ovarian production of estrogen and testicular production of testosterone.
- ❦ There are no known negative effects from the HCG hormone alone.
- ❦ Calorie deprivation *over time* has the *potential* to be harmful.

Summarizing the Physiology of Fat Loss

So far I can summarize the five following strategies and physiological facts that help to regulate fat loss:

- ❦ Eat foods that lower and/or control Insulin.
- ❦ Lower and/or control Cortisol. This means you need to decrease stress. (See Step 2 and Step 6 of the Metabolic Health Protocol.)
- ❦ Avoid foods that promote Inflammation and employ strategies that reduce it.
- ❦ Avoid GRAIN-BASED CARBOHYDRATE foods that contain allergens and particularly lecti
- ❦ Create a Food Lifestyle and improve your relationship with food. (See Step 2—The Metabolic Health Foundation for more information on this often missed component of weight loss and health improvement.)

The simple answer, in terms of the best way to eat, that addresses each of these vitally important components of weight loss, is to AVOID GRAIN-BASED CARBOHYDRATES!

Metabolic Nutrition Introduction

Nutritional science is observed through the lens of current physiological science and the social and even political conditions in which we find ourselves. If we measure the success of the current nutritional advice by existing chronic disease rates, then the science has failed miserably. Additionally, nutritional science does not come equipped with an underlying and unifying paradigm from which it can stand upon. In other words, nutritional science cannot agree on one central theme for its scientific direction. For example, we do not see comprehensive agreement on the concept of how a calorie affects the body. One perspective believes that a calorie is a calorie while another believes that it depends on where that calorie came from, i.e. grain-based carbohydrate, vegetable-based carbohydrate, plant protein, animal protein, etc. Another example would be that "all fats are created equally" and this has been proven false many times over.

> Nutritional science does not come equipped with an underlying and unifying paradigm from which it can stand upon. In other words, nutritional science cannot agree on one central theme for its scientific direction.

This limited scope does not allow us to see the larger picture of human health. Human health and optimal nutrition can be viewed through the consideration and study of an anthropological and archeological perspective. S. Boyd Eaton, a professor at Emory University in Atlanta Georgia, has offered that this perspective provides a unifying paradigm,[25] or scientific foundation, leading to the ability to answer the questions of "What did our ancestors eat that got us here in the first place?"

That rampant chronic disease on the rise is based on a social transition from a hunter-gatherer type diet to our current agricultural based diet that evolved approximately 10,000 years ago. And even more recently, with the industrial revolution, our diets changed even more dramatically. Since the early twentieth century, whole grains have been routinely refined, removing much of their nutritional content, and refined sugar has become a household staple. Jean Bogert, a nutritionist who witnessed the dietary changes of the Industrial Revolution noted, "The machine age has had the effect of forcing upon the peoples of the industrial nations the most gigantic human feeding experiment ever attempted."[26] Currently, the adoption of the FDA Food Pyramid and the diet recommendations of the American Heart Association, both of which promote a high carbohydrate and low fat diet, could be contributing to these chronic diseases of civilization. Even when we think we are eating a good diet we could be fooled, without anyone getting the joke. The diseases we now experience as a result of this nutritional transition include cardiovascular diseases, such as atherosclerosis (hardening of the arteries), hypertension and stroke, cancer, insulin resistance and type II diabetes, obesity, chronic obstructive lung disease such as emphysema and chronic bronchitis, hearing loss and dental caries or cavities.[27, 28, 29]

The following chart compares some of the specific results on the human body of a Paleolithic diet versus a modern contemporary diet. Our ancestors had normal blood pressure, more muscle mass, less body fat, no insulin resistance or diabetes and lower cholesterol levels. They were doing something right.

Table: Ancestral versus Modern Humans

Differences	Contributing Factors	Paleolithic	Contemporary
Blood Pressure Paleolithic: Normotensive through out life cycle Contemporary: Tends to rise with age; many hypertensives	Dietary intake of electrolytes BMI Aerobic Power	$Na+ \ll K+$ Higher Higher	$Na+ > K+$ Higher Lower
Insulin Responsiveness Paleolithic: Nearly all insulin sensitive Contemporary: Many insulin resistant	BMI Body composition Glycemic load Fiber	Lower More muscle, less fat Lower High intake	Higher Less muscle, more fat Higher Low intake
Lipid Metabolism Paleolithic: Lower serum cholesterol Contemporary: Higher serum cholesterol	Saturated fat intake Trans fat PUFA w6:w3 Simple CHO Dietary fiber	Lower Almost nil More About 2:1 Lower Higher	Higher 2% of energy intake Less 10:1 (or more) Higher Lower

Normotensive = normal blood pressure (120/80 or less)

Hypertensive = high blood pressure (greater than 140/85)

$Na+$ = sodium; $K+$ = potassium

BMI = Body Mass Index

Glycemic load = sugar/carb load

serum = blood

PUFA = poly unsaturated fatty acids

CHO = carbohydrate

This chart was adapted from the following article: Eaton SB, Cordain L, Sebastian A. "The Ancestral Biomedical Environment In: Endothelial Biomedicine." W.C. Aird (Ed), Cambridge University Press, 2007, pp. 129-134.

Civilization as we know it today is a relatively new concept. From an evolutionary and historical perspective, our framework of civilization just started a mere 10,000 years ago. And 99.98 percent of our genetic makeup was complete before civilization developed. In fact, the human genome has changed less than 0.02 percent in the last 40,000 years.[30] Along the way we were eating in a particular fashion that has influenced our genetic evolution and established the nutritional requirements for our bodies today.[31] Look at it from the numbers:

> By studying our ancestors of the Paleolithic era from between 1.5 million to 10,000 years ago, we can understand a more complete way of obtaining optimal nutrition, minimizing the risk of chronic disease, and maximizing metabolic health.

100,000 generations of people were hunter-gatherers, 500 generations have depended on agriculture, only 10 generations have lived since the start of the industrial revolution and only 2 generations have grown up with highly processed fast foods. By studying our ancestors of the Paleolithic era from between 1.5 million to 10,000 years ago, we can understand a more complete way of obtaining optimal nutrition, minimizing the risk of chronic disease, and maximizing metabolic health.

The most convincing evidence based on archeological and anthropological studies demonstrates that the diet of our ancestors had the following components: [32, 33]

- 35 percent of dietary energy came from fats, 35 percent from carbohydrates, and 30 percent from protein. Grain-based carbohydrates such as wheat, beans, rice and other cultivated crops were not part of the diet. The typical food pyramid recommendation has the largest percentage of calories coming from grain-source carbohydrates and only 10-20 percent of calories coming from fats. (See Table 1) This is in stark contrast to how our ancestors ate.

- Saturated fats, the incorrectly purported "bad" fats, contributed a substantial 7.5 percent of total energy and harmful trans-fatty acids contributed negligible amounts.

- Polyunsaturated fat intake was high, with an omega 6 to omega 3 (fish oils) fatty acid ratio approaching 2:1, versus the 10:1 ratio of today.

- Cholesterol consumption was substantial, perhaps 480 mg per day. The American Heart Association believes that your cholesterol intake should be between 200 to 300 mg per day to prevent heart disease and keep cholesterol levels in your blood low.

- Carbohydrate came from uncultivated fruits and vegetables, approximately 50 percent energy intake as compared with the present level of 16 percent energy intake for Americans.

- High fruit and vegetable intake and minimal grain and dairy consumption made ancestral diets base-yielding, unlike today's acid-producing pattern.

- Honey comprised 2-3 percent energy intake as compared with the 15 percent added sugars contribute currently.

- Fiber consumption was high, perhaps 100 grams per day, but phytate content was minimal. Phytic acid, found in abundance in many grain foods, interferes with mineral absorption.

- Vitamin, mineral and phytochemical (plant chemical) intake was typically 1.5 to 8 times that of today except for that of sodium, which was generally less than 1,000 mg per day and much less than that of potassium.

Table 1:   Comparison of the current USDA food pyramid versus an ancestral food pyramid

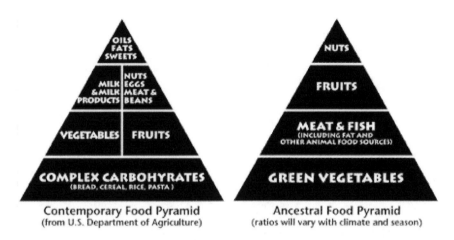

Contemporary Food Pyramid
(from U.S. Department of Agriculture)

Ancestral Food Pyramid
(ratios will vary with climate and season)

This particular anthropological perspective is known as the **Paleolithic Diet** and it will be explained more specifically soon. In summary, simply eat organic healthy meats, organ meats (such as liver), poultry, and fish in abundance, fruits and vegetables of all types, nuts of all types, minimal dairy and avoid grains and other processed carbohydrate sources of all types.

Anthropology is the study of human origin and culture, and it is this approach to the study and understanding of human diet that presents the clear-cut sense for establishing your metabolic health, solving obesity, preventing chronic disease and strengthening the generations. This is not a new concept within science and medicine. Weston A. Price, a prominent dentist from the 1930s, traveled the world and studied the diet and overall health of native peoples culminating in a now renowned legacy and wealth of nutritional knowledge. Current medical science claims that low fat and high carbohydrate diets are traditional and ancestral, but Dr. Price discovered something very different. Various peoples such as the Eskimos of Alaska, indigenous Alpiners and Africans to name a few, all experienced optimal health on plentiful amounts of animal fats and none of these or any studied native peoples on traditional diets consumed low amounts of fat and protein.

Here are some of the highlights of Dr. Price's research:[34]

- All groups studied consumed minerals and fat-soluble vitamins from high vitamin butter or from seafoods, cod liver, seal oil or animal organs with their fat.
- In each diet there was some daily source of raw, unaltered protein from sources such as meats, seafoods, nuts, cheeses, eggs, milk or high quality sprouted seeds. Some sort of sea plant or mineral was a part of most diets. Inland sea deposits of food were treasured and used thriftily.
- Foods were grown on soil that was naturally high in minerals, and no chemical fertilizers or pesticides were used.
- All food was eaten liberally in the natural season in which it grew.
- Sweets (even good, natural sweets) were used rarely or sparingly, only for occasions of ritual, celebration or special feasting. However, there is new research to suggest that some indigenous cultures ate an abundance of raw honey and raw maple syrup.
- Each group observed periods of partial abstinence from food, or regulated periods of under-eating. For some, this came about as a natural result of summer crops being in short supply before the new crops were harvested. For others, certain rituals began or ended with days of fasting. Still others taught the value of periodic under-eating by taboos or other means.
- All ate whole foods, not fractionalized parts of foods. They did not remove the fiber content of their natural foods by refining them. Most foods were eaten raw or very gently and lightly cooked.

How (and What) to Eat Like Your Ancestors

The available evidence and frank common sense shows that we are designed to eat foods that are mostly devoid of grain-based carbohydrates.

Let's explore exactly what this means and how it can be incorporated into your lifestyle to enhance your metabolic health.

The following summary provides an excellent summary that is easy to follow. When in doubt about your diet come back to this table and see how close you are to achieving this nutritional lifestyle. It is provided as a checklist for you to gauge your progress during your journey for metabolic health.

Table 2—Fundamentals of the Hunter-Gatherer Metabolic Diet and Lifestyle Checklist. Let's talk about how you set up this bullet list. Consistency is key.

- Introduce this "lifestyle" slowly.
  - Week 1: Make breakfast and snacks strictly Paleo but keep lunch and dinner as you have normally eaten.
  - Week 2: Make breakfast and lunch and snacks Paleo but allow dinner to contain grain-based carbohydrates. Keep protein and vegetables the focus.
  - Week 3: Move into a complete Paleo lifestyle, but allow one or two meals per week to be whatever you would like. Essentially, maintain a 95 percent Paleo and 5 percent variance with some grain-based carbohydrates. You will be able to maintain the lifestyle in the long run if you allow a transition to take place that has a built-in ability to vary and explore.
- Eat whole, natural, fresh foods. Remember to eat as close to nature as possible as often as possible.
- Keep your calorie ratio about 65 percent animal protein and fat and 35 percent carbohydrates from a large variety of vegetable and fruit sources.
- Eat four to six small meals daily and especially DO NOT skip breakfast. One excellent way to create the practice of small meals is to focus on the traditional three meals daily, breakfast, lunch and dinner, keeping the meals small, and then adding small snacks two to three hours after each main meal.

- Consume a diet high in vegetables, fruits, nuts and berries, avoiding grains and refined sugars. Nutrient-dense fruits and vegetables such as berries, plums, citrus, apples, cantaloupe, spinach, tomatoes, broccoli, cauliflower and avocados are good examples.
- Vegetable to fruit ratio should be about 2:1.
- Choose organic sources of fruits and vegetables.
- It is interesting to note that between 80 and 120 different foods are consumed each day by today's hunter-gatherer societies, containing small quantities of various herbs and wild vegetables. So, again, variety is the key. Be sure to change your vegetable and fruits regularly and follow what is in season.
- Increase consumption of omega-3 fatty acids from fish, fish oil and plant sources.
- Increase consumption of lean protein, such as poultry, fish, pork, game meats and lean cuts of red meat. Cuts with the words *round* or *loin* in the name are usually lean. Limit fatty, salty processed meats such as bacon, sausage and deli meats.
- Chose organic sources of animal proteins that are raised organically and free range. See the Appendix for more information on locations for excellent sources of animal proteins.
- Eat protein at every meal.
- If milk is consumed, chose *raw*, unpasteurized "real" milk sources if possible, from a properly run dairy. (See www.westonapricefoundation.org for more information on real milk.)
- Incorporate olive oil and coconut oil into the diet. Avoid trans-fats entirely and do not fear saturated fat. However, eliminate fried foods, hard margarine, commercial baked goods and most packaged and processed snack foods.
- Drink water. At least half your body weight in ounces daily and then for every six ounces of caffeine or alcohol you consume, you must add eight more ounces of water.
- If sweeteners are desired, use natural sweeteners such as raw honey and dark amber maple syrup sparingly.

- Participate in daily exercise from various activities (incorporating aerobic and strength training and stretching exercises). Outdoor activities are ideal.
- Foods to Avoid
    - All grain-based carbohydrates including wheat, corn, rice, barley, cereals etc.
    - All legumes including peanuts, beans, peas, soybeans, tofu, soy milk and flour.
    - Starchy potatoes including yams, sweet potatoes and Jerusalem artichokes.
    - Yeast, including baked goods, pickled foods, vinegar, fermented foods and fermented beverages such as beer (all contain yeast).
    - Refined sugars of any type.
    - Refined table salt. Use healthy Celtic Sea Salt only.
    - Alcohol. Wine is the best choice and should be limited to six to eight ounces daily or less. No more than eight ounces of beer or four ounces of spirits daily.
    - Pasteurized milk products.
    - Avoid high fructose corn syrup from common sources such as soft drinks and baked goods.
    - Chemical food additives, artificial sweeteners, diet soft drinks and processed foods of any type.

For information on recipe ideas, explore www.thepaleodiet.com and www.paleodiet.com. There is an amazing amount of information on the web for Paleo-style and low-carb diet recipes. The choices are endless. Remember that this nutritional lifestyle has more foods that you can eat versus foods that you should avoid, so it is very difficult to get bored. The limits are only based on your creativity.

The Metabolic Beverage: Water

The importance of water for your entire body, its physiology and metabolism, cannot be overstated. This basic element of nutritional science and practical common sense possesses the innate ability to improve every aspect of your metabolic health. The current paradigm of the science of physiology is based on the study of the "solutes" or the chemicals dissolved in the blood. Little attention is given towards the solvent or the water portion of the blood in the dynamics of all the physiological processes within the body. This paradigm lends itself to a focus on using chemicals, natural or unnatural, to alter the physiology and improve health. This section will provide an overview of the importance of water and the various diseases that it can actually cure, all being largely based on the work of Dr. Fereydoon Batmanghelidj, M.D., an internationally renowned researcher, author and advocate of the natural healing power of water. I encourage you to explore the available scientific research and book, *Your Body's Many Cries for Water*, all available on his website, www.watercure.com. Please see the Appendix for more information.

Water: What, How, When, and Why?

- ❧ Water is constantly being expended by your body through the basic activities of life and the normal physiological processes that make your body work. The average person will lose about three to four liters or ten to fifteen cups of water daily in sweat, urine, bowel movements and even normal breathing.

- ❧ *If you are thirsty, you are already dehydrated.* This is often a shocking realization for many people. The point is to drink water constantly throughout the day to avoid feeling thirsty and therefore avoiding the resultant dehydrated state. Common immediate symptoms of dehydration are fatigue and headaches, which then chronically lead to constipation, halitosis or bad breath and acne. More on disease and dehydration later.

- ❧ *You should drink at least half your body weight in ounces daily and for every six ounces of caffeinated or alcoholic beverage you drink, you should add eight more ounces on top of your main quota.*

- ❧ Based on the unpredictability of municipal water sources at any one time, I believe that everyone should drink filtered water when possible.

❧ To lessen the impact on the environment, avoid plastic disposable water bottles and use a home water filter. By avoiding plastic water bottles, you also avoid harmful estrogen-like compounds called phthalates. Buy a stainless steel water bottle. You will find that the water stays cooler and has a better taste.

❧ Keep your water with you all the time, everywhere you go.

❧ For exercise, you will need about one liter of water for every hour of exercise, and more if you experience hot weather. Be sure to follow your instincts about water intake.

❧ It is an excellent habit to create by starting the day with a large glass of water with a small amount of Celtic Sea Salt added to it. It is refreshing and cleansing and helps to get to your quota of water consumption.

❧ Also, drink water a half hour before and after you eat to support digestion. Constipation is commonly related to and exacerbated by dehydration.

❧ The more you focus on the importance of water, making it a habit, you will begin to notice your body's signals for the need for water.

Remember:

8 ounces is 1 cup

16 ounces is 2 cups which is 1 pint

32 ounces is 4 cups which is 2 pints which is 1 quart

128 ounces is 16 cups which is 8 pints which is 4 quarts which is 1 gallon

Water and Exercise

Although it is extremely important to hydrate while exercising, an excessive amount of water can be dangerous at this time. During intense exercise, the kidneys have difficulty in excreting excess water and it can then move into many body tissues including the brain. This is called water intoxication. The real problem with water intoxication is related to the hyponatremia or lowered sodium levels and other electrolytes in the blood.

When sodium is too low, nerve cells in your body cannot work and this can result in death. This type of water intoxication occurs mostly in marathon runners who are not consuming enough salt/electrolytes along with the water they are consuming. It is very important to have at least one half to one full teaspoon of Celtic Sea Salt with your entire water quota for the day to keep electrolytes up and protect your kidneys.

Water and Disease

Histamine is the major neurotransmitter, or chemical nerve signal, that regulates water intake and its preservation in the body. Unfortunately, histamine has also been viewed as the culprit in many different disease conditions that are actually related to dehydration. Allergies and peptic ulcers are two key examples. Both conditions have excessive histamine production

> When following a low carbohydrate nutritional lifestyle, the initial weight loss is largely due to loss of water, and you need to drink an adequate amount of water in order to avoid dehydration.

during the disease process, but both are related to and can be cured and managed by providing proper hydration. During dehydration, histamine is produced to attempt to hold onto water at all costs. With chronic dehydration, it can lead to allergies and gastrointestinal complaints such as peptic ulcers. And of course, anti-histamines are given believing that the problem is from the histamine, when in fact the histamine is there due to the dehydration. This a common mistake in conventional medicine of treating the symptom and not the cause.

As a result of the role of histamine in water regulation, Dr. Batmanghelidj explains the following adaptive consequences of dehydration: [35]

> - The chronic pains: dyspepsia (ulcer related pain), anginal (chest) pain, rheumatoid joint pain, low back pain, intermittent claudication (muscle cramps) and migraines.
> - Allergies, asthma and pregnancy morning sickness.
> - Essential hypertension (high blood pressure).
> - Insulin resistance or type II diabetes.
> - Chronic Fatigue Syndrome.

Additionally, he lists high cholesterol, heart failure, Alzheimer's disease, strokes, intervertebral disc degeneration, kidney disease in children, insulin dependent or type I diabetes and many other conditions including some psychiatric conditions related to histamine, all being related to dehydration.

Water and Weight Loss

Again, the importance of water for your metabolic health cannot be overstated. For your weight loss goals, water possesses the ability to increase your metabolic rate and decrease appetite. What often seems like hunger signals is actually a signal for water. Always drink water first when you believe you are hungry or are craving something. You will find that often your body is actually craving water.

Water consumption has been shown to have a modest affect directly on basal metabolic rate, or resting metabolism. A recent German study found that after drinking approximately 17 ounces of water, subjects' metabolic rates increased by 30 percent for both men and women. The increases occurred within ten minutes of water consumption and reached a maximum after about thirty to forty minutes.[36] When water is very cold, you can burn between fifty and one hundred calories per day for every half to full gallon of water you drink. This is the process of increasing the metabolic rate.

When following a low carbohydrate nutritional lifestyle, the initial weight loss is largely due to loss of water, and you need to drink an adequate amount of water in order to avoid dehydration. The process of burning calories requires an adequate supply of water in order to function efficiently.

If dehydrated, the liver cannot liberate fatty acids which slow down the fat-burning process. Finally, with a diet that is mostly carbohydrate free but contains substantial fiber from fruits and vegetables, proper hydration is necessary to avoid constipation.

If you wisely chose to make water a part of your daily health regimen, it provides a foundation of support for your metabolic health. This foundation will be what all other health choices and strategies provided in this book will stand upon. So, start drinking water on your way to health today!

Real Milk

There exists a long history of confusion about the benefits and harm of milk. Does it really do a body good? We have been led to believe that it is important for bone growth and development for our children. It is touted as being an excellent source of vitamins and minerals and of course being delicious. But many people understand that it is highly correlated with allergies and negatively affecting immunity, all of which has launched a massive market for milk alternatives such as soy, almond and rice milk. And to make it all more complicated, the question of milk is tightly entwined with political and monetary motivation leaving the consumer with little to believe and even less to help their health. From an anthropological perspective of indigenous cultures around the world today that are still consuming a traditional diet, milk and milk products are part of the diet. However, they are NOT consuming the type of milk we consume in this country.

> Due to the current political control of the American Dairy Association, we are then left with two alternatives: avoid milk all together or continue to drink pasteurized milk hoping that the negative effects will avoid us. But, there is another alternative and it is raw milk.

So, is cow milk causing the negative effects we have traditionally related to it? Yes… and no. The problem with cow milk is the pasteurization process or heat that takes the milk from being a live food with real health benefits to a dead food that has the list of health problems we traditionally associate with milk. Due to the current political control of the American Dairy Association, we are then left with two alternatives: avoid milk all together or continue to drink pasteurized milk hoping that the negative effects will avoid us. But, there is another alternative and it is raw milk.

Unpasteurized, raw and real milk does not have the same negative effects as conventional pasteurized milk. Once milk is heated during the pasteurization process, the natural enzymes and much of the vitamin and mineral content are removed, leaving an unhealthy product. Consuming raw milk can help with your metabolic health.

Pasteurized cow's milk has been associated with a number of health issues:

- Diarrhea, bloating, gas
- Gastrointestinal bleeding
- Allergies and skin rashes
- Colic in infants and recurring ear infections in children
- Increased tooth decay
- Arthritis
- Acne
- Atheroslerosis
- Diabetes
- Cancer
- Here is a summary of some raw or real milk benefits:

COMPARISON CHART BETWEEN RAW AND PASTEURIZED MILKS		
Category Compared	**Raw Milk**	**Pasteurized Milk**
1) Enzymes:	All available. These enzymes are necessary for the actual digestion of the milk and other health-promoting factors.	Less than 10% remaining.
Category Compared	**Raw Milk**	**Pasteurized Milk**
2) Protein:	100% available, all 22 amino acids, including 8 that are essential. This makes the protein profile complete and is excellent for growth and development and maintenance of health.	Protein-lysine and tyrosine are altered by heat with serious loss of metabolic availability. This results in making the whole protein complex less available for tissue repair and rebuilding.
3) Fats: (research studies indicate that fats are necessary to metabolize protein and calcium. All natural protein-bearing foods contain fats.)	All 18 fatty acids metabolically available, both saturated and unsaturated fats.	Altered by heat, especially the 10 essential unsaturated fats.
4) Vitamins:	All 100% available. This includes the Fat and Water Soluble vitamin.	Among the fat-soluble vitamins, some are classed as unstable and therefore a loss is caused by heating above blood temperature. This loss of Vitamin A, D, E and F can run as high as 66%. Vitamin C loss usually exceeds 50%. Losses of water-soluble vitamins are affected by heat and can run from 38% to 80%.
5) Carbohydrates:	Easily utilized in metabolism. Still associated naturally with elements.	Tests indicate that heat has made some changes making elements less available metabolically.
6) Minerals:	All 100% metabolically available. Major mineral components are calcium, chlorine, magnesium, phosphorus, potassium, sodium and sulphur. Vital trace minerals, all 24 or more, 100% available.	Calcium is altered by heat and loss in metabolism may run 50% or more, depending on pasteurization temperature. Losses in other essential minerals too since one mineral usually acts synergistically with another element. There is a loss of enzymes that serve as leaders in assimilation minerals.
NOTE:	Bacteria growth in Raw Milk increases very slowly, because of the friendly acid-forming bacteria (nature's antiseptic) retards the growth of invading organisms (bacteria). Usually keeps for several weeks when under refrigeration and will sour instead of rot.	Pasteurization refers to the process of heating every particle of milk to at least 145° F. and holding at such temperature for at least 15 seconds. Pasteurizing does not remove dirt, bacterially-produced toxins from milk. Bacteria growth will be geometrically rapid after pasteurization and homogenization. Gradually turns rancid in a few days, and then decomposes.

Adapted from: "Supplemental Report in Favor of Grade A Raw Milk: Expert Report and Recommendation." By Dr. William Cambell Douglas Jr., M.D. and Aajonus Vonderplanitz, Scientific Nutritional Researcher. Available: http://www.karlloren.com/aajonus/p15.htm.

Additionally, TSH, or thyroid stimulating hormone, a pituitary hormone that stimulates the thyroid gland, is found in small amounts in unbalanced pasteurized milk. This can contribute to hypothyroidism. Also, another pituitary hormone, ADH, or antidiuretic hormone found in pasteurized cow's milk can lead to water retention. And the pituitary hormone ACTH (adrenocorticotropic hormone) also found in pasteurized cow's milk can stimulate the adrenal glands and lead to Addison's disease or adrenal failure/fatigue.[37]

Is real raw milk safe? Yes. I have consumed raw milk for years and have never had a problem, as have millions of people. The isolated reports of problems with raw milk have been blown out of proportion due to political pressure from the dairy associations.

Where can I get raw milk? There are multiple sources of real milk all over the U.S. and throughout the world. For example, Health Habit Foods located in Phoenix has a ready supply of raw milk from a reputable Arizona farmer. Additionally, explore www.realmilk.com for appropriate sources of certified raw milk in your area.

A final thought on raw or real milk is that you will find, as you explore more details about the Paleo diet that milk products are considered something that our ancestors would not have consumed. There is much debate about this. Many cultures exist today that consume unpasteurized raw milk and benefit greatly from it. I believe that in its raw state, it would have been something that our ancestors could have had some access to. Weston A. Price found this to be true and I believe there is room for raw milk in the diet for those following a more traditional Paleolithic styled diet.

Consuming this form of milk simply tastes better and is clearly better for your health than pasteurized milk, organic or otherwise. I have consumed this type of milk for years, whenever it was available. Purchasing this type of milk sends a message that clearly states your desire to consume foods from sources that are optimal and come from animals that are raised and farmed properly and inevitably more healthy. This is part of the consumer trend towards not just healthier foods, but healthier and more environmentally conscious farming practices.

Paleolithic Salt: Celtic Sea Salt

Just as water is a basic element that is vitally important for our health, so too is salt. However, the type of salt that is being used today in cooking and seasoning is a highly processed junk-food type of salt that would have not been on our ancestors' dinner tables. I believe it is advisable to avoid this type of salt. I disagree that our ancestors would not have had salt in their diets at all, as some in this "Paleo" diet circle contend. Animals will seek out natural salt licks in the wild and humans would have done the same. The negativity associated with salt is actually valid, because that deridement is based on the highly processed table salt that is so often used.

The difference in consumption of sodium and potassium— electrolyte minerals necessary for normal heart function—is especially dramatic. According to Eaton, the typical adult American consumes about 4,000 mg of sodium daily, but less than 10 percent of this amount occurs naturally in food. The rest is added during processing, cooking or seasoning at the table. Potassium consumption is lower, at about 3,000 mg daily.

Salt in its natural whole food state would fit into an original Paleolithic diet. It brings a multitude of health benefits for those seeking optimized metabolic health including:

- Proving all eighty plus minerals and trace elements known to humankind in a complete source benefiting the entire system.
- Stabilizing irregular heartbeats and regulating blood pressure along with adequate hydration.
- Balancing excess acidity of body cells. Acidity is highly correlated with disease.

- Balancing blood sugar levels through mineral balance.
- Vital for generating hydroelectric energy within body cells, which optimizes cellular energy and metabolic health.
- Improving nerve cell communication, optimizing memory and focus.
- Improving digestion.
- Clearing the lungs of excess mucus.
- Improving sinus congestion and health.
- Providing natural antihistamine properties, improving allergies.
- Along with proper hydration, improving muscle cramps.
- Highly cleansing for the entire body.
- Improves sleep by supplying the minerals necessary and also decreases the need to urinate during the night.
- Improves water retention.
- Celtic sea salt has been reported to dissolve kidney stones.
- Enhances immunity and aids healing.
- Helps control saliva and drooling, and even double chin, along with proper hydration.

Celtic sea salt is simply one of the easiest ways to improve your health and I recommend it for all my patients. This whole food, or complete salt, is a truly beautiful salt that provides your body with a multitude of essential minerals to optimize health. Its beauty lies in its simplicity and its inherent chemical properties that literally mimic human life. Simply speaking, the mineral content of whole food sea salt has the same chemical makeup as human blood, lymphatic fluid, and the extracellular fluid that bathes all cells.

Where do you find Celtic sea salt and how do you take it? Most quality health food stores such as Whole Foods carry Celtic sea salt. You can also obtain it online at www.celticseasalt.com.

To enhance your metabolic health, be sure to replace all your table salt use with Celtic sea salt. I always "finish" with this type of salt and avoid cooking with it when possible to avoid destroying the original properties of the salt. However, by all means, cook with it. You will find that food will taste better and you will need less of the salt. If a recipe calls for one teaspoon, use perhaps two thirds of a teaspoon. Celtic sea salt is best kept in a wooden saltcellar or can be kept in a salt mill to grind it as needed for cooking or eating. Finally, add about one eighth to one fourth of a teaspoon of salt to about eight ounces of water in the morning as a cleansing invigorating beverage and the same right before bed to improve sleep.

Metabolic Sweeteners

A low grain-based carbohydrate diet can actually satisfy all of the tastes that humans have the ability to sense, including bitter, sour, pungent (spicy), and even salt and sweet. Actually, primitive diets focused on the sweet taste adding a substantial portion in their diets in the form of honey. The Hazda of Tanzania, the Mbuti pygmies of the Congo, the Veddas or Wild Men of Sri Lanka, the Guayaka Indians of Paraguay, the Bushmen of South Africa and the Aborigines of Australia all consumed honey in large amounts. East coast American Indians consumed plentiful portions of maple syrup, and used it in the production of pemmican. Wild fruits and berries are incredibly sweet at the peak of ripeness, and can be preserved in various ways for consumption throughout the year. Even the fermented foods of the Eskimo are described as tasting sweet like candy.

Many patients have the desire to still add the taste of sweet into their diets. Understanding that sugar is one of the worst things that you could regularly ingest for your overall health and particularly your goals of fat loss, finding suitable alternatives is imperative.

Here is a small list of sweet alternatives:

- **Honey** is one of the best natural alternatives to sugar, possessing a complete array of nutrients along with its sugar content. In fact, honey has a full complement of friendly bacteria that helps with immunity and gut health. It also has anti-viral and anti-bacterial effects, acts as an excellent cough suppressant, and a multitude of other benefits. In small and moderate amounts, its consumption honors the "Paleo" diet concept. Honey contains about 30 percent fructose and it will stimulate insulin production, so should be used sparingly in patients trying to lose weight, but again, do not completely deprive yourself of this. However, when used as a post exercise food or sweetener, the insulin promoting effect will actually be used for muscle growth versus fat storage.

- **Maple syrup** is very similar in its benefits as honey. It has a high mineral content including zinc and manganese and can be used as a sweetener in certain recipes. Just like honey, it should be used sparingly when trying to focus on weight loss.
- **Stevia** is an excellent alternative to sugar and is actually 300 times sweeter than sugar. It is completely devoid of calories and comes from a South American plant called Stevia rebaudiana. This extremely safe sugar alternative has GRAS status (Generally Recognized as Safe) from the FDA. Stevia does not induce insulin and has been used traditionally for diabetes and can actually be added to an insulin resistance nutritional protocol.
- **Xylitol** is a natural chemical compound found in many fruits often derived from the bark of birch trees or the husks of corn. The human body makes several grams of xylitol per day using it in several biochemical processes. There is some research to suggest that it possesses some antibacterial benefits within the oral cavity and the lungs. Additionally, it does not have a significant insulin promoting effect as regular sugar. You can use this as a direct replacement, gram for gram, for sugar and it is found in most health food stores. Be sure to add this, as with any new sweetener, slowly into the diet to avoid digestive upset.
- **Erythritol** is a similar natural sweetener that may be easier for some patients to digest, but is not as sweet as Xylitol.

With all these wonderful alternatives to sugar there is no need to add in the chemical sweeteners such as Sweet-N-Low® (saccharin) and Equal® (aspartame) that both pose too much doubt and suspicion as to possible negative health effects. Both stevia and xylitol can be found in convenient packets and small shaker sized containers.

Metabolic Spices

With all of this discussion about diet, it is important to mention spices, for many different reasons.

- ❧ Utilizing spices enhances the flavor of foods and keeps people interested, especially when they are trying new types of diet lifestyles.
- ❧ The spices listed below are actually considered botanical medicines with an ancient track record of health enhancement.
- ❧ Spices can be taken in a pill form and should then be taken with meals because most spices are fat soluble, which means they are better absorbed along with fats.
- ❧ Many spices have been shown to increase the metabolic rate through thermogenesis and burning more calories.
- ❧ Spices are generally warming to the body.
- ❧ Spices decrease sugar cravings, create a sense of fullness and can even enhance insulin activity.
- ❧ Spices kick-start your metabolic health! So, use them often, explore and experiment, and have fun!

Here is a basic list of spices that can easily be added to many recipes or simply taken in a pill form:

- ❧ Cinnamon
- ❧ Cumin
- ❧ Ginger
- ❧ Turmeric
- ❧ Curry (a combination of ginger, turmeric, cumin)
- ❧ Cayenne pepper
- ❧ Black pepper
- ❧ Chiles (fresh or canned)
- ❧ Chili powder
- ❧ Mustard seed powder

Metabolic Dessert: Cocoa

Here is one item on the dining plate that many people are very excited about. We have heard more and more lately about the wonderful benefits of chocolate, so the secret is out. Cocoa can be very effective in enhancing your overall metabolic health and helping you obtain your weight loss goals. There are two main reasons why I believe cocoa is an important part of any consistent comprehensive diet plan:

1. Its literal herbal actions are biochemically and physiologically profound.
2. It helps to curb food cravings by satisfying not only hunger but providing a psychological benefit.

A Cocoa seed contains oils, tannins and alkaloids, including the much talked about theobromine, and of course caffeine, which both stimulates mental concentration and enhances mood. Cocoa also contains important nutritional antioxidant flavonoids which help to prevent antioxidant or free radical damage that is associated with aging and cancer. Another important component of cocoa is the mood enhancing chemical phenylethylamine (PEA) which is associated with the feeling of being in love. It is also an excellent source of the energy-producing mineral magnesium and other minerals such as copper, phosphorus and potassium.

> Another important component of cocoa is the mood enhancing chemical phenylethylamine (PEA) which is associated with the feeling of being in love. It is also an excellent source of the energy-producing mineral magnesium and other minerals such as copper, phosphorus and potassium.

Cocoa exerts its effects on the nervous system and the heart muscle including expanding or dilating the vessels of the heart, therefore lowering blood pressure. Clinical studies are showing that consuming dark chocolate in the amount of 46-105 grams per day, providing 213-500 mg of cocoa polyphenols, modestly lowers systolic blood pressure by 4.7 mmHg and diastolic blood pressure by 2.8 mmHg in normotensive and hypertensive people.[38, 39] A lower amount of dark chocolate, 6.3 grams daily, providing 30 mg of polyphenols, also decreases systolic blood pressure by 2.9 mmHg and diastolic blood pressure by 1.9 mmHg when consumed for eighteen weeks by patients with prehypertension or mild hypertension.[40] Also, a small amount of evidence is pointing to the benefits of chocolate on overall heart disease and lowering cholesterol levels. [41, 42]

Important information about chocolate:

❧ Be sure to choose chocolate that is at least 70 percent pure cocoa or "dark chocolate" and 100 percent organic to get all the health benefits that are being discussed.

❧ Milk may interfere with the absorption of antioxidants from cacao and lowers the health benefits. Therefore, keep it dark and enjoy it in moderation.

❧ For an even more potent effect, chose the 100 percent cacao beans that are minimally processed, providing a slightly bittersweet taste that is an excellent addition to smoothies.

❧ It is also worth mentioning that chocolate contains caffeine, which could be an excellent addition to your metabolic health journey. However, some people are sensitive to caffeine and its effects, so use with caution.

Frequently Asked Questions
about the Metabolic Paleolithic Diet

Is the low carbohydrate concept a new fad diet?

Although there are many different types of the low carbohydrate diet such as the Zone and Atkins diets, there is nothing new about this concept at all. William Banting, a prominent undertaker from the nineteenth century, wrote a small booklet on the concept of a low carbohydrate diet and he immortalized himself as the Father of the Low Carbohydrate Diet. His small booklet entitled, *Letter on Corpulence Addressed to the Public*, first published in 1863 became an instant success, going into many editions and it continued to be published even after the author's death. Because this diet was so directly opposite to the established medical orthodoxy of the time, Banting was ridiculed, so much so that the term "bantering" comes from his public discussions regarding the topic of the low carbohydrate diet. Despite this ridicule, other physicians of the time experimented with the diet with great success and the diet has never gone away completely.

Will I feel full from the "Paleo" diet if I am not having starches?

You will feel very satisfied because it is easy to get plenty of calories when good fats and adequate protein are abundant in the meal. Also, fats and protein have the ability to provide a sensation of satiety or fullness to your brain and body better than carbohydrates can. Start slowly. Make one meal a day carbohydrate-free and do this for a week to get used to it. Then, the more you find out the wonderful things that you can eat, you will be satisfied beyond your expectations.

Doesn't fat make you fat?

This is an antiquated perspective that was largely touted in the 1980s. Excessive grain based carbohydrates, lack of vitamins and minerals, and lack of exercise are the key factors that are leading to obesity worldwide in industrialized countries.

If I lose weight on a carbohydrate-free diet, is it mostly water weight?

Initially within the first few weeks you will lose some water weight because carbohydrates are aquaphilic or water attracting. Consequently, you will feel less bloated from eating a grain-based carbohydrate-free diet. However, in diet plans that are extremely carbohydrate restricting and limiting, you will have a "flushing out" period and tend to lose even more water weight. The diet plan that is described here is not as radical to your system as other carbohydrate-restricting and calorically-restricting diets. This is a lifestyle, not a diet.

Is the Paleo diet good for my thyroid gland and its function?

There are a multitude of domesticated foods that are now available that are known goitrogens, or foods that lower iodine and cause goiter and thyroid disease even in the presence of adequate dietary iodine. These foods would not have been available in an ancestral diet. [43, 44, 45] These goitrogen foods include millet, maize (corn), soy, cassava, sweet potatoes, lima beans, turnips, cabbage, cauliflower, rapeseed (Canola oil), mustard, onion, garlic, bamboo shoots and palm tree fruit. Although these foods are known to individually have their own health benefits, they should be consumed in smaller quantities by patients suffering from thyroid disease and iodine deficiency. In contrast, traditional societies that eat a largely animal-based diet, similar to the "Paleo" diet, have a very low incidence of iodine deficiency. [46]

What if I have diabetes or insulin resistance?

This is one of the best diets for a patient with diabetes, whether it is type I (insulin dependent diabetes) or type II (non-insulin dependent diabetes or "insulin resistance"). One of the key etiologies or causes of type II diabetes is excessive and prolonged consumption of carbohydrates leading to insulin resistance, so elimination of this will only help maintain blood sugars and prevent the progression into type I diabetes that needs the treatment of insulin. Type I diabetics would likely experience a lowering of their insulin. Be sure to have your medications closely monitored if you are diabetic.

Does this diet help with candida and frequent yeast infections?

Candida is a fungus that naturally occurs in the gut and vagina in limited amounts. This fungus is balanced by normal good bacteria or gut flora. Processed foods and sugars and other grain-based carbohydrates are among the most notorious food sources for the promotion of candida growth. This diet eliminates most of the candida growth promoters. See the section on candida in "Step One of the Metabolic Health Protocol" for more specific information.

Will my cholesterol increase?

The elimination of carbohydrates will generally improve cholesterol and other lipids (fats) in your blood such as triglycerides. Be sure to have your cholesterol monitored by your healthcare professional.

Does eating meat lead to colon cancer and other diseases such as arthritis and osteoporosis?

Remember that our ancestors did not suffer from these diseases. Chronic diseases such as these are relatively new to us, after the trend towards grain-based carbohydrates emerged.

What if I have kidney disease?

It should be noted that this type of diet **does not** cause kidney disease, it just may add an additional burden to a patient with the pre-existing disease. If you have an existing condition of kidney disease, check with your doctor before you make any changes to your diet. In general, if you have an established diagnosis of renal (kidney) disease you should limit your protein intake and increase the amount of fat in your the diet. This will lower the burden on your kidneys and has been shown to at least slow the progression of the disease. Also, the importance of water is that much more key to helping you.

However, if you have normal kidney function, there is really no evidence that a high protein diet causes any problems with the kidneys, as is a usual suspicion among doctors. In a relatively recent review paper in 2002, Eisenstein and Roberts examined the evidence and came to the conclusion that there is little proof for negative effects of high protein diets on renal (kidney) function in people without established renal disease.[47]

What about pregnancy or breastfeeding?

Never change your diet drastically once you are known to be pregnant. The same would go for exercise as well. However, making efforts towards eating a more nutrient dense and clean diet can only enhance and benefit you while pregnant or breast feeding. However, if you are already on a Paleolithic type diet there is no reason to change anything. Be sure to discuss any changes to your diet with your obstetrician.

Should I continue taking my vitamin supplements?

Even with the best diet, in our modern civilization with nutrient-depleted soils, it can be very difficult to get all the vitamins and minerals you need for optimal metabolic health. Also, particular disease processes that may already be preexisting would necessitate additional vitamin and mineral supplementation by your healthcare provider that are acting medicinally for you. Supplements also act as an insurance policy over your normal diet. However, in many cases, once better metabolic health is achieved through this type of optimal diet, one can minimize and streamline their supplement needs to perhaps only a multivitamin and mineral formula. Be sure to consult with your healthcare provider regarding the best choices for you.

What can I do to get over the restrictive nature of this diet?

Most people have about a dozen fruits and vegetables that they are comfortable preparing and eating. Our ancestors would utilize up to around one hundred, depending on the geographical area. The best advice is to have fun and experiment! The more you try, the more you will discover that there are foods you enjoy. Also, try to focus on all the foods that you are allowed to have versus always thinking about the foods that you can't. And when it is socially appropriate, indulge somewhat. This has the psychological approach of keeping you on track so you occasionally allow yourself some reward.

My appetite has increased; won't this just make me gain weight?

Your appetite has increased because your metabolism is increasing and your body is asking for more of the nutrients of which it has long been deprived. Be sure to honor the process and go with it. Also, if you are following the other nutritional advice in this chapter such as keeping your water intake up, then this will help to keep your appetite in check and assist with your weight loss/maintenance goals.

Should I never eat grains at all?

For overall health, disease prevention and enhancing your metabolic health, cereal grains including wheat and corn should be avoided. However, every person is different in the amount they can handle. Work towards eating this way *most* of the time. Try for a 90-95 percent following of the lifestyle and indulge 5-10 percent of the time. If you have insulin resistance, diabetes or gluten sensitivity, then you should avoid grains and other processed carbohydrates as much as possible. If you do add grains in for any reason, keep them whole and as close to nature as possible. Remember, avoid highly processed foods of any type, particularly processed grains.

What if I am a vegetarian?

I have many patients who are vegetarian for many reasons. One typical reason is that they believe the diet is healthier than a diet with animal products in it. Another is simply taste preference and habit. Another common reason for being a vegetarian is the ethical and/or religious implications. If you are a vegetarian based solely on the understanding and belief that it not good for your body to eat meat, then hopefully this chapter and its resources have helped to point you in an alternative direction. If you are a vegetarian based on taste and preference, I would ask you to explore the many different food options that are possible, including an abundance of fruits, vegetables and nuts. Many vegetarians are addicted to processed carbohydrates and derive much of their calories from this source, and often lack the plain fruits and vegetables that are such a key part of our health. If you are a vegetarian that allows milk and eggs (lacto-ovo vegetarian), then you can maintain an excellent Paleolithic diet. All the advice here in this chapter is the same for a vegetarian of this type except the avoidance of the animal meats and the need to focus on raw milk and free-range eggs. So, it will work perfectly!

If you are a strict vegan, for any reason, then I respect this completely and would implore you to follow the proper guidelines of food combining. Also, be sure to eat organic whenever possible and keep your vegetable protein as high as possible. I have provided some resources for vegetarians in Appendix 1.

We are constantly bombarded with information about the best way to eat. Frankly, there is little known about the positive effects of any one particular diet because nutritional science has failed to provide sufficient and consistent information. I have found myself gravitating towards the nutritional lifestyle called the "Paleo" diet due to its underlying paradigm of simple observation of a large human historical picture. This paradigm presents a lens to view not just human nutrition, but human experience. Science can all too often be shortsighted. Traditional medicine is also too often shortsighted. It is possible that optimal human nutrition is best viewed from a study of natural ancestral human behavior while enhanced by the scientific view of human physiology.

With this type of dietary lifestyle, the amount of chronic disease that many in our industrialized nations experience could be eliminated. And of course, for those seeking weight management strategies, the low grain-based carbohydrate diet is suited to achieve rapid and consistent results over time.

Be sure to see the additional comprehensive nutritional advice in Step 2 of The Metabolic Health Protocol. In the section on diet, I offer a fully integrated approach to nutrition including a review of not just what to eat but why, when, and how to eat.

Chapter 5
The Metabolic Exercise Secret

There exists one inevitable truth about exercise… you must do it. There is no way around it. The body is, simply, designed to move. Its very structure begs the unavoidable reality that it must engage itself against the gravitational force it bathes in every day. Movement is the reaction that guides us towards healing. Movement is the force of change, taking us further from the stillness of the preceding moment to the energetic reality of the next, allowing us to come to another unique understanding about ourselves. Physical exercise can be a form of meditation. It always represents the act of doing something to better your individual self and soul. I believe these are some of the metaphors regarding exercise, movement and a healing path, but exercise must be done for practical physiological reasons no matter what.

> The body is, simply, designed to move. Its very structure begs the unavoidable reality that it must engage itself against the gravitational force it bathes in every day.

As you move, you increase your metabolic rate. This is a physical, physiological fact. But certain movements and therefore certain exercises are more effective than others at increasing the metabolic rate. This book has expressed the need to be aware of all the things that increase (or balance) the metabolic rate to direct the physiological state towards health. Hormones affect your metabolic rate. Food affects your metabolic rate. Exercise and your physical routine affect your metabolic rate. Your thoughts even affect metabolic rate. But the common denominator has been the goal to increase the metabolic rate to enhance your health.

This chapter will describe the types of exercise necessary to enhance metabolic health. It is important for patients who have very low metabolisms to start with exercise slowly and begin with light movements like walking and easy yard or house work before advancing steadily towards more advanced metabolic enhancing types of exercise. I use the term "physical routine" to allow the reader to make their own decision about what healthy movements, or exercise, they will engage in. And it is of course always important to state that all patients reading this book consult with a healthcare provider before starting any type of exercise routine. With that said, let's start exploring metabolic exercise.

Cardiovascular Conditioning with Aerobic Exercise

Many patients with low metabolisms, especially including hypothyroid and fibromyalgia patients, have very poor basic cardiovascular conditioning. There exists an immediate need for these patients to engage in some form of aerobic exercise. Many patients tell me that they have trouble getting off the couch to do anything, let alone exercise. I understand this of course, but something will have to be initiated. In the beginning, simply walking around the block for five minutes is the perfect way to start. Often, patients are being helped early on with the newfound hormonal balance and nutritional support that they need, so this provides a slight spark for their bodies to allow the initial engagement of exercise to take place. So, in the beginning of your health journey, you must simply start slow, but please do _start_.

Here are some simple rules for your physical routine in the beginning of your metabolic exercise journey:

- ❧ Keep it simple… remember: "Five minutes is better than no minutes." Simply walking is one of the best exercises that you can engage in.
- ❧ Find something that is FUN. If the gym is boring, don't do it. People often think that to exercise, it must mean going to the gym

and engaging in that specific type of exercise. Yard work, gardening, yoga, Pilates, Zumba, dancing of all types, hiking or any type of movement that keeps you interested counts!

- Find ways to increase activity. Get in the habit of using stairs, walking around the long way when going somewhere, park your car deliberately a little farther, run around with your kids more, walk everywhere you go if you can, get out of your seat to talk to a coworker instead of sending an e-mail, move your body, squirm in your seat: move, move, *move*!

- Keep your exercise SAFE. Don't engage in anything that is not safe for your fitness and skill level. One of the perfect ways to discourage future exercise is to get injured. If you are going to go to a local gym then be sure to find someone to show you around the equipment. Hire a personal trainer for a short period of time, but make sure the trainer has experience with working with someone who has limited experience and minimal fitness. A trainer can be indispensable in revealing to you the world of fitness that can be highly rewarding, motivating and beneficial to your goals of increasing your metabolic health.

- Be sure to warm up properly and stretch before any exercise. This ritual is not just to prevent injury but is an important component to prepare your mind for the upcoming exercise that is to take place. Take your time, breathe and prepare.

Comprehensive, Integrated Exercise

There exists ancient types of exercise incorporating not just physical movement, but also facilitating a mind and spiritual awareness during the process. The two most popular types of exercise in this category are yoga and tai chi chuan. During the actual movements, you practice at truly being aware of your breath, your body and your emotional and spiritual reactions or awareness that begins when doing this type of movement. Specifically, the entire body becomes balanced, even from an endocrine and metabolic standpoint. This type of exercise movement is perfect for beginning a comprehensive mind/body/spirit practice that is so important for your metabolic health. I truly encourage you to explore this type of exercise movement on your own with the understanding that there is a specific type for your needs, whether you are physically fit or not.

High Intensity, Short Duration Exercise:
The Metabolic Health Answer for Fat Loss

This section is for patients with a fitness experience that is of a moderate or advanced level. Normally this is a patient who has engaged in fitness for at least a year, who has perhaps been to a personal trainer for several sessions, or who has the past foundation of fitness experience as an athlete. If this does not yet fit your particular fitness level yet, then focus on the recommendations in the section above, build up your stamina and experience, then by all means start exploring this wonderful type of exercise. Your healthcare provider who is guiding you in enhancing your metabolic health can help to clinically determine if you are prepared for the next step. Finally, this section is particularly for the patient who has been exercising while focusing on their metabolic health and not achieving the fat loss that they are expecting. Read on....

There are three main types of exercise, light intensity, moderate intensity, and high intensity. The easiest way to distinguish these three types is based on your ability to speak during the exercise. During light intensity exercise or activities, you can easily hold a conversation with little to no straining. While engaging in moderate intensity exercise, you can still hold a conversation, but with some level of difficulty. High intensity exercise makes it almost impossible to talk. When performing high intensity exercise to an all out maximum, it is literally impossible to talk.

Intensity levels of different activities and exercises can also be based on Metabolic Equivalent, or MET. One MET is equivalent to the amount of energy or calories your body uses per minute while at rest, equating to approximately sixty calories per hour for a woman and seventy for a man. MET levels increase as the intensity of your activity or exercise increases.

Some examples of the various intensities of activities and exercises and their relative MET:[48]

Physical Activity	MET
Light Intensity Activities	< 3
Sleeping	0.9
Watching television	1.0
Writing, desk work, typing	1.8
Walking, 1.7 mph (2.7 km/h), level ground, strolling, very slow	2.3
Walking, 2.5 mph	2.9
Moderate Intensity Activities	3 to 6
Bicycling, stationary, 50 watts, very light effort	3.0
Walking 3.0 mph	3.3
Calisthenics, home exercise, light or moderate effort, general	3.5
Walking 3.4 mph	3.6
Bicycling, <10 mph (16 km/h), leisure, to work or for pleasure	4.0
Bicycling, stationary, 100 watts, light effort	5.5
Vigorous Intensity Activities	> 6
Jogging, general	7.0
Calisthenics (e.g. pushups, sit-ups, pull-ups, jumping jacks), heavy, vigorous effort	8.0
Running, jogging in place	8.0
Rope jumping	10.0

Patients often lament that no matter how much exercise they do on a daily and weekly basis, and even after many months of exercising religiously, they do not reap the benefit of weight loss they used to experience when they first started the exercise program. This can be due to a few reasons. Sometimes patients have unreasonable expectations, but I find this to be the rare exception. Also, fat weight will not come off easily for patients with low metabolisms and in hypothyroidism, sex hormone imbalances, fibromyalgia, chronic fatigue, and related hypometabolism conditions. But more often, patients will describe the intense and often excessive amount of cardiovascular/aerobic exercise they are performing. *And it is this excessive amount of cardio that is causing the problem of not being able to lose body fat.*

When you continue doing cardiovascular exercise to excess for weight loss, you become more efficient at burning fat. When first reading this, it sounds exactly like what you would want. But "efficiency" in this case refers to the body's way of actually preserving fat.

Cardiovascular exercise, performed in the typical fashion by most people, is a LOW INTENSITY, LONG DURATION exercise. This means, for example, that you get on the treadmill, walk at a good pace where you can still hold a conversation, and keep going for thirty minutes or more. The intensity is low and the duration is starting to get long. This type of cardiovascular exercise is working on conditioning your heart and blood vessels, which is a wonderful thing. But I assure you, it is not the main reason why my patients are engaging in this type of exercise. They are performing cardiovascular exercise to help them burn fat.

> When you continue doing cardiovascular exercise to excess for weight loss, you become more efficient at burning fat. When first reading this, it sounds exactly like what you would want. But "efficiency" in this case refers to the body's way of actually preserving fat.

And the secret here is that the more low intensity, long duration exercise you perform, the more your body thinks it needs to conserve its fat stores to have the energy to go for a long time. In essence, your body is lowering its metabolism to become more efficient at burning fat, which is the exact opposite of what you are trying to accomplish.

I have seen countless examples of patients who perform excessive amounts of cardiovascular exercise, lose a little weight initially, and then continue to literally "spin their wheels" and either not lose anymore weight or actually start to gain weight. This can be very frustrating for someone who is very dedicated to physical exercise but does not get the results they want, which is normally losing body fat and gaining muscle tone.

How does a high intensity, short duration exercise routine affect your metabolic health and hormonal physiology? If you are looking for an activity that enhances the production of your own hormones, then here is a summary of the hormonal benefits of high intensity, short duration exercise:

- **Increased testosterone**, which in turn increases overall metabolism, improves protein synthesis and the repair of body tissue and increases lipolysis, or the breakdown of fat storage in the body.

- **Increased human growth hormone (HGH)** levels which have the function of increasing muscle and bone mass, promoting a healthy immune system, improving pancreatic function and increasing lipolysis or fat burning.

- **Temporarily increases cortisol** from the adrenal glands, which in turn increases lipolysis and an enzyme called Lipoprotein Lipase or LPL, which in turn utilizes triglycerides as energy in the muscles. The effects of cortisol are enhanced particularly in the presence of HGH and testosterone.[49, 50, 51]

- **Insulin,** a potent fat storage hormone, **is decreased**, while **glucagon,** the antagonist to insulin that takes glucose or sugar out of fat storage, **is increased**. Overall **lipolysis (fat burning) is therefore increased**.

- **Increased adrenaline and noradrenaline**, which are potent energy producing hormones that increase anti-inflammatory cytokines such as IL-6 and IL-10 and also increase glycolysis or the breakdown of sugar for energy lipolysis.

- **Decreased ghrelin,** a recently discovered hormone that is responsible for increasing appetite.

- **Increased adiponectin**. This hormone is very important in fat loss regulation and has many specific functions, maintaining proper uptake of glucose out of the blood and into body cells, assists insulin to do the same, breaks down fats in the blood, clears triglycerides and protects blood vessel linings, lowering the formation of atherosclerotic plaque formation. In short, this hormone will lower the risk of insulin resistance and diabetes.

- ❡ **Increased lactic acid**, as a result of oxygen debt from this type of exercise, further stimulates the production and activation of testosterone and HGH.[52, 53, 54, 55, 56, 57]
- ❡ **Dopamine is increased** which is an important neurochemical involved in sleep and mood stability.
- ❡ **TSH or thyroid stimulating hormone is increased** which stimulates the activity of the thyroid gland to produce more thyroid hormone, increasing overall metabolic rate.

Keep in mind that low intensity, long duration exercise, such as cardiovascular exercises performed in excess, has the opposite effect with the hormones listed.

Another excellent effect of this type of exercise is a stimulated metabolism for a longer period of time after the actual exercise. High intensity exercise increases what is known as Excess Post-exertional Oxygen Consumption (EPOC), which means the amount of oxygen being used which indicates a higher overall metabolic rate and fat burning capacity. (See the information on page 240 on the ReeVue® machine that measures Resting Metabolic Rate.) Metabolic rate is increased up to sixteen hours after high intensity, short duration exercise and even up to forty-eight hours after in men.[58, 59] Cardiovascular exercise does not have the same metabolic boosting impact for that long after exercise. [60, 61]

> Metabolic rate is increased up to sixteen hours after high intensity, short duration exercise and even up to forty-eight hours after in men. Cardiovascular exercise does not have the same metabolic boosting impact for that long after exercise.

So, what is the end result of this very particular hormonal profile created by high intensity, short duration exercise? With an exercise routine that is less time consuming, you can get a more balanced, muscular, strong and lean body more efficient at burning fat, that possesses a higher metabolism with improved thyroid health, lowered inflammation throughout the body therefore protecting joints, muscles, and internal organs, lowered insulin resistance which protects against developing diabetes, improved cardiovascular health and an improved sense of mental and emotional well being. With a consistent high intensity, short duration exercise routine, you are one significant step closer towards experiencing metabolic health.

How Do I Perform High Intensity, Short Duration Exercise?

High intensity, short duration exercise is an excellent solution to improve the ability to lose body fat and improve the conditioning of the heart, in a *shorter* time frame for the busy person. Another name for this type of exercise is HIIT or High Intensity Interval Training. The method of this exercise is to keep intensity up for short bursts followed by rest periods.

This type of exercise also does not necessitate belonging to a gym, which many of my patients do not want to do. High intensity training can be done in the home or outside at a park, or in your own backyard. However, you may chose to find a personal trainer who understands this concept and can lead you in designing routines and give you a better feel for how to keep your intensity up when you train.

Here are four ways to get you started in the right direction.

❧ You can utilize different movements that you find interesting and fun. Almost any movement can be done with high intensity. Remember that *intensity* of the movement is the key. For example:
  - Sprinting/Walking
  - Stationary bike
  - Jumping Jacks
  - Jumping rope
  - Weight training

- With weight training, use compound movements that utilize as many joints in the exercise as possible, such as squats or overhead presses. Then, you can also incorporate hybrid movements by combining traditional exercise movements into one exercise, such as a squat combined with arm curls. This also has the added benefit of taking old movements and giving them a fresh and fun makeover.

- To keep the intensity up, alternate between all out exertion of your chosen exercise and then recovery. Here's how:

  - Beginners: (new to this type of exercise) Exert yourself for 30 seconds in your exercise of choice, then recover for 120 seconds. Repeat this 6-8 times.

  - Intermediate: (training for about one month) Exert for 30 seconds, then recover for 90 seconds. Repeat this 8-10 times.

  - Advanced: (training for over three months) Exert for 30 seconds, then recover for 60-90 seconds. Repeat this 8-10 times.

- Keep your exercise time to forty minutes or less. In fact, when you first start utilizing high intensity exercise, ten to twenty minutes can be extremely beneficial. Remember to warm up and cool down before and after your exercise, and include light stretching once you are warmed up and at the end of the routine. You only need to exercise two to four times per week. Be aware that the increased metabolic rate is lasting well past your time spent exercising. And, keeping your overall exercise to under forty minutes keeps cortisol levels down and testosterone and human growth hormone up. Good Luck!

Section 3
The Metabolic Sovereign:
Your Thyroid Gland and
its Hormonal Power

Introduction

Thyroid disease is a worldwide epidemic, presenting itself very commonly in my practice. I have found that the thyroid gland and its proper function is a key element to anyone's metabolic health. This section will reveal what the thyroid does and what happens when it is not working properly. You will understand that the thyroid is the very seat of metabolism, orchestrating the production and delivery of one of the most important hormones in your body, and influencing and maintaining all other tissues. When it dysfunctions, the results range from mild to devastating, leading to the common conditions of hypothyroidism (low thyroid function) or hyperthyroidism (high thyroid function), both of which cause many untoward problems. And much more....

You will also discover a detailed explanation of thyroid laboratory analysis, with what could be a very refreshing approach to these elusive numbers, as some of the text will offer an alternative opinion rooted in science and keen observation.

One of the most important aspects of the thyroid reveals its nature as a reservoir for iodine. We will explore this key thyroid element and vital nutrient revealing its long history for helping not just with thyroid disease, but the entire body. Iodine deficiency could very well be at the root of the rampant thyroid problems many doctors see. And, when employed correctly, iodine may offer a viable solution for both preventing and treating thyroid dysfunction.

Chapter 6
Thyroid Anatomy, Physiology, Thyroid Hormones and Related Laboratory Analysis

Your thyroid gland is one of the most important, vital glands in your body. It secretes a set of hormones that are vital to your entire body. Each of your cells need thyroid hormone to properly develop and to optimally function. That statement bears repeating: *Every cell in your body, head to toe, inside and out, needs thyroid hormone to function properly*. So, you can see how the thyroid hormones in your body, when not in the correct balance, can lead to so many different symptoms in so many different body parts.

> The take home message is this: If a hormone physiologically affects every cell in your body, and that hormone is out of balance, it therefore has the potential to be associated with almost every symptom one could imagine.

The take home message is this: If a hormone physiologically affects every cell in your body, and that hormone is out of balance, it therefore has the potential to be associated with almost every symptom one could imagine. Let's explore the unique nature of the thyroid gland and its hormone.

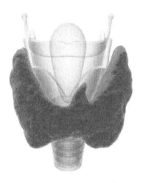
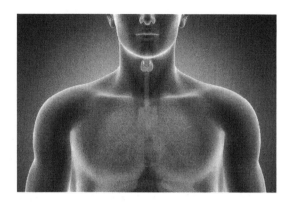

Thyroid Anatomy

- The thyroid gland is a brownish-red gland located at the front of the lower neck, about the level of the thyroid cartilage or Adam's apple on either side of the trachea or windpipe.
- The gland may have an H or U shape formed from two lobes and a connecting piece of thyroid tissue called the isthmus.
- Each lobe is about 5 to 6 cm long (or about 2.5 to 3 inches) and weighs about 30 grams in adults. It is usually heavier in women.
- The thyroid gland has an incredible amount of blood vessels traveling to and from it, retrieving precious nutrients and blood from the gland and delivering the all-important thyroid hormone to the rest of the blood circulation. In fact, ounce for ounce, the thyroid has a larger blood supply than the kidneys.
- The thyroid is composed of two primary cell types, each with its own function.

     1. Follicular cells and follicles: these spherical follicular cells trap iodine   from the blood to produce thyroid hormone. Within these cells is another feature   known as colloid, which serves to store the materials for thyroid hormone production such as the amino acid tyrosine and a very important thyroid protein called thyroglobulin (TG) which directly participates in the production of thyroid hormone. Thyroglobulin and thyroid peroxidase (TPO) interact with the amino   acid tyrosine and the mineral iodine to

produce T1 and T2 thyroid hormones, which have little to no cellular potency. But one T2 combines with another T2 to produce the most abundant thyroid hormone, T4 or thyroxine. T2 and T1 will combine to produce the most potent and active form of thyroid hormone, T3 or triiodothyronine.

2. Parafollicular cells are found interspersed within the follicular cells. These cells produce calcitonin, which is partially responsible for calcium regulation.

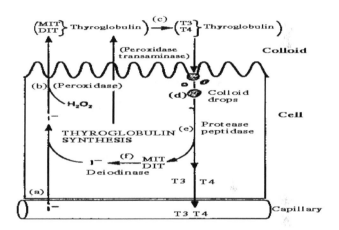

Seeing your thyroid gland

In a mirror, you can easily see the basic location of the thyroid gland in relationship to some basic anatomical landmarks. The thyroid gland rests within what is called the "thyroid bed."

- The thyroid bed is within the borders of the Adam's apple that is at the top, the collarbone at the bottom, and the thick muscles that connect to the collar bone that lie on either side of the trachea or windpipe.

- An enlarged thyroid is known as a goiter and your doctor can help you determine its size if you believe it is enlarged.

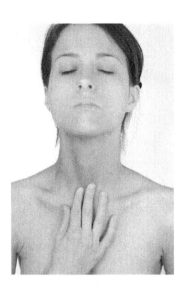

Feeling your thyroid gland

Find your Adam's apple with your fingers of each hand and then travel slowly down on each side of your trachea to just above the clavicle or collarbone. The muscles just off to the side, the sternocleidomastoid muscles, slightly cover each lobe, so gently slipping your fingers under those muscles can get you a better feel. The centerpiece, called the isthmus, can be felt easier if you swallow because the gland tends to ride up a little from under the collarbone. If you don't feel your thyroid, don't worry. It is not the most obvious gland to feel, even for trained physicians. But have fun... it's *your* thyroid, so check it out!

Your Thyroid Hormones

Now that you know more about the anatomy of the thyroid gland and where it is located in your neck, let's explore the actual hormones that the gland excretes. The action of all of your thyroid hormones are a cascade of events that start with your hypothalamus in your brain, then your pituitary gland, then your thyroid gland itself, and finally the target tissues of your body. This is a finely orchestrated process that keeps thyroid hormone levels at normal production.

Normal Thyroid Hormone Production and Regulation:
- Your hypothalamus senses if levels of thyroid hormone are low and secretes thyroid releasing hormone (TRH).
- TRH stimulates the anterior pituitary gland which secretes thyroid stimulating hormone, TSH.
- TSH stimulates the thyroid gland to produce thyroid hormone.
- Thyroid hormone exerts its effects on the body cells and the available thyroid hormone sends a negative feedback loop signal to the hypothalamus that decreases the amount of TRH and/or TSH.
- There are two principle hormones that the thyroid gland synthesizes: T4 and T3. The primary hormone that is synthesized by the gland is **thyroxine** (levothyroxine) or **T4**. It consists of a central tyrosine molecule with four attached iodine molecules, hence its name T4. Thyroxine is considered a pro-hormone because it is inactivated and does not have any direct physiological effect on body cells. Thyroxine or T4 is converted by the body cells when one iodine molecule is cleaved off, forming **triiodothyronine** or **T3** the active hormone. The T3 that is converted from T4 is what actually gets into each cell of the body to make it function optimally. T3 is the actual hormone that has the ability to enhance the function of its target cell. And remember, those target cells mean every cell in your body.
- Upon entering the cell, T3 connects with its receptor within the nucleus of the cell and directly affects the DNA of that cell at the genomic or gene level.

The following list describes some of the basic, yet vital, actions of thyroid hormone within the body:
- In the form of ATP, or adenosinetriphosphate, within each cell, it allows that cell to function and develop optimally.
- Assists in bringing sugar (glucose) into the cell.
- Stimulates amino acids from proteins in the diet to transport into the cell.
- Assists fats to be metabolized.
- Enhances vitamin metabolism.

- Improves the liver's ability to make sugar (glucose) and to eliminate excess cholesterol, bringing down cholesterol levels in the blood.
- Stimulates neurochemicals in the brain such as serotonin, dopamine and norepinephrine which enhance and regulate mood as well as stimulate the natural production of human growth hormone.
- Decreases substance P, a molecule in the body associated with increased pain sensation.

    Here is a list of how thyroid hormone helps the body in general:
- Increases basal (resting) metabolic rate.
- Increases energy and recovery from exercise.
- Stimulates heart tissue and enhances cardiac output.
- Enhances overall metabolism making it easier to maintain a normal weight.
- Vital for normal development in children.
- Maintains fertility and pregnancy.

So, what does this all mean? Thyroid hormone comes down to one concept in general: metabolism. Health, in general, relates back to optimal metabolism. If the metabolism within a cell or body organ is diminished, then the health of that cell or organ is diminished, which can lead to a multitude of symptoms and disease processes.

Thyroid Hormone Physiology and Laboratory Analysis

It is important to review some of the basics of the various thyroid hormones that many patients will see on laboratory analysis. There is much confusion about which thyroid hormone values to measure as well as what are the accepted ranges.

Radioimmunoassay (RIA) is the main type of thyroid hormone testing used today. It was discovered by Dr. Solomon Berson and Dr. Rosalyn Yallow. Both were awarded the 1977 Nobel Prize in Medicine for this achievement that changed the study of thyroid disease as well as the entire field of endocrinology. It was their contributions to the accuracy, convenience and cost of these tests that was commended. However, the interpretation of these tests by thyroidologists and endocrinologists is still left to debate and concern.

TSH or Thyroid Stimulating Hormone aka Thyrotropin

TSH is a hormone produced by the pituitary gland in the brain that acts as a messenger that stimulates the actual thyroid gland itself, increasing its activity to produce thyroid hormone. When the pituitary senses the levels of thyroid hormone, such as thyroxine (T4) and triodothyronine (T3), are low it sends additional messages to stimulate the thyroid to increase production. When the thyroid gland increases production of the thyroid hormones T4 and T3, it down-regulates the amount of TSH messages. This is a delicate balance that keeps TSH relatively low and thyroxine (T4) and liothyronine (T3) adequately high, all assuming that the thyroid gland is functioning properly.

- ❧ In overt hypothyroidism (low thyroid function), the TSH value is increased and the T4 and T3 values are relatively low.
- ❧ In overt hyperthyroidism (high thyroid function), the TSH becomes very low and the T4 and T3 values are high.

Problems with the TSH Test

I can think of no other laboratory value that has caused so much confusion regarding thyroidology than the notorious TSH test and results. In fact, this confusion has led to a lot of unnecessary suffering for multitudes of patients. People sometimes ask me why I became interested in treating the thyroid. I always explain that I did not go to the thyroid… *the thyroid came to me*, in droves of menopausal

> I can think of no other laboratory value that has caused so much confusion regarding thyroidology than the notorious TSH test and results. In fact, this confusion has led to a lot of unnecessary suffering for multitudes of patients.

and hypothyroid women who were poorly regulated on their low dose T4 levothyroxine thyroid medication (or on none at all), all tightly packaged in the confusion and ineptness of the interpretation of the TSH reading by their doctors.

Once I saw this confusion and so many people suffering, I undertook a quest to discover how to help. This book is a limited compilation of the fruits of that endeavor. But it was the TSH test results that I found to be the most egregious

The blind adherence to the TSH value and the resulting medication dosage was what was keeping people unhealthy.

and outrageous from a scientific, rational and clinical perspective. The blind adherence to the TSH value and the resulting medication dosage was what was keeping people unhealthy.

TSH Detecting Hypothyroidism

The most current type of TSH test is a Third Generation TSH Assay which is purported to be the most sensitive assay available at detecting TSH in the blood. This is true but it does not give any additional ability to diagnose hypothyroidism than previous generation assays. This newer Third Generation TSH Assay is more sensitive at detecting *lower* amounts of TSH, but does not help to further sensitively detect hypothyroidism. For example, a second generation TSH assay may have reported the value at 2.5 uU/mL, where the newer Third Generation would report the value at 2.56 uU/mL, giving a slightly more specific number, but doing nothing in terms of helping with the diagnosis and course of treatment for hypothyroidism.[62, 63] However, having a sensitive TSH assay can help to detect very low amounts of TSH in the case of hyperthyroidism (high thyroid function).

Current Ranges for TSH

It is important to understand that the TSH value expresses disease potential and does not give a direct diagnosis of thyroid disease. It is a tool that must be wielded correctly by a rationally thinking healthcare diagnostician. In the right hands, its value (within the context of the larger diagnostic picture) can help establish the correct diagnosis of thyroid disease or exclude it. There are certain clinical circumstances where the TSH will be within a normal range but the patient presents with clear symptoms of being hypothyroid. In this case, a trial of thyroid hormone is a safe, clinically rational and humane course of action.

> There are certain clinical circumstances where the TSH will be within a normal range but the patient presents with clear symptoms of being hypothyroid. In this case, a trial of thyroid hormone is a safe, clinically rational and humane course of action.

There are times when the TSH can be slightly out of the range and the patient exhibits absolutely no clinical signs or symptoms of hypothyroidism. In this case, a conservative approach towards offering thyroid hormone should be exercised, being sure to monitor other facets of the metabolism. In short, the TSH must be taken with the proverbial grain of salt by both the clinician and the patient, being sure to exercise pure rational judgment each and every time.

The normal ranges for TSH have serially lowered since its popular use in the 1980s. Here are some of the most current ranges:

- Conventional laboratory ranges for TSH depend on the state you live in. The value can range from 0.45 to upwards of 6.0 uU/mL. This means that hyperthyroidism (high thyroid function) is considered when the value is below 0.45 uU/mL and hypothyroidism (low thyroid function) will not be considered until the value is above 6.0 uU/mL.

- The American Association of Clinical Endocrinologists uses a range of 0.3 to 2.5 uU/mL.
- The American Thyroid Association wants to "treat" the TSH in hypothyroidism to a range below 2.0 uU/mL.
- A large British community study helped to codify a more effective range of 0.3 to 2.0 uU/mL. This is the range I use. This study demonstrated that people with a TSH above 2.0 have a greatly increased risk of future hypothyroidism.[64, 65]

Treating the TSH

Patients are all too often told, by both conventional and even alternative practitioners alike, that the goal of thyroid hormone treatment is to give just enough thyroid hormone medication to make the TSH fall within normal ranges. The problem with this approach is that keeping the TSH within the normal range does not necessarily make the hypothyroid patient free of their signs and symptoms of their hypothyroidism. Additionally, the course of treatment will depend on if the doctor uses more currently accepted ranges of the TSH value. Giving a small amount of thyroxine (T4) in many cases will easily keep the TSH normal, but the patient is still symptomatic and suffering. Many physicians believe that if the TSH is kept within a normal range then they have sufficiently done their job, regardless of what the patient continues to express symptomatically. This dogmatic and tyrannical approach to thyroid treatment is a direct result of the unwavering belief in the clinical relevance of the TSH value. All physicians should treat the patient and not just treat the TSH.

> **All physicians should treat the patient and not just treat the TSH.**

Doses of Thyroid Hormone "Suppressing" the TSH Value

When patients are given a dose of thyroid hormone medication necessary to eliminate their signs and symptoms of hypothyroidism and hypometabolism, it very often will result in a "suppressed" TSH value, or a value that is very low and under the range. Many doctors wrongly interpret this value as automatically indicating that a patient is on too much thyroid hormone. These well-intentioned doctors warn of cardiac problems or heart attacks and bone loss. These body responses are all possible if someone has too much thyroid hormone in their system, but a suppressed TSH does not automatically mean that it is happening or will happen. In fact, most of the time it will not. But doctors continue to parrot the same general misinformation under the false premise that the TSH value will always tell you exactly what is going on in a patient's body.

There are two important terms that are often misrepresented by both physician and patient alike. Defining them will help to explain why confusion exists about the TSH.

- Hyperthyroidism. This term indicates that the thyroid gland is, by itself, functioning high, leading to high levels of circulating T4 and T3 thyroid hormone that lead to actual tissue over-stimulation resulting in "thyrotoxicosis." Typically, test results show that the TSH is very low and the thyroid hormones T4 and T3 are high.

- Thyrotoxicosis. This relates to actually being in the state of over-stimulation from either too much thyroid hormone medication or thyroid hormone being produced by an overactive thyroid gland. This results in such signs and symptoms as rapid heart rate, palpitations, continuous sweating, limb shaking and body tremors, anxiety, eyelid retraction and eye bulging.

The important distinction between these two terms is that hyperthyroidism is defined by the laboratory values and does not necessarily indicate that the person's body is over stimulated or in tissue thyrotoxicosis. However, doctors usually automatically confuse the two definitions which leads to the assumption that if the TSH is low and/or T4 and T3 is high, then that person is both hyperthyroid and is experiencing thyrotoxicosis. The message here for both the patient and the doctor alike is to clinically assess actual thyrotoxicosis using clinical signs and symptoms and to reference the laboratory values as being suggestive only of hyperthyroidism.

If a hypothyroid patient taking thyroid hormone medication understands what to look out for in terms of the signs and symptoms of overstimulation, then the associated risks are very low. If a patient experiences these symptoms, then the dose is simply lowered and the effects will quickly abate.

For a list of signs and symptoms of thyroid overstimulation, see Overstimulation by Thyroid Hormone Evaluation Form in Appendix 6.

Your Thyroid Hormones and Related Laboratory Analysis

When you undergo blood tests for your thyroid function your lab report gets sent to your doctor for interpretation. You can see a copy of your results if you wish. Once you get your report home, you can decipher it with the help of this book. Here is a list of the categories of the most common thyroid tests. Below the list are paragraphs that help to explain the name of and the reason for the test,

> If a hypothyroid patient taking thyroid hormone medication understands what to look out for in terms of the signs and symptoms of overstimulation, then the associated risks are very low.

the scoring range and additional details that are useful to both doctor and patient in achieving health. An asterisk is next to the thyroid tests I find to be most useful. The others are listed based on how commonly they are ordered.

- ❧ Total T4
- ❧ Free T4
- ❧ T3 Uptake
- ❧ Free Thyroxine Index
- ❧ Total T3

- Free T3
- Reverse T3
- Anti-TPO
- Anti-TG
- TSI (or TSH receptor antibodies)
- TRH

TOTAL T4. Remember that T4 or levothyroxine is the main hormone produced by the thyroid gland. It consists of a central tyrosine molecule surrounded by four iodine molecules. It is considered a prohomone because it is the inactive form of thyroid hormone. It is not until T4 is converted into T3 that it is capable of affecting cells. T4 is the typical hormone medication most conventional physicians prescribe, such as the common generic levothyroxine or one of the two commonly prescribed T4 medications Synthroid® or Levoxyl®. When you see "Total T4"on your lab report, with the range being 4.6 to 12 mcg/dl you are getting a direct measurement of the actual amount of T4 in the blood at any one specific time. If the value is low, it may indicate hypothyroidism; if high, perhaps hyperthyroidism.

FREE T4. Another score is Free T4 and the range is 0.7-1.9 ng/dl. This means that thyroxine or T4 travels in the blood bound to a protein called Thyroxine Binding Globulin or TBG. When thyroxine or T4 is attached to TBG, it is not capable of getting directly into cells to be converted to active triiodothyronine or T3. At times, TBG is high due to the use of certain medications such as estrogen, or can be high due to genetic traits. Free T4 is a measurement of unbound and readily available T4. If this value is low, it could indicate hypothyroidism or possibly too low of a dose of thyroid hormone. If it is high, it could indicate the opposite.

T3 UPTAKE. This is one of the most confusing tests to explain and understanding the particulars here is not overly important, as this is not a test I recommend. Your T3 Uptake (range: 25-35 percent) score is an indirect measurement of T4, <u>not</u> T3, as is often misunderstood by clinicians. The test utilizes radioactivated T3 to bind sites on a Thyroxine

Binding Globulin (TBG) molecule. The remaining unbound sites left on the TBG give an indirect measurement of T4. If the value is low, it could indicate hypothyroidism, and if high, hyperthyroidism.

FTI. In the Free Thyroxine Index (FTI) or T7 category, the range is 0-25 pmol/L or 0.7 –2.1 ng/dL. The FTI is a calculation using the results from the T3 uptake test and total T4 test and provides only an estimate of the level of free T4 in the blood. It is rarely used because the Free T4 and T3 can be measured directly. If the value is low, it could indicate hypothyroidism. If the value is high, then hyperthyroidism could be likely.

TOTAL T3. Triiodothyronine or liothyronine, T3, is the active form of thyroid hormone, producing at least four times the amount of affect on the body cells than levothyroxine (T4). It is composed of a central tyrosine molecule and three iodine molecules. The common T3 medication prescribed in the U.S. is Cytomel®, but it is rarely given by endocrinologists or primary care doctors. T3 is found in desiccated thyroid hormone medications such as Armour® and Nature Throid®. T3 can be compounded by a compounding pharmacy into a prescription medication also. This active hormone has the most success at making hypothyroid patients well. There are three types of T3 lab results:

- Total T3 (range: 80-200). This is the direct measurement of the total amount of T3 in the blood at a given time. If the level is low, then hypothyroidism is possible and if high, hyperthyroidism is possible.

- Free T3 (range: 0.2 – 6.5 ng/dL or 2.3 to 4.2 pg/mL). This lab value is very similar in function as the Free T4. This test is a direct measurement of the amount of unbound T3 in the blood, "free" from being bound to TBG. If the value is high, it could indicate hyperthyroidism, and if low, hypothyroidism.

- Reverse T3 (range: 0.2 – 0.7 nmol/L). The molecule of "reverse T3" is a mirror image of the main T3 molecule. Since reverse T3 (rT3) is an opposite replica, it is not as active. During starvation diets followed by obese patients, the rT3 will increase. However, in catabolic states such as cirrhosis of the liver, starvation and insulin dependent diabetes, the rT3 will decrease.[66] (Note: I have found very little clinical use for the Reverse T3 test. Most often, patients score in the normal range and thus it would not provide any additional clinical relevance to my approach towards any hypothyroid patient or hypometabolic patient. E. Denis Wilson, M.D has coined the term "Wilson's Temperature Syndrome" and has utilized the rT3 test and the basal body temperature test to justify the use of thyroid hormone, making the rT3 test and the view that rT3 increases during stress, both very popular among alternative health care practitioners. I have the greatest respect for any healthcare practitioner who is willing to think outside of convention when that thinking is sound and rational, particularly with thyroid hormone treatment. However, I have not found Wilson's treatment protocol to be effective and convenient for my patients.)

ANTI-TPO. Thyroid peroxidase (TPO) is a necessary enzyme component for producing thyroid hormone. A lab result for TPO shows a score <35. An autoimmune reaction can occur whereby the body produces antibodies against itself and can target the thyroid gland and the thyroid peroxidase enzyme, thereby lowering the overall function of the thyroid gland. The Anti-TPO antibody is the most common antibody measured to detect the presence of what is known as Hashimoto's Autoimmune Thyroiditis. This antibody "blocks" thyroid production.

ANTI-TG. Thyroglobulin is a protein that is used in the production of thyroid hormone. Just as in the anti-TPO situation above, antibodies can also be produced from the immune system against the thyroglobulin protein indicating an autoimmune (self attacking) reaction and the likelihood of Hashimoto's thyroiditis. When completely normal, the lab results will show this test as an Anti-TG with a range of <35. When abnormal, the number will be higher than 35 and can even be over 1000 when there is a significant immune reaction. Both the Anti-TPO and Anti-TG antibodies are not typically checked by most doctors, but can be useful in detecting both Hashimoto's disease (hypothyroidism) and Graves' disease (hyperthyroidism). This antibody "blocks" thyroid production, so it is important to decrease the autoimmune response in the body if this anti-TG antibody is present.

TSI (or TSH receptor antibodies). The range for TSI (thyroid stimulating immunoglobins, also known as TSH receptor antibodies) show a scoring range from <2 percent activity up to <130 percent activity. These are specific antibodies that target the TSH receptor of the thyroid cell, thereby stimulating the thyroid gland excessively, which results in overproduction of thyroid hormone. This leads to hyperthyroidism or high thyroid function. TSI antibodies are very specific to the diagnosis of hyperthyroidism. As a result, this antibody stimulates thyroid production. Ideally, the TSI score should be practically zero. The value could be up to 100 percent or more and the patient may not present with any signs or symptoms of hyperthyroidism. If you have the presence of TSI antibodies, then you should be closely monitored. Be sure to refer to Chapter 8 on iodine.

Note: Patients will often have both thyroid stimulating and thyroid blocking antibodies present. If they are both in equal amounts, the patient could be in a normal thyroid state. If the TSI stimulating antibodies are higher, then hyperthyroidism or Graves' disease ensues. If the Anti-TPO and Anti-TG blocking antibodies are more abundant, then Hashimoto's hypothyroidism occurs.

TRH (Thyrotropin [TSH] Releasing Hormone) Stimulation Test [67]

Here is another type of test for thyroid function. It is ordered when thyroid dysfunction is assumed clinically, but traditional thyroid tests are normal and therefore not helpful. This test is not commonly ordered by most physicians because it is a more complicated test, but it can yield fruitful results. TRH is a hormone that comes from the hypothalamus in the brain. It is a hormone signal that targets the anterior pituitary gland instructing it to release thyrotropin or TSH. And of course, TSH then stimulates the thyroid gland to secrete thyroid hormone.

Interpretation of the TRH Stimulation Test

In the TRH Stimulation Test, the first step is to obtain a baseline TSH value blood sample. After that, the clinician injects a harmless medication that mimics TRH, known as an analog, into the test patient intravenously. The TRH analog should tell the anterior pituitary to produce additional TSH. If the anterior pituitary is working properly there is a *significant rise in TSH* within thirty minutes and this is determined with another TSH blood sample. The resulting interpretations are listed below:

- Normal: A TSH response of less than 20 uU/mL but greater than 8.5 uU/mL, above the baseline TSH value.

- Central (Hypothalamic) Hypothyroidism: This type of hypothyroidism (low thyroid function) derives from a lack of communication of the hypothalamus to the pituitary gland. And remember, the pituitary is responsible for secreting TSH (Thyroid Stimulating Hormone) which then stimulates the thyroid gland to produce thyroid hormone. In the TRH stimulation test, the TSH response will be greater than 20 uU/mL above the baseline TSH value. When the TSH response from the pituitary gland is exaggerated from the injected TRH analog, then it could indicate that natural TRH, usually coming from the hypothalamus in the brain, is usually low in this patient, disallowing normal stimulation of the anterior pituitary to produce adequate TSH which would in turn produce normal thyroid hormone from the thyroid gland.

- Overt (Primary) Hypothyroidism: The TSH response will be greater than 20 uU/mL above the baseline TSH value. If a patient has a baseline TSH above 2.0 uU/mL accompanied by clinical signs and symptoms of hypothyroidism, and the injected TRH analog produces an exaggerated TSH response greater than 20 uU/mL above the baseline TSH, then this is indicative of low amounts of circulating thyroid hormone. When the circulating amounts of thyroid hormone are low, then the injected TRH will stimulate an excessive amount of TSH because there are inadequate amounts of thyroid hormone to counteract the TSH. Remember, when thyroid hormone levels are high, TSH goes down by a negative feedback loop at the anterior pituitary level. If thyroid hormone levels are low, TSH should go up and will definitely go up uninhibited when a TRH analog is administered.

  ❧ Pituitary Hypothyroidism: This occurs when the TSH response is less than 8.5 uU/mL above the baseline TSH value. If a patient has a baseline TSH of 1.0 uU/mL or less and presents with clinical signs and symptoms of hypothyroidism, then a blunted response to TRH could indicate a dysfunction of the pituitary. This indicates that the anterior pituitary gland that secretes TSH cannot produce enough TSH to stimulate production of thyroid hormone from the thyroid gland. In this case, the thyroid gland is functioning normally, but there is not enough stimulus from TSH from the pituitary gland to produce a thyroid hormone producing response from the thyroid gland.

The TRH Stimulation test can be very useful for patients who have a baseline TSH above 2.0 uU/mL and/or the presence of thyroid antibodies (i.e. anti-TPO, anti-TG) accompanied by clinical signs and symptoms of hypothyroidism. Very often, these patients are denied thyroid hormone treatment when in fact the condition of hypothyroidism does exist, but conventional testing is unable to correctly make the diagnosis.

Does Thyroid Laboratory Analysis Test Thyroid Function?

Conventional thyroid labs provide a snapshot in time of the amount of thyroid hormone in your blood, measured as T4 and T3. It is assumed that if the levels of thyroid hormone are either high or low, there is an abnormality in the function of the thyroid. This is true only if you are NOT on thyroid hormone medication, and even then it will not give the full picture of thyroid function. I am always concerned about the function and health of a particular endocrine organ, such as the thyroid, but I am even more concerned about the effect of that endocrine organ's hormone on the body.

If a patient is taking thyroid hormone medication, then the assessment of the levels of TSH, T4, and T3, DO NOT assess the function of the thyroid. Rather, it is a measurement of the levels of the thyroid hormone medication only—without exact determination of the effect of that hormone on its target tissues in the body. So, patients and doctors alike will say something like, "Let's check your thyroid function to adjust the medication," when in fact this is not actually what the thyroid labs do. This is an extremely important point to stress for the patient who is trying to grasp the concept of improving their metabolism versus simply improving their thyroid function.

Is Thyroid Hormone Testing Useful?

Once a patient is on thyroid hormone, thyroid hormone laboratory testing is of limited value.[68] Be sure to understand that I mean "limited" value versus "no value." Thyroid testing can occasionally catch variances in thyroid hormone medication assimilation and absorbability and it can certainly help to catch if a patient is actually compliant with their thyroid hormone dosage, as the levels will change drastically in patients who do not follow a regular schedule of taking their medication. Hashimoto's thyroiditis, a thyroid inflammatory process related to low thyroid function, also presents with fluctuating inflammatory flare-ups that will cause the TSH to rapidly increase and necessitate a thyroid hormone dose increase.

If thyroid labs are being used to determine dose at all, then the following two considerations are reasonable, but are by no means absolute and determinant of health:

- Keep the TSH below at least 2.0.
- Strive for a Free T3 and Free T4 to be towards the high end of the range.

Thyroid labs, therefore, have their merit in an overall *limited* clinical capacity. Most often, once a patient finds a perfect dose of thyroid hormone medication, the TSH becomes suppressed and even the Free T3 and Free T4 can become elevated or altered right away. In the end, following a patient's measurable and perceivable body response to thyroid hormone will provide the most relevant clinical data to guide the clinician towards the optimal thyroid hormone dose.

Medications That Interfere with Thyroid Function Tests

There are many different medications that interfere with thyroid function testing. Here is a list organized by mechanism: [69]

- Drugs that reduce thyroid hormone concentration
  - Suppression of TSH
    - Dopamine (Levadopa® for Parkinson's disease)
    - Glucocorticoids (prednisone)
  - Reduction of TBG level
    - Androgens (testosterone, DHEA)
    - Glucocorticoids (cortisol, steroids)
  - Impaired protein binding
    - Salicylates (aspirin)
    - Diphenylhydantoin   (anti-seizure drug)
    - Furosemide (diuretic)
  - Impaired thyroid hormone production or secretion
    - Propylthiouracil (anti-thyroid drug)
    - Methimazole (anti-thyroid drug)

- Lithium (anti-psychotic drug)
- Drugs that raise T4 concentration
  - Increase in TBG level
    - Estrogen
    - Tamoxifen (breast cancer drug)
  - Impaired T4 to T3 conversion
    - Amiodarone (high blood pressure drug)
    - Ipodate sodium (contrast medium for x-rays)
    - Iopanoic acid (iodine containing contrast medium)
    - Propranolol (high blood pressure drug)
    - Glucocorticoids (cortisol, steroids)

Timing for thyroid testing

It is very important for patients who are taking thyroid hormone medication to avoid the medication for at least three to four hours before having their blood drawn for thyroid hormone testing. If thyroid hormone is taken directly before the blood draw, then the Total T4 and T3 and Free T4 and T3 can be high and thus yield a false reading. Other factors such as the time of the day and the point in the menstrual cycle have no major bearing.

Chapter 7
Hypothyroidism, Hyperthyroidism and Related Diseases

Why do we have a thyroid gland?

What is the real reason or purpose we have a thyroid gland? The simple answer to a complex and vital situation is this: *To collect iodine to be delivered to the rest of the body.* Typically, it is perceived that the thyroid gland collects iodine solely for the sake of the thyroid gland itself, when in fact it is collecting iodine to be delivered to the whole body in the form of thyroid hormone (T4, T3, and even T2) with a concentrated physiological effect of increasing overall metabolism.

> **What is the real reason or purpose we have a thyroid gland? The simple answer to a complex and vital situation is this:** *To collect iodine to be delivered to the rest of the body.*

Aquatic life in general has no need for an organ like the thyroid gland to concentrate iodine because aquatic life is constantly bathed in iodine. As life evolved to a terrestrial, land based existence, the need to concentrate iodine arose, and therefore the thyroid evolved. Aquatic life uses a gastric or stomach pump to get iodine into circulation. And the thyroid and gastric (stomach) cells share the same morphology from an embryological (fetal development) perspective.

Thyroid hormone is by weight only 1/30th of the total amount of iodine in the body. This suggests that iodine has roles in other tissues in the body and also suggests that thyroid hormone and its related receptors have a concentrated biological and physiological effect on body tissues. Sabastiano Venturi, one of the foremost biologists in the study of iodine, summarized, "Evans et al. [70] reported that 5 milligrams of potassium iodide (daily injected) acts as 0.25 micrograms of L-thyroxine (T4) in recovering the impaired functions of many organs of thyroidectomized rats. Furthermore, Wolff [71] reported that two patients with goiter and hypothyroidism have been described in whom the ability to concentrate iodide was lost in the thyroid (and in gastric mucosa and salivary gland); both patients were treated with large doses of iodide alone: both responded well (regarding to growth, BMR (Basal Metabolic Rate), cholesterol, etc.). This suggests strongly that while iodides are always necessary, the *thyroid hormones are not indispensable for living organisms.*" [72] [Emphasis added.] This means that iodine, in the correct form and amount, possesses the potential to sustain the same biological effect as thyroid hormone.

We have learned from previous chapters that the body possesses a relatively small organ with a tremendous relative blood supply for the sole purpose of making sure humans concentrate and store iodine for producing thyroid hormones. We can now additionally add that the thyroid has the purpose of creating thyroid hormone to actually *deliver* iodine, with a concentrated biological and metabolic effect, to the entire body. We know that thyroid hormone affects every cell in the human body and, as we will soon learn, all cells in the body need iodine, and certain tissues even concentrate iodine similarly to the thyroid gland. In the next chapter, the role of iodine and how it benefits health will be explained in detail.

HYPOTHYROIDISM
The Symptoms and Signs of
Hypothyroidism (Low Thyroid Function)

Hypothyroidism presents as a multitude of clinical signs and symptoms. In fact, the condition of hypothyroidism has been dubbed "the great pretender." The condition is both elusive and straightforward. The examination of a hypothyroid patient takes an attentive ear and an open mind. The signs and symptoms of hypothyroidism are many and not all patients will present the same way. If the condition is in the early stages, there can be very few signs and symptoms. Or at other times, it can be a singular *related* condition such as menstrual irregularities that have the clinician and patient chasing the wrong underlying cause or missing it altogether, not realizing that it is a manifestation of lowered metabolism and hypothyroidism.

Patients often ask me what the symptoms of hypothyroidism look like. They ask how they would know if they had hypothyroidism. The easiest way to answer the question is through understanding this one simple concept: Thyroid hormone is needed by every cell in your body for proper and optimal function. Thyroid hormone, when either in excess or deficiency, may result in a multitude of dysfunctions in every organ tissue, every organ system, and virtually the entire body. Since every body cell is affected by thyroid hormone there are a multitude of symptoms that relate to its imbalance.

Let's start with the thorough checklist, then I will elaborate on some of the more common symptoms one-by-one. But first, here is the difference between a symptom and a sign:

- A *symptom* is something that is subjectively felt or sensed by the person experiencing it that is not necessarily observable by anyone else. For example, pain. It may seem to a doctor that someone is experiencing pain, but the doctor could not be certain of this.
- A *sign* is something the patient experiences that an outside observer can actually see and perhaps measure. For example, swelling of the legs or dry skin are observable and measurable phenomena.

Both signs and symptoms have tremendous usefulness in both the diagnosis and treatment of hypothyroidism. Far too often, signs and symptoms are ignored by most doctors. This is for a few reasons. Symptoms are not considered objective enough to be scientific due to the possibility of the patient not reporting their experiences correctly. It is of course possible that someone would not report symptoms completely accurately, but to throw out this valuable information and not allow it to guide clinical judgment is foolish. Also, if a physician has developed a good rapport with his patient, the subtleties of what a patient is trying to communicate can be discerned. But learning this about each patient takes time and thoroughness.

This brings me to my next point. Considering symptoms and signs takes considerable time that most doctors are not willing or able to take. Even a measurable sign, something that a doctor could see and follow its course, such as skin dryness or changes in an EKG or something as easy as checking the Achilles reflex on the ankle with a reflex hammer, seems to take too much time for most doctors. Another difficulty in watching for measurable signs related to hypothyroidism is that the signs could be related to other diseases. This is true, but that is what being a doctor is all about, *knowing the difference*. No single clinical test is perfect when diagnosing and monitoring hypothyroidism, or any disease process.

In short, signs and symptoms of hypothyroidism are invaluable for both diagnosis and treatment follow up. If a doctor is not willing to listen and keenly observe what can be completely obvious, then it is time to seek a doctor who will listen and pay attention to the patient's overall physicality and attitude.

Common Symptoms of Hypothyroidism

These are the things that you may feel which are impossible or extremely difficult to measure. There may be some overlap with the signs of hypothyroidism:

- Anxiety
- Choking sensation
- Constipation
- Decreased sweating
- Depression
- Difficulty in swallowing
- Dizziness
- Dry mucous membranes
- Easy emotional upset
- Emotional instability
- Fatigue
- Fineness of hair
- Heat intolerance
- Impotence
- Insomnia
- Joint pain
- Lethargy
- Loss of appetite
- Low endurance
- Low motivation

- Low sex drive
- Muscle pain
- Nervousness
- Non-restful sleep
- Numbness or tingling
- Obsessive thinking
- Pain at the front of the chest
- Painful menstruation
- Poor concentration
- Poor memory
- Poor vision
- Pounding heart beat
- Prolonged or heavy menstrual bleeding
- Sensation of cold
- Shortness of breath
- Slow speech
- Slow thinking
- Vague body aches and pains
- Weakness
- Weight gain unexplainably
- WorryingCommon Signs of Hypothyroidism

These are the things that you and your doctor can observe. There may be some overlap with the symptoms of hypothyroidism.

- Bluish or purplish coloration of the skin, nail beds, lips, mucous membranes (cyanosis)
- Brittle nails
- Cardiac enlargement on x-ray
- Changes at the back of the eye
- Coarse skin
- Cold skin
- Dry ridges down nails
- Dry skin
- Dry, coarse, brittle hair
- Fineness of hair
- Fluid accumulation in the abdomen (ascites)
- Fluid around the heart (pericardial effusion)
- Hair loss
- Hearing loss
- Indistinct or faint heart tones
- Listless, dull look to the eyes
- Long-normal intervals on EKG
- Low basal temperature
- Nonpitting edema of the ankles
- Paleness of skin
- Paleness of skin Low QRS voltage on EKG
- Pounding heart beat
- Protrusion of one or both eyeballs (exopthalmos)
- Slow heart rate despite low aerobic fitness
- Slow pulse despite low physical fitness

- Slow relaxation phase of the knee or ankle reflex
- Slow speech
- Slow thinking
- Sluggish movements
- Sparse eyebrows, particularly the outer third
- Swelling around the eyes

- Swelling of the ankles
- Swelling of the face
- Thick tongue
- Thick, scaling skin
- Voice hoarseness
- Wasting of the tongue
- Weight gain (unexplainable)

After L.J. DeGroot, P.R. Larsen, S. Refetoff, and J.B. Stanbury: *The Thyroid and Its Diseases*, 5th edition. New York, John Wiley & Sons, Inc. 1984, pp.577-578.

* From Lowe, J.C.: *The Metabolic Treatment of Fibromyalgia*. McDowell Publishing Co., L.C., Boulder, 2000.

- R.L. DeGowin and E.L. DeGowin, *Bedside Diagnostic Examination*, 3rd edition. New York, MacMillan Publishing Co., Inc., 1976, p. 860.

* From Honeyman, G.S. and Lowe, J.C.: *Your Guide to Metabolic Health*. Boulder, McDowell Health-Science Books, 2003.

The Underlying Mechanism of Related Hypothyroid Diseases: Respiration

When cells dysfunction, particularly to the point of cancer, those cells have an altered cellular respiration or insufficient oxygen. Many other diseases are now known to be caused by respiratory defects including inflammation, lowered immune function and autoimmunity, degenerative diseases and aging, and all involve altered cellular respiration and oxygen debt. Thyroid hormone is a key hormone for cellular respiration. When thyroid hormone is low, or its absorption is altered in the body resulting in impaired cellular respiration, a multitude of conditions and diseases result.

Common Health Conditions and Diseases of Hypothyroidism

This section will review a multitude of common health conditions and diseases that are intimately related with hypothyroidism (low thyroid function), thyroid disease in general, and ultimately *slow metabolism*. The relationship with these conditions should make the physician treating these conditions take a closer look at thyroid function and the state of metabolism as it relates to thyroid hormone medications. I see many of the following conditions in people who either have not yet had the proper diagnosis of hypothyroidism or in patients who are already diagnosed with hypothyroidism but are inadequately treated with low doses of synthetic thyroid hormone medications. I am convinced that a multitude of common health conditions that many people continue to suffer with or who are at a very high risk of having, are due to undiagnosed or poorly treated thyroid disease. If you are already taking thyroid hormone and you have one or more of these conditions and are on medications to control them, it could be due to the wrong type of thyroid medication and/or an inadequate dose. Or, if you have one or more of these conditions, and you are not yet diagnosed with hypothyroidism, then this helps to point to the diagnosis of hypothyroidism, even if your thyroid lab results are normal.

Heart Disease

The association with heart disease and thyroid disease is commonly understood. It is related in overt hypothyroidism (low thyroid function), subclinical hypothyroidism and hyperthyroidism (high thyroid function). This section focuses on hypothyroidism. Arteriosclerosis (hardening of the arteries), high cholesterol, high blood pressure and heart electrical conduction problems like atrial fibrillation are all associated with hypothyroidism.

The general effects of hypothyroidism (low thyroid function) on the cardiovascular system involve a complicated compensatory process of increasing some aspects of heart physiology and decreasing others in an attempt to maintain overall cardiovascular normalcy. But this compensation ultimately results in problems which include:

- A 50-60 percent higher systemic vascular resistance or high blood pressure.
- Lowered cardiac output or "efficiency" of the heart muscle.
- Lowered size of the heart and decreased effectiveness to contract properly.
- Lowered systolic blood pressure (top number) and increased diastolic blood pressure (bottom number).
- The heart rate or pulse is lowered, which is a sign of *lowered* metabolism and *poor* heart efficiency; not having good fitness.

It is important to note that in early mild to moderate hypothyroidism, which often goes undetected, the blood pressure is initially low for years, such as 90/60, which begins to rise steadily into high blood pressure. I have had many patients tell me that they have followed this pattern.

In subclinical hypothyroidism, or mild hypothyroidism, where only the TSH value is mildly elevated and some or many symptoms present, the long-term risk of cardiovascular disease is increased.[73, 74] Treating subclinical hypothyroidism also helps to lower the inflammation causing substance known as homocysteine[75, 76] as well as the inflammatory blood marker CRP or C-reactive protein.[77] Helping to lower both of these blood markers decreases the overall risks of cardiovascular disease. This is an extremely important factor in deciding if thyroid hormone treatment is warranted, as disease prevention is always to be clinically considered.

> It is important to note that in early mild to moderate hypothyroidism, which often goes undetected, the blood pressure is initially low for years, such as 90/60, which begins to rise steadily into high blood pressure.

Atherosclerosis and High Cholesterol

Atherosclerosis is a disease that results in the hardening of the arteries. When inflammation is present in and around the blood vessels, cholesterol sticks to the walls and hardens over time, leading to blood vessel narrowing, lowered blood flow and increased risk for heart attack and stroke.

Broda Barnes M.D., a well-known thyroidologist, found that when the thyroid glands of rabbits were removed, they developed atherosclerosis, just as hypothyroid patients did.[78] By the mid-1930s, it was generally known that hypothyroidism caused cholesterol levels in the blood to increase and this was viewed medically as a diagnostic sign of hypothyroidism.

Your body is always making cholesterol. It is a vital substance needed for cell-to- cell communication and hormone synthesis. However, as your metabolism lowers in hypothyroidism, your liver cannot clear the cholesterol at the same rate in which your body is making the cholesterol, and the net effect is an increase in the cholesterol levels in your blood. Restoring the metabolism with the assistance of proper thyroid hormone treatment can often very easily lower cholesterol levels and allow patients to be free from cholesterol medications.

> Restoring the metabolism with the assistance of proper thyroid hormone treatment can often very easily lower cholesterol levels and allow patients to be free from cholesterol medications.

Hypertension (High Blood Pressure)

Thyroid hormone is responsible for helping blood vessels to dilate.[79] In hypothyroidism, lowered thyroid hormone levels increase blood vessel resistance and this results in increased blood pressure. Hypothyroidism can also lead to the abnormalities in how sodium is retained in the body—increased sympathetic nervous responses (the fight or flight response), and decreased kidney function and filtration—all contributing to hypertension.[80, 81, 82]

As mentioned before, hypothyroidism can result in both low and high blood pressure, depending on the timing of the hypothyroid diagnosis and general genetic tendencies towards high blood pressure. Through the work of Broda Barnes M.D. and recently with current research,[83] evidence shows the relationship between hypothyroidism and high blood pressure. However, a paradox does exist with high blood pressure occurring in both hypothyroidism (low thyroid function) and hyperthyroidism (high thyroid function). When both of these thyroid conditions are corrected, normal blood pressure can often be reestablished.

> A paradox does exist with high blood pressure occurring in both hypothyroidism (low thyroid function) and hyperthyroidism (high thyroid function). When both of these thyroid conditions are corrected, normal blood pressure can often be reestablished.

Atrial Fibrillation

The top two smaller chambers of the heart are known as the atria. Your heart sends electric signals to these chambers to make the atria contract to allow blood to be pumped through the heart and the rest of the body. When the electrical signals to the atria are too rapid, it results in rapid contraction leading to a fluttering sensation in the chest and poor blood circulation through the heart and body. This heart condition is typically related to hyperthyroidism[84] (high thyroid function) but is also related to hypothyroidism and too little thyroid hormone.[85, 86] Even though the relationship to atrial fibrillation and hypothyroidism is not as common, it should be considered carefully.

Autoimmune Conditions

The most common reason for hypothyroidism in the United States is Hashimoto's thyroiditis, an autoimmune condition that results in the overall dysfunction of the thyroid gland.[87] Graves' disease is the most common form of hyperthyroidism and is also related to an autoimmune condition. These autoimmune conditions are the result of antibodies or small proteins made by the immune system that attack the thyroid gland leading to actual destruction of thyroid cells and altered synthesis (lowered in hypothyroidism and increased in hyperthyroidism) of your thyroid hormones.

What is important to understand in this section is that there are other autoimmune conditions that result in the body that are also caused by or are related to the presence of antibodies. There are different types of antibodies that are normally associated with particular diseases. However, if a patient has the presence of one type of antibody, it increases the likelihood of having other autoimmune antibodies for other disease conditions. This is important to note because if you have one or more types of known and diagnosed autoimmune conditions, it increases the likelihood of having other types of autoimmune conditions, such as Hashimoto's thyroiditis or Graves' disease and the often resulting altered thyroid function.

Here is a list of some autoimmune conditions that may alter thyroid function:

- SLE (Systemic Lupus Erythematosus)
- Sjogren's Syndrome
- Multiple Sclerosis
- Lichen Sclerosis
- Type I Diabetes
- Rheumatoid Arthritis

Fibromyalgia: The Elusive Thyroid Disease

This section on fibromyalgia was contributed by Cristina Romero-Bosch N.M.D. Fibromyalgia is another condition related to thyroid disease. Dr. Bosch, a specialist in fibromyalgia and metabolic conditions, presents how these two seemingly separate conditions are actually one and the same.

This controversial condition was first recognized by the American Medical Association as recently as 1987. Fibromyalgia (FM) is defined by the presence of widespread body pain and tenderness with often debilitating fatigue and depression, sleep disturbance and often irritable bowel symptoms.[88] In the 1990s, John Lowe D.C., with his

> In the 1990s, John Lowe D.C., with his research team and Professor Jean Eisinger, simultaneously began to define fibromyalgia as a thyroid hormone deficient or resistant condition.

research team and Professor Jean Eisinger, simultaneously began to define fibromyalgia as a thyroid hormone deficient or resistant condition.[89] It is currently a condition that is ineffectively treated and at times even ignored. Despite being present in approximately 2 percent of the general population, many patients still find proper diagnosis and treatment elusive.

The diffuse pain of fibromyalgia is identified as a series of painful points on the body called trigger points. A doctor, such as a rheumatologist, makes the diagnosis of fibromyalgia based on the presence of eleven of eighteen specific trigger points that elicit pain when pressed. The diagnosis also includes six months or more of persistent related signs and symptoms. Another significant complaint is extreme fatigue. Fibromyalgia is often found in conjunction with a diagnosis of chronic fatigue. FM may also result in sleep disturbance, weight gain, skin complaints, and irritable bowel syndrome, to name a few. Cognitive dysfunction is evident by anxiety, depression, and a common brain fog referred to as "fibro fog." Symptoms are extremely varied in intensity but often render the patient handicapped by interfering with normal daily activities.

Doctors often have difficulty in agreeing on a diagnosis for fibromyalgia due to a lack of significant supportive laboratory evidence. Due to fibromyalgia's nonspecific presentation, it is often considered a diagnosis of exclusion or a diagnosis made when no other disease process is found.

Fibromyalgia's widespread effects and cryptic presentation of minimal abnormal lab findings makes it challenging to treat through conventional methods of anti-depressants and muscle relaxants. Therefore, it is necessary to identify the underlying cause to effectively treat this complicated disease. At the core of fibromyalgia lies either undiagnosed or poorly treated hypothyroidism or resistance to what thyroid hormone is present in the body. The estimated incidence of hypothyroidism in patients who have FM is higher than in the general public. The reported incidence of primary hypothyroidism in the general non-elderly U.S. population varies between 1[90] and 5 percent.[91] Laboratory thyroid function testing suggests that the incidence of primary hypothyroidism in FMS is significantly higher, 10 to 13 percent.[92, 93, 94]

Thyroid hormone resistance means body cells cannot use the thyroid hormone effectively even though adequate thyroid hormone levels are present. It is similar to type II diabetes, or insulin resistance, where insulin is present in adequate amounts but is unable to do its job effectively, resulting in elevated sugar levels.

We have also learned of other underlying factors that worsen or complicate the severity of many patients' fibromyalgia. The most common of these factors are low cortisol, abnormal daytime/nighttime cortisol levels, poor blood sugar regulation, sex hormone imbalances, pro-inflammatory diets, nutritional deficiencies, low physical fitness and adverse effects of a

> **At the core of fibromyalgia lies either undiagnosed or poorly treated hypothyroidism or resistance to what thyroid hormone is present in the body.**

variety of prescription drugs. Clinical evaluation exposes the almost identical symptom presentation between the patient populations. By properly assessing the patient's metabolic and endocrine functioning, which is almost invariably low in patients with fibromyalgia, a diagnosis and course of effective treatment becomes possible.

The ultimate result of FM and thyroid hormone resistance is a lowered metabolism called hypometabolism. Hypometabolism

> Most hypothyroid or fibromyalgia patients will not recover if their thyroid hormone treatment includes the use of a T4-only product. Most patients find greater success on a product containing the active form of thyroid hormone called T3.

can only be determined by measuring basal metabolic rates, assessing nutritional status, through analysis of blood thyroid hormone levels beyond what is often done conventionally, by thorough clinical examinations of medical history and by observing symptoms and signs. This type of complete examination is often ignored in favor of using a simple blood test that measures the TSH level and then using the lab result as sole indicator of thyroid health. It is this mainstream practice of relying on a TSH reading alone to evaluate thyroid function that has resulted in many patients inaccurately being dismissed by their physician as having "normal" thyroid function and has left countless FM patients without relief.

When undergoing proper metabolic evaluation and treatment, the patient must use a holistic metabolism-raising approach that includes thyroid hormone replacement, diet modifications and nutritional support, exercise, mental and emotional support, soft tissue manipulative medicine, and when medically appropriate, avoidance of metabolism lowering medications such as pain medications and antidepressants.[95] It is through appropriate hormonal support coupled with a holistic, comprehensive approach, that the patient achieves full body recovery.

Many fibromyalgia patients are already being treated for hypothyroidism with thyroid hormone medication in the form of inactive T4, most commonly by Synthroid® or synthetic levothyroxine. If you are a patient being treated for hypothyroidism, you should not be satisfied with the use of a thyroid product containing only T4. Most hypothyroid or fibromyalgia patients will not recover if their thyroid hormone treatment includes the use of a T4-only product. Most patients find greater success on a product containing the active form of thyroid hormone called T3. A common thyroid hormone medication that has been proven in decades of successful treatment is natural desiccated thyroid in products such as Armour® thyroid or Naturethroid®. At times, plain synthetic T3 is necessary for fibromyalgia patients to achieve full recovery.

Fibromyalgia, although presently considered an incurable condition, has the potential to be effectively controlled. Focusing treatment on the underlying cause of the hypometabolism, rather than attempting to dissect the condition into seemingly unrelated symptoms with ineffective drug therapy, will help ensure successful and permanent results. Patients and physicians must understand that fibromyalgia is ultimately a hypometabolic condition dependent on diminished thyroid hormone levels or a resistance to the hormone that is present. Fibromyalgia patients must remain hopeful and understand that the condition can be treated effectively if the hypometabolic state is properly addressed.

Possible Symptoms of Fibromyalgia

- Feeling of pain, burning, aching, and soreness in the body.
- Headaches, tenderness of the scalp, pain in the back of the skull.
- Pain in the neck, shoulder, shoulder blades and elbows.
- Pain in hips, top of buttocks, outside the lower hip, below buttocks, and the pelvis.
- Pain in the knees and kneecap area.
- Fatigue, unrefreshing sleep, waking up tired, morning stiffness.
- Insomnia, frequent waking, difficulty falling asleep, or falling asleep immediately.

- Raynaud's phenomenon (where your hands feel cold, numb, or turn blue, when exposed to temperature changes).
- Irritable bowel syndrome, diarrhea and constipation, bloating, cramping.
- Balance problems.
- Orthostatic hypotension—when you stand up, your blood pressure drops, which can make you feel faint, dizzy, nauseous, your heart rate drops and you can even faint.
- Restless leg syndrome.
- Sense of tissues feeling swollen.
- Numbness, tingling and feeling of cold in the hands and feet.
- Chest pain, palpitations.
- Shortness of breath.
- Painful menstrual periods.
- Anxiety, depression and "fibrofog," the term used to describe the confusion and forgetfulness, inability to concentrate, difficulty recalling simple words and numbers, and transposing.

Adrenal Dysfunction

Thyroid disease, particularly low thyroid function, has an intimate relationship with the adrenal glands. If hypothyroidism exists, then the adrenals must work harder to maintain energy throughout the body. Over time, the adrenals may become dysfunctional or exhausted. Additionally, the main adrenal hormone cortisol is needed to stimulate the production of cellular receptors for T3. Remember, T3 is the active form of thyroid hormone that is needed to induce proper cellular function. Without the ability to absorb T3, the body will not get what it needs and the system can become toxic from unutilized T3. Be sure to refer to Chapter 9 on Adrenal Dysfunction.

Depression and Emotional Disturbances

It has been known for years about the relationship of depression to low thyroid function. Not long after hypothyroidism was first identified officially in England in 1873, it was understood that mental disorders accompany the condition. Psychiatric circles utilized thyroid hormone in the past with great results, until the advent of newer psychotherapeutic drugs took over.

The brain has multiple receptors for thyroid hormone. When thyroid hormone is low or high, it can cause an inability to focus and understand complex questions and tasks. Additionally, the psychological symptoms can range from mood swings, anxiety, and irritability to hallucinations and psychotic episodes. However, when a patient presents with hypothyroidism, depression may or may not be the most prominent feature. If a patient presents with depression, the hypothyroidism may or may not be discovered, leading to the use of psychotropic drugs only with treating the underlying cause of the depression.

The use of T3 by psychiatrists has been noted to be effective for depression.[96] However, all too often, the dose would not be increased to a point of elimination of symptoms or at least for any consistent duration of time, leading to the additional need of psychotherapeutic drugs. The key to helping with many cases of depression is to treat the underlying hypometabolic state comprehensively and allow for adequate thyroid hormone dosing to be applied to the clinical situation.

> **The key to helping with many cases of depression is to treat the underlying hypometabolic state comprehensively and allow for adequate thyroid hormone dosing to be applied to the clinical situation.**

Menstrual Difficulties

There are many different ways in which a woman's menstrual cycle can be altered. Here are some quick definitions:

- ❦ **Dysmenorrhea** is the medical term for painful periods.

- **Oligomenorrhea** refers to cycles longer than thirty-five days—or only four to nine periods per year.
- **Polymenorrhea** refers to repeated cycles of less than twenty-one days, or menstruation at two to three week intervals.
- **Metrorrhagia** refers to bleeding at irregular intervals, such as between menstrual periods. Metrorrhagia can range from light spotting, to continuous bleeding for weeks.
- **Menorrhagia** refers to a very heavy or excessive period.
- **Anovulatory Bleeding** refers to uterine bleeding occurring without normal ovulation mid-cycle, leading to lowered progesterone levels and abnormal bleeding, particularly metrorrhagia.

Any of these menstrual difficulties can occur in a woman with thyroid abnormalities. Most dysfunctional uterine bleeding occurs in hypothyroidism or low thyroid function at about one in four, but hyperthyroidism or high thyroid function also contributes at a slightly lower rate.

The cause of dysfunctional uterine bleeding, particularly menorrhagia and metrorrhagia, is related to the following conditions that occur in hypothyroidism: [97, 98]

- Reduced levels of SHBG (Sex Hormone Binding Globulin), a protein that carries sex hormones in the blood.
- Decreased levels of estrogens and testosterone.
- Reduced levels of follicle-stimulating hormone (FSH) and leutinizing hormone (LH). These pituitary hormones stimulate the production and balance of sex hormones at the right time during the menstrual cycle.
- Clotting difficulties due to decreased levels of the clotting factors VII, VIII, IX, and XI made in the liver.
- Decreased metabolic clearance rates of androstenedione and estrone through the liver. This leads to high amounts of both androstenedione and estrone in the blood. Androstenedione is a potent hormone like testosterone and estrone is a particular type of estrogen that in high amounts is associated with breast and uterine abnormalities.

> ❧ Hyperprolactinemia, or excess levels of prolactin, may present as infertility, oligomenorrhea or amenorrhea. High levels of prolactin may lead to breast milk leakage called galactorrhea. High levels of prolactin are associated with hypothyroidism. If levels are in excess of 100 ng/dL, then an MRI should be ordered to rule out a pituitary tumor, which can result in excessive excretion of prolactin. If you are hypothyroid and have bleeding difficulties, then be sure to have your prolactin levels checked.

Understand that these uterine bleeding problems can also occur in a woman in peri-menopause or for other gynecological issues. Be sure to check with your healthcare provider if your dysfunctional uterine bleeding occurs for longer than a few weeks.

When adequate thyroid hormone replacement is given in hypothyroid patients with dysfunctional uterine bleeding, the problem can be corrected. It is also important to note that when iodine is deficient in the body, the ovary has difficulty functioning properly which could lead to dysfunctional uterine bleeding and particularly anovulatory bleeding. Be sure to have your healthcare provider discuss proper iodine replacement, particularly if you are on thyroid hormone replacement medication.

Infertility

The relationship of infertility and thyroid disease, particularly hypothyroidism, has been long understood. Unfortunately, this is overlooked by many doctors as a prime reason for the inability of a woman to get pregnant. But the association is very clear. An opinion statement issued by Obstetrics and Gynecology was very clear about the association of hypothyroidism and infertility concluding, "Awareness of the thyroid status in the infertile couple is crucial, because of its significant, frequent and often reversible or preventable effect on infertility."[99]

As explained in the above section, hypothyroidism influences ovarian function by decreasing levels of SHBG (Sex Hormone-Binding Globulin) and increasing the secretion of prolactin. Both of these factors interfere with the ability of proper sex hormone balance to take place to allow fertilization and implantation. Once the hypothyroidism is corrected, the odds of getting pregnant and staying pregnant greatly increase. Be sure to have your thyroid checked if you plan

> **Once the hypothyroidism is corrected, the odds of getting pregnant and staying pregnant greatly increase.**

on getting pregnant and throughout your pregnancy.

For male infertility, thyroid function was classically thought to have little to do with the ability of the testicles to produce sperm and enhance fertility. In the past two decades, the research has helped to demonstrate that hypothyroidism can affect sperm count and the quality of sperm,[100] but controversy still remains. Either way, men should consider having their thyroid function tested appropriately if they are trying to conceive.

Anemia

This is one of the most common diseases associated with hypothyroidism, occurring in 20-60 percent of the cases.[101] One of the general reasons for the relationship of anemia and hypothyroidism is the impaired gut absorption that often results in the low thyroid patient. Iron, vitamin B12, folate and other nutritional factors can be poorly absorbed through the gut leading to the different anemias. Pernicious anemia, which is B12 and folate deficiency, occurs twenty times more frequently in patients with hypothyroidism than in the normal population. This type of anemia may result from the insufficiency of the thyroid hormones themselves versus poor nutrition intake or absorption. If you are hypothyroid, proper thyroid hormone medication is of course indicated, but supplementing with B12, whether orally or with an injection, is a good idea to help with a diagnosed condition of anemia.

Thyroid hormone is responsible for stimulating the production of another hormone called erythropoietin that stimulates the production of red blood cells. If thyroid hormone is deficient, then the lowered erythropoietin cannot make adequate red blood cells.

I see the association of anemia and hypothyroidism often in my practice. It is very important to have your iron and ferritin levels checked routinely if you are hypothyroid or suspect you are hypothyroid. Ferritin is the storage form of iron and is more accurate at gauging your stores of iron than simply looking at the iron level.

Gastrointestinal Conditions

Inadequate thyroid hormone from hypothyroidism can lead to many different problems with the gastrointestinal system including poor digestion and slow transit time. GERD (Gastro-Esophageal Reflux Disease) is a common condition that is also related to hypothyroidism. Stomach emptying time is often slower in a hypothyroid patient. This allows the acidic stomach contents to travel back up through the esophagus leading to irritation.

> One of the most common GI complaints in a hypothyroid patient is chronic constipation. Due to the overall lowered metabolic rate, the motility and movement of the bowels is slowed.

One of the most common GI complaints in a hypothyroid patient is chronic constipation. Due to the overall lowered metabolic rate, the motility and movement of the bowels is slowed. Irritable bowel syndrome (IBS) is also commonly associated for similar reasons.

Insulin Resistance and the Metabolic Syndrome

Insulin is responsible for shuttling glucose (sugar) from the blood into the cells of the body. When insulin become unable to do its job due to excessive carbohydrate intake and other factors, the excess sugar stays in the blood damaging blood vessels and eventually gets stored as fat, increasing obesity. The condition is related to increased abdominal fat, high blood pressure, high cholesterol and can eventually lead to diabetes.

It is very well known and accepted that in overt hypothyroidism (elevated TSH with very low free T4 and free T3), there is a direct correlation to insulin resistance. In fact, to be hypothyroid is to be automatically insulin resistant to some degree.[102, 103, 104] And in subclinical hypothyroidism (elevated TSH value with normal free T4 and free T3), a correlation exists comparable to overt hypothyroidism.[105] Even when thyroid hormone levels are on the low end of normal, there is still a strong correlation with insulin resistance and increased cholesterol.[106] When thyroid hormone levels are optimized along with a comprehensive metabolic enhancing regimen of diet and exercise, insulin resistance can be corrected.

Obstructive Sleep Apnea and Snoring

Approximately forty million people suffer from this debilitating condition in the U.S., but only about 600,000 are actually properly diagnosed.[107] Obstructive Sleep Apnea (OSA) affects millions of Americans and is associated with an increased risk for death and disease. Patients with this condition suffer from fatigue, nighttime snoring, lowered libido, memory loss, depression, headache and obesity. It seems that obesity and insulin resistance are key factors in sleep apnea. Hypothyroidism seems to complete the overall picture here.

One of the reasons that OSA occurs may be due to extra swelling in the structures of the face and throat. In fact, eye and whole body swelling are common in OSA patients[108] and these are also very common hypothyroid signs. Obesity is also related to OSA and of course this is related to insulin resistance and hypothyroidism.

> **The best course of action when treating OSA should be to correct the metabolic dysfunctions comprehensively, treating the hypothyroidism if present and eliminating the insulin resistance and excessive weight.**

The best course of action when treating OSA should be to correct the metabolic dysfunctions comprehensively, treating the hypothyroidism if present and eliminating the insulin resistance and excessive weight.

Carpal Tunnel Syndrome

The carpal tunnel refers to the narrow region on the palm side of the hand near the wrist where the "median nerve" travels through. In carpal tunnel syndrome, the nerve becomes trapped and leads to pain and dysfunction in the wrist and hand. In hypothyroidism, the two key dysfunctions of swelling and decreased nerve conduction help lead to the condition of carpal tunnel syndrome. The swelling places pressure on the median nerve causing pain, and the decreased nerve conduction further exacerbates the problem. Depending on the extent of the carpal tunnel syndrome, proper treatment of hypothyroidism can eliminate the condition.

Plantar Fasciitis

This is a painful inflammation of the thick connective tissue on the bottom of the feet. The pain is usually felt on the underside of the heel and is usually worse in the morning. Movement can be restricted and the condition is very debilitating for many patients. What is not commonly known or understood is that this condition is related to hypothyroidism.

In hypothyroidism, there is an increase in the levels of hyaluronic acid which accumulates in many body tissues including the skin, joints and the connective tissues of the body such as the plantar fascia which can lead to

> In hypothyroidism, there is an increase in the levels of hyaluronic acid which accumulates in many body tissues including the skin, joints and the connective tissues of the body such as the plantar fascia which can lead to pain and diminished flexibility and movement.

pain and diminished flexibility and movement.[109] When thyroid hormone bathes this affected connective tissue, hyaluronic acid levels decrease, and the connective tissue will return to a normal structure and function.[110] I have had many patients gain relief from this condition once proper thyroid hormone replacement was prescribed.

Hashimoto's Thyroiditis

This condition is one of the most prevalent autoimmune conditions, and is the most common cause of hypothyroidism. In the U.S. it is estimated annually to be 3.5 cases per 1,000 in women and 0.8 per 1,000 in men. Simply speaking, this form of low thyroid function is a condition where the body's immune system attacks the proteins and structures of the thyroid gland itself, leading to its slow destruction, and overall lowered thyroid function.

Antibodies

The cells of the immune system normally produce specialized proteins that attack foreign invaders called antibodies. In Hashimoto's, the immune system produces specific antibodies that can be measured in the blood: Anti-TPO and Anti-TG antibodies. Normally there can be very low amounts of these antibodies present, but this condition can make them increase drastically in amount.

A simple blood test can determine the presence of these antibodies. If you have these antibodies detected above the normal range, and you have other signs and symptoms of hypothyroidism, then treatment should be considered.

HYPERTHYROIDISM

This section largely focuses on hypothyroidism, or lowered thyroid function and slow metabolism. However, the opposite can occur in the thyroid leading to hyperthyroidism, or high thyroid function. The overall incidence of hyperthyroidism is estimated between 0.05 and 1.3 percent, with the majority being subclinical hyperthyroidism, where only the TSH is affected and the patient has no or limited symptoms. The incidence of hyperthyroidism is approximately five to ten times less than hypothyroidism.[111] With that understanding, it is important to be aware of the condition so proper treatment can ensue.

The Symptoms of Hyperthyroidism

- Nervousness
- Anxiety
- Increased perspiration (sweating)
- Heat intolerance
- Tremors and shaking
- Hyperactivity
- Palpitations
- Weight loss despite increased appetite
- Reduction in menstrual flow or skipping periods

The Signs of Hyperthyroidism

- Hyperactivity
- Elevated heart rate (tachycardia) or
- Atrial fibrillation (A-fib, heart arrhythmia)
- Elevated blood pressure
- Warm, moist, and smooth skin
- Lid lag (The upper eye lid does not follow the motion of the eye.)
- Upper eyelid retraction leading to constant stare
- Visible tremor (hands or head)
- Muscle weakness

Graves' Disease

Graves' disease is an autoimmune condition and is the most common form of hyperthyroidism. It is distinguished by the presence of circulating antibodies, including common autoimmune antibodies such as those associated with lupus and rheumatoid arthritis, as well as anti-thyroid peroxidase (anti-TPO) and antithyroglobulin (anti-TG) which are also seen in hypothyroidism. However, the most important autoantibody is thyroid-stimulating immunoglobulin (TSI). TSI antibodies act like thyroid-stimulating hormone (TSH) and create a constant stimulation to the thyroid gland to overproduce thyroid hormone. This leads to an enlarged thyroid gland.

Hormone Alterations in Hyperthyroidism

❧ Lowered levels of the stress hormone cortisol by increased clearance through the liver.

❧ Increased levels of estrogen in men, sometimes leading to gynecomastia (breast enlargement).

❧ Increased SHBG (Sex Hormone Binding Globulin) levels that lead to increased estrogen and testosterone in both men and women.

Thyroid Nodules: Benign and Cancerous

Thyroid nodules are very common. Many people can have one or two simple thyroid nodules and most are benign. Only about 0.004 percent of these are cancerous in the American population.[112] Reasons for these benign nodules are largely unknown, but iodine deficiency is one likely possibility. This concept is discussed in the chapter on iodine on page 160. Factors associated with a benign thyroid nodule include:

❧ Family history of autoimmune disease such as Hashimoto's thyroiditis or Graves' disease

❧ Family history of benign thyroid nodule or goiter

❧ Already diagnosed thyroid disease such as hypothyroidism or hyperthyroidism

❧ Pain or tenderness associated with nodule

❧ Soft, smooth, and mobile nodule

Consider these factors if you have been diagnosed with thyroid nodules. Factors associated with a cancerous thyroid nodule include:

❧ Younger than twenty years or older than seventy years

❧ Male

❧ Difficulty swallowing or speaking

❧ History of neck irradiation, such as frequent x-rays

❧ Previous history of thyroid cancer

❧ Firm, hard, or immovable nodule

❧ Swelling in the glands along the neck

Chapter 8
Iodine for Your Thyroid and Beyond

Introduction

"All truth goes through three stages. First, it is ridiculed. Then it is violently opposed. Finally it is accepted as self-evident." —Schopenhauer

In the never-ending attempt to discover simple, effective and safe medicines that truly react at the causal level of disease, a fork in this road of discovery brought me to iodine. And in my quest to better understand why thyroid disease plagued so many of my patients, I again was led to iodine. Without a doubt, our environment plays a role in our present state of health and how it specifically affects the thyroid gland. Our inadequate nutritional state greatly contributes to the lowered function of the thyroid. But specifically, one key nutrient may lie at the core of most of the reason why we see so much hypothyroidism not only in this country, but in the world. That one nutrient is iodine.

Most people have heard of iodine. It is found in iodized salt in the famous navy blue containers. Mom used to slather the liquid form of iodine on our scrapped knees with a "this will make it better" sting, leaving an interesting orange stain on our skin. It is found in foods like ocean fish and you may even have had to be injected with or had to drink a particular type of iodine used in medical imaging tests. But iodine does much more.

Iodine has had a long historical use in the field of medicine. More than a hundred years ago, iodine was called "The Universal Medicine" and was used for just about everything. Albert Szent Györgyi, the Nobel Laureate and physician who discovered Vitamin C in 1928, was quoted saying: "When I was a medical student, iodine in the form of KI [potassium iodide] was the universal medicine. Nobody knew what it did, but it did something and did something good. We students used to sum up the situation in this little rhyme: *If ye don't know where, what, and why, Prescribe ye then K and I.*"[113]

K and I refers to potassium iodide or Lugol's solution, a medicinal form of iodine that has been widely used since 1829. Iodine has a long history of medical use, spanning over three generations of physicians. Despite this understanding and knowledge of effectiveness and safety, the dawn of patented medicines made many simple remedies including iodine, fall to the wayside.

Iodine as an Element

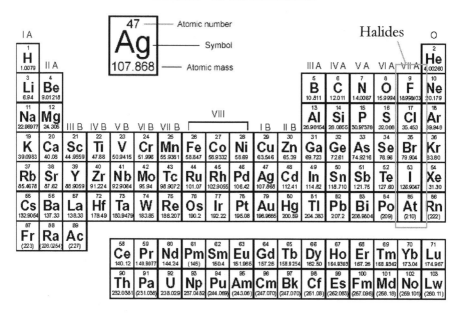

Iodine is positioned on the Periodic Table of Elements in a special grouping called the halogens. These negatively charged ions are similar in atomic structure and share similar properties. It is important to show that the halogens are elements found commonly in our environment. In decreasing reactivity, these elements are fluorine, chlorine, bromine, iodine, and astatine. The higher an element is on the Periodic Table, the more reactive it is. This is important because fluorine, chlorine, and bromine are all more reactive than iodine and will displace and compete with iodine in our bodies and our diets. And we are insulted with excess fluorine, chlorine, and bromine in our drinking water, diets, and environment on a daily basis.

Different Forms of Iodine

Following is a summary of the differing forms of iodine. Not all forms of iodine are good for us. You will notice that the "good" kind of iodine is actually termed "inorganic" and the unfavorable kind of iodine is termed "organic." This is one of the rare times when the term "organic" is not good for you.

The element iodine exists in nature as:
- Inorganic sodium and potassium salts of iodates (IO3-)
- Iodides (I-)
- Inorganic diatomic iodine (I2)
- Organic monatomic iodine (C-I)
  - Natural sources of iodine[114]
- Atmospheric air (major reservoir but extremely dilute at 1 mcg per cubic meter)
- Oceans (major reservoir but very dilute at 0.05 mcg/ml of sea water)
- Sea vegetables
  - Kelp (contains over 400 mcg per ¼ cup or 20 grams)
  - Sea algae (up to 0.5 percent wet weight being reported in red algae[115])
- Sources used for iodine production: caliches (sodium nitrate deposits), oil wells, and deep well water.
  - Forms of Iodine Used in Clinical Medicine[116]
- Inorganic
  - Nonradioactive (Non-toxic)
    - Iodides (SSKI—Saturated Solution of Potassium Iodide): 100 g KI/100 ml [1g/ml], One drop = 0.5 mg iodide.
    - Lugol's solution: 5 mg iodine/7.5 mg potassium iodide, 2 drops (0.1 ml) = 12.5 mg iodine/iodide = One tablet Iodoral® or iThroid®.

- Tincture of Iodine (Used in hospitals as an antiseptic, as in the product Povidone)
- Radioactive Iodides used for diagnostic and therapeutic purposes (Toxic)
- Organic
  - Naturally Occurring (Non-toxic at normal physiological levels)
    - Thyroid Hormones
    - Thyroidal Iodolipids
  - Man Made (Highly toxic)
    - Radiographic Contrast Media
    - Iodine-containing drugs (Amiodorone, a high blood pressure medication)

Where is all the iodine?

The World Health Organization (WHO) has revealed many global health problems as they relate to iodine deficiency. In fact, iodine deficiency is the world's greatest single cause of preventable mental retardation.[117] We see iodine deficiency as a public health problem in at least fifty-four countries resulting in an overall decreased childhood survival rate in these areas. Simply solving the iodine deficiency in these areas decreases the infant mortality rate by 50 percent.[118, 119, 120]

It is important to note that we do not see severe iodine deficiency at the same rate of occurrence as expressed in the above paragraph. However, in the U.S., the National Health and Nutrition Examination Survey (NHANES) conducted a broad national survey for nutritional status initially from 1971-1974 (NHANES I) and then reported data from 1971 to 2000 (NHANES II).[121, 122, 123] They reported that the proportion of the U.S. population with moderate to severe iodine deficiency (defined as <50 mcg/L in urine) has increased over 400 percent in the past twenty years.[124] So, the problem is growing and these data do not include "mild" iodine deficiency.

Clearly, there is a deficiency of iodine in this country and even worldwide. But why?

- ❧ It seems that Americans are consuming less iodized salt than in the past.
- ❧ There have also been political movements to lower the amount of iodine in salt and other food sources such as baked goods, further compounding the deficiency.
- ❧ Of the amount of iodized salt that we do consume, most of it is not absorbed, further driving the deficiency lower.
- ❧ The final blow to our deficient iodine state comes in the form of environmental factors, such as the previously mentioned halides, that further displace what little iodine is available to us.

What about iodine intake in other countries?

The Japanese people consume a daily average of 4.6 gm of seaweed and they are one of the healthiest people on earth.[125, 126, 127, 128] This amount of seaweed comes out to an average of about 13.8 milligrams of iodine, some ninety times higher than the U.S. RDA of 150 micrograms. The Japanese have the lowest overall risk of cancer and the lowest incidence of endemic goiter and hypothyroidism.[129, 130] This is an important point as many opponents of the use of iodine in larger milligram amounts insist that too much iodine will cause goiter, hyperthyroidism (high thyroid function) and hypothyroidism (low thyroid function).

Finland added iodine to their dairy feed and animal salt and the following past several decades have shown a decrease of cardiovascular mortality by over 50 percent, and life expectancy increased by five years. This addition of iodine to their food chain brought them to having the highest iodine intake of all European countries.[131, 132]

> The Japanese have the lowest overall risk of cancer and the lowest incidence of endemic goiter and hypothyroidism.

What about iodized salt?

We would think that since iodine is added to salt, we would get enough iodine. This is not the case. First of all, salt intake has decreased since the 1980s when it was incorrectly correlated with hypertension (high blood pressure) in the majority of people. Additionally, there simply is not enough iodine in salt to achieve whole body sufficiency. There is enough, however, to prevent goiter…theoretically. Iodized table salt contains 75 mcg of iodine per gram of salt. Americans ingest an average of 10 grams of salt, so that would give us about 750 mcg of iodine daily, more than enough for the prevention of goiter that only needs 50 mcg of iodine daily. However, drop for drop, there is 30,000 times more chloride than iodide in iodized salt. Since chloride and iodide are similar in atomic structure, classified in the group called halides, they strongly compete for absorption and inevitably only 10 percent of the iodide in iodized salt is bioavailable and actually absorbed.[133] This would be about 75 mcg of iodine, just above the amount needed to prevent goiter and only half of the U.S. RDA of 150 mcg. We will see that the U.S. RDA for iodine is inadequate for full body iodine sufficiency.

The Iodine Competitors: The "Other" Halides

Remember iodine's position on the periodic chart? Iodine shares a commonality with the other halides: fluorine, chlorine, bromine and finally astatine. Their common relationship causes them to jockey for position within our bodies. Fluorine, chlorine and bromine will almost always win over iodine. This means that if they are present in our bodies in a significant abundance over iodine, then iodine will have difficulty being absorbed and influencing our body positively. This section lists common sources of these other competing halides to illustrate why we are seeing more iodine deficiency that leads to thyroid dysfunction. We should take the opportunity to avoid exposure to these halides when possible to optimize iodine utilization for the body.

Here are some common places we find bromine, chlorine and fluorine and how they affect the thyroid gland and our health.

Bromine

Bromine is a common water sterilizer used in pools and as a fumigant for agricultural crops. It is also a fumigant for termites and other pests. Bromine has replaced iodine in bakery products since the 1980s.[134] (One slice of bread used to contain the RDA for iodine of 150 mcg.) It is also found in soft drinks in the form of polybrominated diphenyl ethers. In the past, bromine was used in medicine as a sedative and for seizures, but the toxicity of the drug fortunately phased out its use. However, it is still present in some medications such as the popular asthma medications Atrovent® Inhaler and Spray, ipratripium nasal spray, Pro-Panthine, and Spiriva® Handihaler.[135]

Bromine is a known goitrogen, or substance that is known to interfere with thyroid function and in excessive intake will lead to hypothyroidism.[136] It has no known physiological benefit to the human body. In fact, low amounts of bromide have shown to induce goiter even in the presence of adequate amounts of iodine to prevent goiter.[137, 138, 139] Bromine intoxication has also been shown to produce a multitude of psychological problems such as schizophrenia, hallucination and delirium.[140]

> Bromine is a known goitrogen, or substance that is known to interfere with thyroid function and in excessive intake will lead to hypothyroidism.

Chloride

Chloride is very important for our bodies, helping with a multitude of cellular processes. However, the oxidized form, known as chlorine, is a toxic element. Chlorine is used in the manufacture of chlorinated organic chemicals, plastics and chlorinated lime. Other uses include water purification, shrink proofing wool, in flame-retardant compounds, processing of some foods, as a bleaching agent and in pulp and paper manufacturing. It is used as a post-harvest disinfectant for fruits and vegetables, or as a disinfectant in human drinking water treatment systems, swimming pool water systems, industrial ponds and sewage systems. Chlorine may also be used as an algaecide in commercial and industrial water-cooling tower systems.[141] Simply, chlorine is everywhere and this is a direct toxic burden to our bodies and our thyroid gland, displacing iodine and competing with its absorption.

One of the worst sources of chlorine in our environment is perchlorate, which consists of one atom of chlorine and four atoms of oxygen. It is naturally occurring and is also man-made, commonly as jet fuel. This toxic substance has been associated with thyroid cancer, goiter, hypothyroidism, menstrual irregularities and immune problems.[142] It has been shown to inhibit the sodium-iodide symporter (NIS), the cellular component vital for bringing iodine into cells.[143] With this in mind, conventional medicine once used potassium perchlorate as a treatment for hyperthyroidism (high thyroid function) to deliver high doses of chlorine that competed with iodine absorption and arrested complete thyroid function. Fortunately, its use was discontinued when the toxic effects of the treatment were realized.

Most of the perchlorate contamination in the U.S. is attributed to its use as an oxidizer and primary ingredient in solid rocket fuel. The majority of sites where perchlorate was detected as a contaminant in groundwater are associated with the manufacturing or testing of solid rocket fuel by

> One of the worst sources of chlorine in our environment is perchlorate, which consists of one atom of chlorine and four atoms of oxygen. It is naturally occurring and is also man-made, commonly as jet fuel. This toxic substance has been associated with thyroid cancer, goiter, hypothyroidism, menstrual irregularities and immune problems.

the Department of Defense (DOD), and by the National Aeronautics and Space Administration (NASA), and with the manufacture of ammonium perchlorate.[144] The inevitable exposure to perchlorate that so many Americans have experienced has shown increases in breast disease, hypothyroidism, immune system problems, mental retardation in newborns, poor fetal and neonatal development and thyroid cancer.[145]

Fluorine

Fluoride is yet another prominent culprit in displacing the available iodine in your body. As another halide, fluoride is competing with iodine receptors in the thyroid gland and the rest of the body, and therefore inhibits the ability of the thyroid to concentrate iodine.[146] And just as the other halides described above, fluorine has been shown to be more toxic to the body if an iodine deficiency is present.

Fluoride use and exposure is a major health issue. The rampant use of sodium fluoride in municipal water sources has been a major cause for alarm. Fluoride has been linked in government and scientific reports to a wide range of harmful health effects, including bone and tooth decay including dental and skeletal fluorosis, bone pathology, arthritis, osteoporosis, Alzheimer's disease, memory loss and other neurological impairments, kidney damage, cancer, genetic damage and gastrointestinal problems. [147]

At least 22 percent of all American children now have dental fluorosis as a result of ingesting too much fluoride, according to The Centers for Disease Control (CDC). Fluorosis is the discoloration and, in advanced cases, the pitting of teeth. That rate may be as high as 69 percent in children from high socioeconomic-status families and those who live in fluoridated

> **At least 22 percent of all American children now have dental fluorosis as a result of ingesting too much fluoride, according to The Centers for Disease Control (CDC).**

communities, according to a July 1998 report from The American Academy of Pediatric Dentistry and corroborated in several reports published since 1995 in the *Journal of the American Dental Association.*

Calcium fluoride is naturally occurring, but sodium fluoride is a waste product of the aluminum industry that is added to our water and therefore found in our foods and beverages. Sodium fluoride has never received FDA approval from the U.S. Food and Drug Administration. It is listed as an unapproved new drug by the FDA, and as a contaminant by the EPA. The issue of fluoridation in the water and food supply and its potential negative affects on health is large and ominous. I recommend exploring www.flouridealert.org for detailed information. Using reverse osmosis and activated alumina water filter systems will eliminate fluoride from the water. A Brita® water filtration system will not remove fluoride effectively. Spring water is also a good choice as it contains very low levels of fluoride. Other common fluoride sources include toothpaste and processed beverages such as soda and reconstituted juice.

Many patients come to me having already been prescribed SSRI (selective serotonin reuptake inhibitors) antidepressants such as Paxil® and Prozac®. These medications contain fluoride. Asthma medications such as Flonase® and Flovent® also contain fluoride.

As we can see, there are multiple sources of these toxic halogens competing with iodine absorption and interfering with our health. But there is always something that can be done. First of all, avoid the common sources of these halogens to the best of your ability. We can always

> **Many patients come to me having already been prescribed SSRI (selective serotonin reuptake inhibitors) antidepressants such as Paxil® and Prozac®. These medications contain fluoride. Asthma medications such as Flonase® and Flovent® also contain fluoride.**

take steps to decrease our exposure to any toxic element in our personal environment and lower our overall toxic burden. As suggested earlier, use filtered and bottled water to drink and cook in and fluoride free toothpastes. Consider alternative water cleansers for pools and hot tubs. Also, the use of iodine, in its proper medicinal amount, will help to displace the presence of these toxic halogens and other toxic substances. As a result, the proper use of iodine becomes protective from the inevitable insult of these toxic elements. So, read on....

The Thyroid Gland and Iodine Deficiency

There are various disease processes that arise in the structure of the thyroid gland itself with deficiency of iodine.

Goiter

Goiter is the enlargement of the thyroid gland, most often due to iodine deficiency, hypothyroidism and a swelling process called thyroiditis. Doctors often believe that TSH (Thyroid Stimulating Hormone) is mostly responsible for the thyroid growing in size, but goiter development correlates better with low thyroidal iodine than with elevated TSH levels from a clinical perspective.[148] Elevated TSH levels induce thyroid hypertrophy or an actual enlargement of the gland, where intrathyroidal (inside the thyroid gland) iodine deficiency induces thyroid hyperplasia (an increased number of thyroid cells).

In the case of an iodine-deficient goiter, iodine supplementation abolishes not only hypertrophy (enlargement of the gland), but also hyperplasia (increased number of cells) of the thyroid gland. On the other hand, suppression of TSH with thyroid hormone such as with levothyroxine

> **Suppression of TSH with thyroid hormone such as with levothyroxine (T4) will correct the hypertrophy, but NOT hyperplasia if there is intrathyroidal iodine deficiency.**

(T4) will correct the hypertrophy, but NOT hyperplasia if there is intrathyroidal iodine deficiency.[149] This is an extremely important concept. This supports the reason why iodine therapy should be included in the treatment of thyroid disease such as goiter and/or hypothyroidism. Merely suppressing TSH to correct the enlargement of the thyroid, or to provide a dose large enough to eliminate hypothyroid signs and symptoms, will not always work if there is still underlying iodine deficiency.

Thyroid Nodules

Thyroid nodules are very common and I have many patients that come to me with this diagnosis. Most thyroid nodules are solitary and benign (non-cancerous), but they do increase the risk of having or developing hypothyroidism or hyperthyroidism. This condition also suggests that the thyroid is in the beginning stages of a nutritional deficiency. It has been shown that thyroid nodules have significantly less iodine within them compared to surrounding normal thyroid tissue. Benign (non-cancerous) thyroid nodules contain 56 percent of the iodine content as compared to normal thyroid tissue and malignant (cancerous) thyroid nodules which contain only 3 percent. Selenium, another important nutrient for thyroid function, has also been shown to be low in both malignant and benign nodules.[150] It has been shown that malignant thyroid nodules contain 68 percent less selenium as compared to normal healthy thyroid tissue.[151] It is important to supplement with selenium and focus on getting enough in the diet; about 200 to 400 mcg of selenium daily supports optimal thyroid function.

Thyroid Cancer and Iodine

When available iodine in the diet is lower, the incidence of thyroid cancer is generally higher. There has been evidence to show that when iodine content is low in the thyroid gland, the overall thyroid cell proliferation (growth) is higher, leading to a cancerous situation. When iodine is present in the thyroid gland in sufficient amounts, iodine attaches to lipids, or fats, normally found in the thyroid gland and elsewhere in the body. This process is called "iodination of lipids" and requires iodine in an amount at least double the RDA (Recommended Daily Allowance), which would be at least 800 mcg daily.[152] These iodinized lipids are protective to the thyroid gland and the rest of the body.

You may ask: besides my thyroid gland, what else in my body needs iodine? Every cell in your body needs and utilizes iodine. When at full iodine sufficiency, approximately 1.5-2.0 grams is stored in the entire body. Your thyroid has about 50 mg, muscle tissue about 650 mg, and fat tissue holds about 700 mg of iodine. It has been shown that breast tissue, white blood cells (leukocytes), ovaries, testicles, thymus, adrenal tissue and prostate tissue all concentrate and metabolize iodine in a very similar way that the thyroid concentrates iodine.[153]

Iodine Intake and Breast Cancer

Iodine deficiency has now been shown in a multitude of scientific studies to be correlated strongly with breast cancer. An excellent study conducted by Wiseman concluded that there is a single causative element in the majority of cases: iodine deficiency.[154] And other researchers agree with this conclusion.[155, 156, 157, 158, 159, 160]

Populations have been studied across the world for iodine intake and the incidence of breast cancer and it is clear that the lower the amount of iodine in the diet, the higher the risk for breast cancer and vice versa.[161, 162] Japan and Iceland have the highest iodine intake in their diets and they enjoy the lowest risks for breast cancer. Mexico and Thailand have the lowest intake of iodine and they suffer the highest risk of breast cancer for any country.[163] We have also seen thyroid size to be larger, indicating goiter and

> **Populations have been studied across the world for iodine intake and the incidence of breast cancer and it is clear that the lower the amount of iodine in the diet, the higher the risk for breast cancer and vice versa.**

iodine deficiency, in women with breast cancer.[164] The amount of iodine required to prevent goiter is very low: in the range of the 150 mcg U.S. RDA. Delange has reported it be as low as 50 mcg to prevent goiter.[165] It should be made clear that the amount of iodine needed to prevent breast cancer and other breast changes, such as fibrocystic breast disease, has been shown to be at least twenty to forty times the amount needed to prevent goiter.[166,167] Another study by Giani, *et. al.* demonstrated an association with breast cancer, Hashimoto's thyroiditis and simple goiter— all conditions associated with iodine deficiency. The study examined one hundred patients with breast cancer and one hundred matched controls without breast cancer. Hashimoto's thyroiditis was present in 2 percent of the control group compared with 13.7 percent in the group with breast cancer, and simple goiter was present in 11 percent of controls compared to 27.4 percent of the patients with breast cancer.[168]

Thyroid Hormone Medication and Breast Cancer

It is important to note that there have been recent studies showing that women taking thyroid hormone have a possible increased risk of developing breast cancer.[169] The link here could be iodine deficiency, and the failure to add iodine supplementation along with thyroid hormone administration. Eskin clearly showed that hypothyroidism by itself was not the cause of breast cancer, but rather the deficiency of iodine.[170] But why does iodine become deficient when thyroid hormone is administered?

When you must take thyroid hormone, it increases the overall metabolic processes within all cells, increasing your need for a multitude of vitamins and minerals, including iodine. In other words, as the metabolism increases, the need for iodine increases. As the metabolism increases with the use of thyroid hormone, the utilization of ATP, the body's energy powerhouse within cells, increases. With lowered available ATP, the body has more difficulty uptaking and utilizing iodine. During this deficiency, the thyroid and breast tissue increase in size in an attempt to capture more iodine.[171] By adding iodine supplementation with the use of thyroid hormone treatment, the health of the thyroid gland and other body structures such as breast tissue are more optimized and protected.

Estrogen Replacement Therapy, Breast Cancer and Iodine

Since 2002, the Women's Health Initiative study changed forever the way we view estrogen, announcing that the use of synthetic estrogens and progestins are linked to an increased risk of breast cancer and blood clots. Since that time, confusion of epic proportions has littered and confused the minds of physicians and patients alike. In my practice, I have used natural bioequivalent estradiol with thousands of patients with great success, without an increased incidence of breast cancer or any other associated malignancy or disease complication. When using estrogen replacement therapy, in any form, a complete therapeutic approach using vitamins and minerals, particularly iodine, should be considered. If an iodine deficiency is present, estrogens have the ability to increase the likelihood of malignant changes within the breasts of animals.[172, 173] Iodine has been found in the terminal and intralobular duct cells of breast tissue, which comprises an overall minimal amount of breast volume. However, it is in these specific areas that both fibrocystic changes and breast cancer malignancy take place.[174] And when iodine is deficient, it renders these areas more sensitive to estrogens.[175]

Iodine has also shown to be effective at metabolizing or eliminating circulating estrogens in the body. Recent studies with iodine by Stoddard on breast cancer cells have demonstrated that the genes responsible for properly metabolizing estrogens are enhanced in the presence of sufficient iodine.[176] This information may suggest an

> By adding iodine supplementation with the use of thyroid hormone treatment, the health of the thyroid gland and other body structures such as breast tissue are more optimized and protected.

importance of properly correcting an iodine deficiency while on estrogen replacement therapy.

Iodine and Fibrocystic Breast Disease

Fibrocystic Breast Disease (FBD) is a condition where the breasts contain varying sized painful cysts. The overall structure of the breast tissue changes including hyperplasia and mostly fibrosis or hardening. The disease is widespread and increasing in prevalence, affecting approximately 80 percent of North American women compared to only 3 percent in a report from 1928.[177] These cysts are often painful and can fluctuate in size and shape throughout the menstrual cycle. FBD is considered to be a benign condition, but there is mounting evidence showing that it is a precursor to breast cancer.[178, 179] A new study published in March of 2009 showed that women with dense breasts have a relative risk ratio of 4.03 for developing breast cancer. This means that women with dense breasts have a four-fold increased likelihood of developing breast cancer.[180]

Typical treatments for FBD are the use of oral contraceptives (birth control pills) to suppress ovarian production of estrogen as well as dietary modifications that include elimination of caffeine, chocolate and avoiding processed foods containing trans fatty acids. Also helpful are the additions of essential fatty acids such as fish oil or evening primrose oil, and improving the overall nutritional profile to include many vitamins and minerals. These strategies are surely helpful, but I have found that many patients still have the painful cysts in their breasts. Iodine has been shown to help with FBD and I have seen this in private practice.

Hyperthyroidism (High Thyroid Function) and Iodine

There has been a long historical use of high doses of iodine to treat hyperthyroidism (high thyroid function) also commonly known as Graves' disease. From Massachusetts General Hospital to the Mayo Clinic, the early twentieth century had many successes with treating hyperthyroidism safely and effectively, and either preventing surgery or at the very least lowering the mortality associated with surgery for hyperthyroidism. The daily amount of iodine used in the form of Lugol solution for Graves' disease ranged from one drop (6.25 mg) to thirty drops (180 mg). [181, 182, 183, 184, 185, 186, 187, 188, 189]

By the mid to late 1940s, a new drug type became available for the treatment of hyperthyroidism. The anti-thyroid, goitrogen drugs thiourea and thiouracil, which eventually evolved into the more powerful versions we are familiar with today (the thiionamides: methimazole, carbimazole, and propylthiouracil).[190] Interestingly, one year after the first anti-thyroid drug was introduced, the first article on the negative effects of iodine was published[191] beginning a new age of medical "iodophobia" or fear of iodine. By the late 1940s, even more articles were published on iodophobia[192, 193] and the positive effects of the use of anti-thyroid drugs.[194]

By the 1960s and 1970s, mixed reports surfaced regarding the ineffectiveness of the use of the anti-thyroid drugs resulting in a high incidence rate of remission back into hyperthyroidism.[195, 196] By the 1980s, thyroidologists began using iodine again, but unfortunately they were using the more detrimental radioactive version. Currently, the only conventional options for hyperthyroidism offered are anti-thyroid drugs, radioactive iodine or surgery, all of which come with their common side effects and high rate of either remission back into hyperthyroidism or over treatment into inevitable hypothyroidism.[197]

Iodine, in the form of Lugol's solution, Iodoral®, or iThroid®, has the potential to be effective in the treatment of hyperthyroidism. Of course, as with any advice in this book, you must consult with a healthcare professional to consider your options and if iodine treatment is something that you think may help, you must work closely with a healthcare provider well versed in the use of iodine and additional natural modalities to enhance the effectiveness of the iodine treatment.

Subclinical hyperthyroidism is a version of hyperthyroidism that has a very low, suppressed Thyroid Stimulating Hormone (TSH) lab result, with high end normal or normal levels of T4 and/or T3, and limited signs and symptoms of the actual disease of hyperthyroidism. (Refer to Chapter 7 for more information on hyperthyroidism.) The daily dose would range from 6.25 mg to 180 mg iodine in the typically used form of Lugol's solution. A dose of 90 mg was shown to be successful as much as 90 percent of the time.[198] Iodine supplementation can achieve very good responses in these cases and I have seen this many times. Overt hyperthyroidism presents with actual signs and symptoms of the disease and the response to iodine supplementation is still effective, but must be treated even more carefully.

Hypothyroidism (Low Thyroid Function) and Iodine

Iodine has been historically used for the treatment of hypothyroidism (low thyroid function).[199] Essentially, the symptoms of hypothyroidism are the same for iodine deficiency. With the condition of subclinical hypothyroidism, a more mild form of hypothyroidism, the TSH (Thyroid Stimulating Hormone) value is elevated above the normal range, but the remaining thyroid hormone values such as total T4 and T3 and free T4 and T3 are normal. The symptoms of subclinical hypothyroidism are usually less severe, but they can also be very debilitating. Often, patients will be put on typical thyroid hormone medication, natural or otherwise, at that point. A more conservative approach may be to add iodine first with a complete nutritional guidance plan, such as what is described in the Metabolic Health Protocol in Section 5, before implementing thyroid hormone treatment, then retest and reassess the clinical situation in the future. If the hypothyroidism is still present or in the future gets worse, then thyroid hormone treatment can be added.

It is not uncommon when taking natural thyroid hormone in a sufficient enough dose to eliminate the signs and symptoms of hypothyroidism that TSH (Thyroid Stimulating Hormone) becomes low or suppressed. It has been mentioned in Chapter 6 that a lowered TSH is not necessarily a problem and it certainly does not indicate that too much thyroid hormone is being taken. However, a lowered TSH, or TSH suppression, while on thyroid hormone may be important if an iodine deficiency is present. A recently published study in 2005 by Bruno et. al. showed that TSH suppression lowered the function of the NIS (Sodium Iodine Symporter) that shuttles iodine into the cell, which can lead to iodine deficiency.[200] Another study by Okerlund reported that thyroid hormone therapy and irradiation of the thyroid gland cause a depletion of iodine from the thyroid gland. Taking thyroid hormones for three or more months resulted in very low levels of iodine in the thyroid gland. Okerlund concludes, "The finding that previously irradiated thyroid glands are sometimes iodide depleted, coupled with the observation that the iodide depleted gland in experimental animals is physiologically more sensitive to the effects of pituitary thyrotropin (TSH), may lead to changes in the understanding of radiation-induced thyroid disease and to changes in the clinical management of at least some of these patients, who are known to be at high risk for thyroid tumor development."[201]

Okerlund is suggesting that patients on thyroid hormones who are also receiving radioiodide or radiation therapy should be supplemented with iodine as a preventative measure against the carcinogenic effect of these interventions in iodine depleted thyroid glands.

If a patient is in need of a large enough dose of thyroid hormone to eliminate his or her signs and symptoms, and at the same time TSH is suppressed, then adding iodine in conjunction with thyroid hormone treatment can help keep the thyroid gland healthy and functioning properly. Additionally, since iodine increases TSH, which in turn stimulates the NIS (Sodium Iodide Symporter) to shuttle available iodine into cells, then iodine supplementation along with thyroid hormone treatment has the potential to increase the TSH from suppression into potentially more normal ranges.

Hashimoto's Thyroiditis and Iodine

Hashimoto's Thyroiditis is an autoimmune (self-attacking) process resulting in the production of antibodies to TPO (thyroid peroxidase) that in effect, attack the thyroid gland, leading to an inflammatory response in the thyroid gland and resultant hypothyroidism, or low thyroid function. It is a poorly understood process overall, but much research has been undertaken in the attempt to understand it.

Many doctors have held the antiquated view that iodine supplementation will lead to Hashimoto's and also make the existing condition worse. This could not be further from the truth. In fact, iodine deficiency coupled with the presence of goitrogens, will lead to the condition.[202, 203, 204, 205] As this chapter has explained, the prevalence of goitrogens in our diet and environment is very high, and the incidence of iodine deficiency in general is also very high. We have seen the incidence of Hashimoto's thyroiditis and its related hypothyroidism rise in this country over the past forty years as the levels of iodine have slowly gone down.

> If a patient is in need of a large enough dose of thyroid hormone to eliminate his or her signs and symptoms, and at the same time TSH is suppressed, then adding iodine in conjunction with thyroid hormone treatment can help keep the thyroid gland healthy and functioning properly.

If a patient presents with laboratory values that show elevated antibodies (anti-TPO and anti-TG), but TSH and other parameters are within normal limits, then ensuring adequate iodine and proper antioxidant supplementation, such as magnesium, vitamin C, and others, should be administered to prevent the further destroying oxidation process from taking place. Guy Abraham, M.D., elaborates on the mechanisms

> Many doctors have held the antiquated view that iodine supplementation will lead to Hashimoto's and also make the existing condition worse. This could not be further from the truth. In fact, iodine deficiency coupled with the presence of goitrogens, will lead to the condition.

of autoimmune thyroiditis and its relationship to goitrogens and not the iodine itself: "Experimentally induced autoimmune thyroiditis in laboratory animals by acutely administered iodide required the use of antithyroid drugs, essentially goitrogens, to produce these effects. These goitrogens induced thyroid hyperplasia and iodide deficiency. Antioxidants either reduced or prevented the acute iodide-induced thyroiditis in chicks and mice." [206]

I suggest that any patient who has Hashimoto's thyroiditis consider iodine supplementation along with their thyroid hormone treatment to enhance overall outcomes and improvement of the condition. Additionally, all steps should be made to avoid as many of the known goitrogens that are described in this chapter as well as in other places in this book. And of course, this iodine supplementation should be included along with a comprehensive nutritional supplementation, and overall lifestyle protocol to enhance your metabolic health.

Iodine and Detoxification

Iodine supplementation results in detoxification of the body of the toxic metals aluminum, cadmium, lead, mercury, and arsenic. These observations were made by physicians who used iodine during the early twentieth century. Iodine supplementation has been confirmed in initial studies by Guy E. Abraham, M.D.[207] Iodine therapy has been shown to detoxify the body of the harmful halides such as fluorine, perchlorate, and bromine.[208] When using iodine in the proper amounts, you can displace these halides from cells and flush them from the body. The more of these halides you have in the body, the more need for iodine in general due to competition for absorption. Remember that these halides are some of the major culprits that lower the overall amount of iodine in your body. We always want

> Iodine supplementation results in detoxification of the body of the toxic metals aluminum, cadmium, lead, mercury, and arsenic.

to do our best to avoid exposure of these toxic elements; however, it is not always possible. It is a goal to ensure that there is a sufficient amount of iodine in the body to properly compete with these harmful substances.

If you have had exposure in the past to these metals or halides, and iodine therapy is started, a physician should be monitoring your progress closely. Often, as the metals are being eliminated, detoxification reactions can take place that should be encouraged and supported through proper supplementation, but closely monitored.

Where Do I Get Iodine?

The diet should include iodine rich foods such as sea vegetables like kelp and seaweed that are commonly served in Japanese restaurants that serve sushi. Seaweed contains more available iodine than any land-based plant. The seaweeds with the most available iodine are the giant kelps of the northern hemisphere such as from the coasts of Maine and California because they contain 1000-2000 ppm (parts per million). But Icelandic kelp contains a record-breaking 8000 ppm and Norwegian kelp contains 4000 ppm. The seaweeds with the least amounts of iodine are nori at about 15 ppm and sargassum at about 30-40 ppm.

Seafoods such as cod, sea bass, perch, and haddock provide some dietary iodine. Dairy products are also a rich source of iodine, particularly yogurt. Common land-based vegetables that are a good source of iodine include asparagus, dulce, garlic, lima beans, mushrooms, sesame seeds, spinach, summer squash, Swiss chard, and turnip greens. These food sources are an excellent start, but to achieve the therapeutic effects of iodine that are described in this chapter will require larger amounts that are obtained only with supplementation.

The RDA for iodine is woefully low. The RDA states women and men should have at least 150 mcg of iodine daily.

> Iodine therapy has been shown to detoxify the body of the harmful halides such as fluorine, perchlorate, and bromine.

During pregnancy the amount jumps to 220 mcg daily and during lactation the recommendation is 290 mcg daily.[209] What you need to know is that because the official guidelines on iodine from the RDA are so low, you may not be getting enough iodine to maintain your health.

How much should I be taking?

Guy E. Abraham, M.D., the foremost authority on the use of iodine, recommends at least 12.5 mg daily, which is in the range of the traditional dose of Lugol's solution of 0.1 ml and 0.3 ml (or two to six drops)[210] and very close to the 13.8 mg amount that mainland Japanese ingest daily. It is also recommended that the body must achieve a full sufficiency that takes, on average, a dose of 50 mg daily for approximately three months. This "50 mg" dose is a very important concept as it relates to iodine cellular physiology. To achieve the maximum transport of iodine across the membrane of the cell of approximately 600 mcg per day, the serum or blood must contain the correct concentration of iodine at 10^{-5} to 10^{-6} M (Molar). And 50 mg of iodine per day can reach 10^{-5} M concentration in the blood.

Whole body sufficiency of iodine can be achieved in most cases in about three months using 50 mg of iodine/iodide in a form such as Iodoral® or iThroid®. According to Abraham, using one tablet a day may require up to eighteen months to two years to achieve full body sufficiency in some patients.

I recommend the following dosing strategy for patients seeking optimization of their thyroid gland and their entire body utilizing iodine. It is designed to start the loading process slowly to assess tolerance of the iodine and any possible side effects.

First initial dose [on the first day]: ¼-½ tablet or one capsule to assess tolerance.

1st Week: One tablet or capsule daily (12.5 mg)

2nd Week: Two tablets or capsules daily (25 mg)

3rd Week: Two tablets or capsules in the morning and one tablet or capsule in evening (37.5 mg)

> 4th Week: Two tablets or capsules twice daily (50 mg) for three
> months, then reduce to one maintenance tablet or capsule daily
> 12.5 mg)
> Maintenance Dose: One tablet or capsule (12.5 mg) daily
> Note: Iodoral® is an enterically coated tablet produced by Optimox, and
> iThroid® is a capsule produced by RLC Labs. Both are excellent products.
> For patients with particularly sensitive stomachs, they should consider
> using the Iodoral® due to the special coating it contains. However, the
> majority of patients have no problem with the iThroid®, but it should be
> taken with meals to avoid any possible stomach irritation.

It is also important to state that hypothyroid patients already prescribed and taking thyroid hormone may experience signs and symptoms of over-stimulation due to the improvement of the function of their thyroid glands. Your healthcare provider will need to adjust your thyroid hormone medication. I find this occurring in about 10-20 percent of my patients and I consider it an excellent effect. The use of iodine in conjunction with thyroid hormone allows patients to keep their overall dose of thyroid hormone at a minimum, while still achieving the results of sign and symptomatic relief for their metabolic health.

Why Are Doctors Afraid of Using Iodine?

As has been noted, Guy E. Abraham, M.D. coined the term "medical iodophobia" which refers to the fear that so many doctors have of using iodine, even though it was safely done for so many years in the past. Throughout this chapter I have focused on a multitude of examples of scientific research, empirical evidence, and historical use of iodine in milligram doses with excellent outcomes and safety. But in the conventional medical model that is propagated by the sale of synthetic medications by the pharmaceutical companies, basic elements such as iodine in the use of medicine and healing are often shut down by medical doctors. This is true of many natural substances that were once used successfully in healing.

One area of misconception is the relationship of iodine containing drugs, such as amiodarone, causing ill effects. Abraham elaborates on this:

"The severe side effects of iodine-containing drugs have been attributed to inorganic iodine (the healthy iodine we are discussing here), even though published studies clearly demonstrate that it is the whole organic molecule (like that found in iodine-containing drugs) that is cytotoxic (cell toxic)...." [211] Additionally, Phillipou, et. al., is quoted saying, "We can, therefore, conclude that the effect of amiodarone, benziodarone, sodium iopanate, and other iodine containing substances with similar effects is due to the entire molecule and not to the iodine liberated. It should be noted that the cytotoxic effect of amiodarone in all cultures is also due to the *entire molecule* and not to the iodine present in it." [212]

Iodine Urine Testing

To assist the clinical outcomes for some patients using iodine, a convenient and accurate iodine urinalysis test was created by Guy E. Abraham, M.D. The majority of Americans who test will be found deficient in iodine. This iodine test is a simple twenty-four hour urine collection that is then sent out for analysis. Abraham, Brownstein, and Flechas have reported that over 90 percent of those they tested were deficient in iodine. In order to achieve full body sufficiency of iodine, 50 mg of iodine daily for three months is the average necessary to achieve success. However, some may need more time and possibly larger doses. In those occasions, iodine testing is very helpful to gauge the rate of success that a patient is experiencing.

Possible Side Effects with Iodine Use

It is very important to note that the thyroid gland itself has a self-protective mechanism that allows only a certain amount of iodine to be absorbed in a day. This amount is limited to a maximum of 0.6 mg/day when 50 mg or more elemental iodine is ingested.

I have been fortunate to observe only occasional side effects in my patients with the use of Iodoral® at doses up to 50 mg daily for three or more months. But these are mild and easily remedied by decreasing the dose or in very rare cases, avoiding the iodine all together. I have also had patients come to me already on doses this high or even higher for years with no ill effects. However, I have had some patients experience side effects on rare occasions, but they were easily remedied by reducing the dose to a tolerable level and/or enhancing detoxification. Abraham, Brownstein, and Flechas have reported the following possible side effects:

- ❧ Acne-like skin lesions in certain areas of your body
- ❧ Unpleasant brassy and metallic taste
- ❧ Increased salivation and sneezing

Based on the experience of many different clinicians with several thousands of patients on Iodoral®, with daily amounts ranging from 6.25 to 50 mg for up to three years, the incidence of the above side effects has been estimated at 1 percent.[213, 214] Abraham explains that, "Iodine supplementation induces a detoxification reaction in some patients with high bromide levels including increased body odor and cloudy urine. The body odor lasts one to two weeks, but the cloudy urine may last several months before clearing up."[215]

In any detoxification process, it is important to provide the body with the needed elements to enhance the detoxification that is taking place. Increased water intake, use of healthy, unprocessed salt, higher amounts of magnesium up to 1,200 mg daily, adequate amounts of vitamin C and an overall full nutritional supplementation and diet program all under the guidance of a healthcare provider well-versed in this arena, will assist in any possible detoxification reaction. This book provides the information necessary to guide you through possible roadblocks to your progress.

There is no one thing that answers the questions about all of our ailments all of the time, and iodine is no exception. However, I see iodine as an integral part of enhancing overall metabolism and improving outcomes for patients with thyroid disease. Iodine levels in human beings are slowly going down and our exposure to goitrogens is steadily on the rise, greatly contributing to the cause of the thyroid disease epidemic we find ourselves in. Take this simple, yet profound step by adding iodine to your supplement regimen and start enhancing your metabolic health now.

Section 4
Completing the Metabolic Triad:
Thyroid, Adrenals and Sex Hormones

Introduction

This section will explore two of the most important aspects of your hormonal and metabolic health: your adrenals and your sex hormones. In fact, the thyroid, adrenals, and sex hormones all dance around one another in dynamic interplay, with one depending on the other for proper function.

In Chapter 7, you were introduced to the expertise of Dr. Cristina Romero-Bosch where she discussed fibromyalgia and its relationship to lowered metabolism. Now she will take you on a journey of exploration through the complex and often overlooked world of the adrenals. She will lay out the groundwork of understanding the basics of the adrenals and follow up with specific treatment options in Step 6 of The Metabolic Health Treatment Protocol in Section 5. I will take up the pen again in Chapter 10 of this section and lay down a foundation of understanding female menopause and male andropause and the functions of the sex hormones. And again, the treatment options for menopause and andropause will be provided in Step 4 of The Metabolic Health Treatment Protocol.

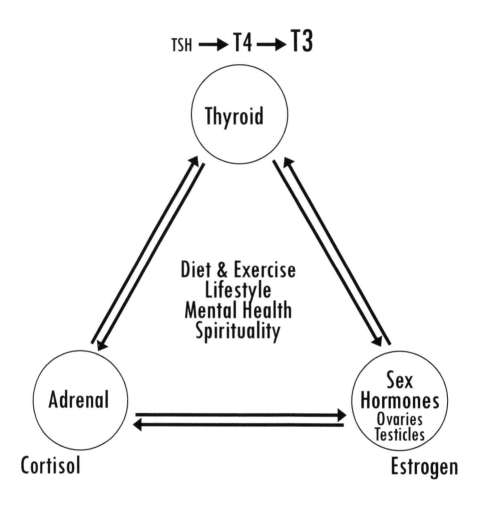

Chapter 9
Adrenal Dysfunction: An Overview

Introduction

Before you study with me the adrenal glands and preservation of their health as well as their potential fatigue syndromes, I must thoroughly discuss the notion of stress, stressors, and stress induced illnesses. Together we will explore the interrelationship between the metabolism of adrenal hormones, the prevalence of stress and the symptoms that warn of oncoming disease. Understanding the detrimental effect prolonged stress has on general health is the essential starting point for preventing adrenal disease and sustaining metabolic transformation. At the end of this chapter, you will be armed with the information necessary to take daily action in preserving adrenal health by understanding how medically supervised rehabilitation is possible for restoring already dysfunctional adrenals, and how taking such actions positively affects your holistic metabolic goals.

Remember that disease can be simply thought of as dis-ease, a lack of ease. The body, as all things in nature, seeks to be in a state of equilibrium. Any force pushing against this tendency towards balance causes dis-ease. With this awareness, adrenal disease can be avoided or at minimum repaired. For this

> Remember that disease can be simply thought of as dis-ease, a lack of ease. The body, as all things in nature, seeks to be in a state of equilibrium. Any force pushing against this tendency towards balance causes dis-ease.

reason a chapter on adrenal health and dysfunction must begin with a strong foundation in understanding and thereby preventing stressors from causing dis-ease.

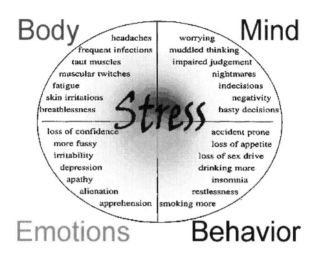

Stress: What Is It?

I am certain that we can all claim to know stress well. It is an unwelcome companion in our daily life. And despite the frequency of stress in life, it has been a difficult concept for biologists to define. Stress can be the cause, or force, towards change, or the resulting adaptation itself. It is this adaptation, or even the *failure* to adapt, that can lead to diseases produced by stress. The difficulty with defining stress is that it is relatively intangible and highly subjective. Stress can be real, like a physical injury or trauma, grief over the passing of a loved one or being stuck in traffic and late for an appointment, but it can also be perceived as the anticipatory anxiety before a public speech or first date. One official definition for stress is, "Any physical, emotional, or chemical factor that cause bodily or mental tension and may be a factor in disease causation." [216]

We must also distinguish between stress as defined above, and stressors. Merriam-Webster's defines a stressor as "a stimulus that causes stress." [217] This subtle distinction is important as it will help us segue into how we can manage our stressors by minimizing our stress.

The concept of a stressor leading to stress is an empowering one as it illustrates the individual's ability to control their response to stressors that may be out of their control. In other words, the things (stressors) that most cause us stress often do so because we feel we cannot control them. Despite the fact of our inability to control a stressor, our response to that stressor, defined as both our physical and emotional stress, is *entirely* within our control.

Recognizing a stressor is the initial step for controlling your stress response. There are four commonly found characteristics that identify an event as stressful: a new experience, the unpredictability of outcomes, actual physical threat and the feeling of not being in control.

Dr. Hans Selye was an endocrinologist and a pioneer in the study of stress and its subsequent effects on health. He extensively studied the presence of biological stressors (internal) or prolonged environmental stressors (external) that result in adverse biological effects.[218] His observation that stressors can clearly result in degenerative diseases launched extensive research and exploration into the effect of stress on hormones and the subsequent development of diseases. These explorations led doctors and scientists alike to recognize that stress induced diseases ranged from peptic ulcers to cancer, and must therefore be at the forefront of medical concern.

Selye's book, *The Stress of Life*, published in 1978, brought the concept of stress and its relationship to health to the consciousness of not only the scientific community, but to the public as well. Dr. Seyle's research exposed a common subset of physiological responses, or symptoms, to recurrent stressors. These outcomes were stomach ulcers, shrinking (atrophy) of lymphatic organs (such as the spleen and thymus gland) and growth (hypertrophy) of the adrenal glands.

Selye developed a three-stage process he called General Adaptation Syndrome (GAS)[219] which is explained below:

- ❧ Stage One: **Alarm**. Reaction-increased adrenal response and activation of the sympathetic nervous system. The demand for cortisol increases. Can be referred to as "Sympathetic Overdrive."

● Stage Two: **Resistance**. Adrenal hormones are excessively stimulated resulting in water, electrolyte, and carbohydrate metabolism being affected in attempt to re-establish balance. Cortisol begins to be produced at irregular and extended intervals. Can be referred to as "Adaptation."

● Stage Three: **Exhaustion**. The adrenal glands are no longer able to satisfy the need for hormone production; the adaptation cannot be sustained. Hormones, principally cortisol, are not produced in adequate amounts. Can be referred to as "Adrenal Fatigue."

An alternative to describing the GAS process is what I list here as the Four Stages of Adrenal Health:

● Healthy Adrenal Glands. Hormones are produced at appropriate levels and cortisol function follows healthy circadian rhythm.

● Dysfunctional Adrenal Glands. Hormones are produced at appropriate levels or in excess and cortisol's release does not follow healthy circadian rhythm. Complete repair is probable.

● Fatigued Adrenal Glands. Hormones, principally cortisol, are not produced at sufficient levels and cortisol's release does not follow healthy circadian rhythm. Complete repair is probable.

● Insufficient Adrenal Glands. Adrenal hormones are not meeting basic physiologic needs and circadian rhythm is not relevant. Complete repair is improbable.

It can be said that no one is spared exposure to stressful situations because stress is a common social experience. Stress varies from daily assaults like traffic jams and the frequent absence of a healthy breakfast, to unexpected and severe trauma. Our bodies undergo a cascade of hormonal, neuro-chemical and physical reactions in attempt to maneuver, adapt, and survive these stress-induced reactions. It has been concluded that as our systems become overburdened by frequent stress, our predisposition to dis-ease becomes more likely and the adaptive changes to the initial stressor may become pathologically permanent.[220]

Therefore, the more stressors one is exposed to, the less effective a person becomes at controlling their stress response. If it is acknowledged that many external stressors are beyond our control, then it must so too be recognized that preventing stressors we can control becomes vital for our health. A disregard for a healthy lifestyle increases the chance of adrenal dysfunction from fatigue to complete insufficiency, by neglecting the responsibility of avoiding daily stressors.

In 1967, in an attempt to measure life changes and their effect on health, psychiatrists Thomas Holmes and Richard Rahe evaluated over 5,000 patients to establish a correlation between stressors and the onset of illnesses. A significant positive correlation was found proving the theory that an increase in stressors, even positive ones, could predispose individuals to illness.[221]

Despite the negative connotation associated with the word "stress," Holmes and Rahe recognized that almost one-third of stress inducing life events (stressors) are usually classified as *positive* changes. This vital establishment emphasizes the importance of learning how to cope with stressors as a method of minimizing the burden on our adrenals verses the common approach of expecting that stressors should be completely eliminated. Because stress is so subjective, intangible and difficult to define, an attempt to eliminate all stress from our lives would not only be challenging, but may result in depriving ourselves of many of life's accomplishments. That is, if some of the stress-inducing life events are positive, like getting married, giving birth or achieving professional success, then we would be doing ourselves a disservice if we put energy into the elimination of all such stressors.

We must understand our perception of stress. If we identify life-changing events as stressful, they carry the emotional and chemical power to catalyze our stress response. Recognizing stressors and improving our techniques for dealing with them would allow us to confront life's challenges with minimal detriment to our general health and maximum experience. It has been shown that those who evaluate life challenges with a positive affect significantly reduce negative biological responses. Believing stressors are exciting and new can reduce adverse effects on adrenals and promote positive physical health outcomes.[222] Essentially, one man's stress can be another man's adventure.

The purpose of transforming our metabolic health is to achieve *true* well-being through understanding ourselves, having power over our lives, and being actively engaged in the joy of living. This is partially achieved through a constant effort to move away from the notion that life, mostly overwhelming and stressful, is beyond our control. Implementation of techniques that allow one to view possibility and opportunity in daily challenges results in healthy adrenals, optimal metabolism, and enduring personal transformation.

> We must understand our perception of stress. If we identify life-changing events as stressful, they carry the emotional and chemical power to catalyze our stress response. Recognizing stressors and improving our techniques for dealing with them would allow us to confront life's challenges with minimal detriment to our general health and maximum experience.

Stress Induced Diseases

Now that we have begun to understand how prolonged stress leads to illness it's time to improve stress response tendencies and avoid controllable stressors. This section will focus on the daily responsibilities we have for protecting our adrenal health. Daily responsibilities help to engage your consciousness in the life you live and remind you that you are in control of your life and not simply an observer. Persistent demands on your stress response can lead to malfunctions in the hormonal system that responds to stressors.[223] That is, when bodies are consistently requested to release stress-hormones, eventually the system is exhausted and it ceases to cooperate. In essence, we damage the "pump" and deplete the "tank."[224]

These *persistent* demands of stress on the body system are less commonly due to unexpected, traumatic events, but instead are predominantly simple and easily avoidable daily habits. Regulation of blood sugar, diminishing general inflammation in the body, and management of mental and emotional stress would be the three basic quotidian changes that would significantly reduce

> When bodies are consistently requested to release stress-hormones, eventually the system is exhausted and it ceases to cooperate. In essence, we damage the "pump" and deplete the "tank."

stress hormone demands, aid in preservation of adrenal function, and reduce risk of illness.

- **Blood sugar management:** Cortisol stimulates release of glucose (sugar) from storage in the cells to help increase blood sugar to generate energy.[225] Avoiding extended periods of fasting will provide sufficient glucose in the blood and help prevent unnecessary release of cortisol to stimulate gluconeogenesis (formation of glucose from storage). Blood sugar control is a keystone to decreasing frequent demands on our stress hormone system. When you eat regularly you are not requiring the release of sugar from storage as you are getting it from a meal. This reduces one of cortisol's main daily tasks— blood sugar regulation.

- **Mental-emotional stress management:** Extensive research demonstrates the relationship between emotional stressors and the increased release of cortisol.[226] But, research also demonstrates that having *perceived emotional* control over stressors significantly reduces the release of cortisol and improves health outcomes.[227] Evidence suggests that there are significant correlations between positive psychological states and health outcomes, indicating that positive emotions and sense of control over situations increases immune function and reduces susceptibility to disease.[228] When you approach daily challenges as opportunities for growth and not burdens you immediately reduce demand for cortisol. If you are not "stressed out" by a challenge then there is little need for cortisol. You are not eliminating the challenge, but eliminating the perception of burden.

● **General inflammation:** Cortisol is your primary immune and inflammation regulating hormone. By mistreating your body through poor diet and lifestyle you are pushing your tissues into a constant inflammatory stage. This constant inflammation further demands cortisol from the adrenals in an attempt to reduce the tissue damage. A poor diet deprives your body of nutritional anti-inflammatory nutrients and assaults your body with inflammatory chemicals. Inactivity increases release of inflammatory hormones. Physical activity decreases mortality rate even in those that are overweight or obese.[229] Think of these contrasts:

● Twinkie vs. Apple
● Soda vs. Water
● Watching TV vs. Hiking
● High Intensity Exercising vs. Regular Exercising

The stress induced diseases can start as early as birth. Consider that often women are already in an adrenal-fatigued state when they conceive a child.[230] Many women will note that although they feel exhausted during the first and second trimester, the third trimester comes with a feeling of strength and clarity that they haven't felt in a long time. It is during the third trimester that the placenta along with the adrenal gland plays a major endocrine role for both the mother and the child.[231] The child is therefore providing the mother with an increase in adrenal hormones,[232] but is also "sharing" adrenal production. It is theorized that this results in newborns with adrenal reserves already utilized.

It then follows that we create hectic lifestyles with little regard for daily rest, joy, physical activity, and proper digestion and elimination. These are the pillars for adrenal fatigue and subsequent metabolic dysfunction.

How many of these sources of chronic stress relate to you?

Mental & Emotional:	Blood Sugar Regulation:	Inflammation:	Others:
• Anger • Worry • Fear • Grief • Bitterness • Hopelessness • Guilt • Depression • Anxiety • Job/performance demands • Financial pressures • Relational conflict	• Skipping meals • Calorie deficit dieting • High carbohydrate intake • Alcoholism • Nutritional deficiencies	• Surgery • Trauma • Injury • Infections • Inhalant allergies • Food sensitivities • Constipation • Crohn's Disease • Colitis • Celiac • Arthritis • Toxins; heavy metals, molds, chemicals	• Temperature extremes • Sleep deprivation

Diseases of Underactive Adrenals

The intention of this section is to familiarize you with the adrenal glands so that you may better preserve their health, optimize your well-being, and allow for personal transformation. This chapter on adrenal health focuses mostly on underactive adrenal diseases, adrenal dysfunction, and adrenal fatigue. However, it is necessary that you understand the fourth stage of adrenal health—adrenal insufficiency. Adrenal insufficiency is an endocrine disorder in which the adrenal glands do not produce sufficient adrenal hormones. Adrenal insufficiency can be primary or secondary and is often further classified as congenital, from birth, or acquired, occurring later in life.

Addison's Disease—Primary Adrenal Insufficiency

Primary adrenal insufficiency, also called Addison's disease, occurs when the adrenal glands are damaged and therefore do not produce sufficient cortisol and often insufficient aldosterone.[233] This rare disease process is a result of a damaged adrenal gland, most commonly of autoimmune origin, and it is found in approximately four out of every 100,000 people with no specific gender or age association. Patients with Addison's disease often lead normal lives if they manage their disease through appropriate medical attention. President John F. Kennedy had Addison's disease. [234]

Secondary Adrenal Insufficiency

With secondary adrenal insufficiency, the lack of adrenal hormones is a result of the pituitary gland not producing enough adrenocorticotropic hormone (ACTH) or a lack of secretion of corticotrophin-releasing hormone (CRH) from the hypothalamus. ACTH is responsible for stimulating the adrenal glands to produce cortisol. With decreased stimulation there is a decrease of cortisol production. If diminished cortisol activity persists, the adrenal glands can atrophy (shrink). Secondary adrenal insufficiency is much more common than Addison's disease.

Although adrenal insufficiency is not a common dysfunction it can be fatal if not properly addressed and treated. Conventional treatments of these conditions involve medications to replace mineral, sugar, and cortisol activity. Prednisone, close electrolyte monitoring, and blood sugar controlling agents are typically used.

The symptoms accompanying either form of adrenal insufficiency present similarly to adrenal fatigue such as feelings of fatigue, possible hyperpigmentation or darkening of the skin particularly around the genitalia and areola, salt cravings, weight loss, possible abdominal pain or recurrent nausea and vomiting, and/or a general feeling of weakness. Weight loss is related to the fatigue and weakness and is a predominant sign in adrenal insufficiency. And as also seen with adrenal fatigue, patients may have difficulty maintaining blood sugar and easily get hypoglycemia. Blood pressure will often run low or may decrease with a change in postural position such as going from lying to sitting. This orthostatic change in blood pressure and pulse are considered cardinal signs of adrenal insufficiency. Many patients will also report loss of body hair. However, many of these symptoms can be found with adrenal fatigue, thyroid dysfunction or other metabolic disorders.

Diseases of Overactive Adrenals

Overactive adrenals are adrenal glands that are producing an excess of adrenal hormones. Remember that the adrenal gland produces your androgen (sex) hormones, your cortisol hormone, and your aldosterone (electrolyte) hormone. When aldosterone is produced in excess it can lead to difficulty controlling blood pressure as a result of electrolyte imbalance. When electrolytes are not well-controlled blood pressure and heart health is impaired as well as muscle health. Insufficient potassium, as found in cases of overactive adrenals, can lead to muscle cramping, spasms or even paralysis.

When the androgenic hormones are produced in excess in females, male sex characteristics are displayed. An increase in androgen production can result in male-patterned baldness, deepening of voice, acne, unwanted hair growth, and may result in abnormal genitalia formation in female fetuses.

When cortisol is produced in excess, a condition known as Cushing's syndrome[235] occurs. The symptoms of overactive adrenal glands may resemble other endocrine medical conditions. Always consult your physician for a diagnosis.

Cushing's Syndrome

Cushing's syndrome is a hormonal disorder of excess adrenal gland secretion and can be considered the opposite of Addison's (cortisol deficiency).[236] Cushing's, also known as hypercorticolism, is caused by prolonged periods of excess cortisol secretion. Like adrenal insufficiency, Cushing's syndrome is also quite rare, but mostly affects those between the ages of twenty and fifty. It may also be identified in children that have slow growth rates and who are obese. Cushing's will be more prevalent in those already suffering from obesity, type II diabetes, and high blood pressure (hypertension).

This syndrome will present with increase in body fat deposits especially around the face, neck, and torso, but unlike with general obesity the arms and legs remain slender. Cushing's results in discoloration of the skin, but is less a hyperpigmentation and more an increase in pink-purple stretchmarks and easy bruising. So, too, Cushing's patients will often be quite fragile and break bones and skin easily and then suffer from poor wound healing. This level of adrenal dysfunction will eventually affect menstruation, fertility, and even erectile function.

Like with adrenal insufficiency, Cushing's can mimic symptoms of other endocrine disorders like hypothyroid, metabolic syndrome, or polycystic ovarian syndrome (PCOS). Symptoms found in Cushing's that are common to many hormone dysfunctions are severe fatigue, weak muscles, blood sugar dysregulation (high blood sugar verses the low blood sugar from Addison's), excess hair growth and irritability, anxiety or depression as well as abnormal cholesterol readings. And most Cushing's patients will present with a fatty hump between the shoulders and of course have abnormally elevated cortisol.

Many people develop Cushing's syndrome because they take glucocorticoids for extended periods of time. These medications (such as prednisone) are steroid based hormones that are chemically similar to naturally produced cortisol and are used commonly to treat asthma, rheumatoid arthritis, lupus, and other inflammatory diseases. Glucocorticoids are also used to suppress the immune system after transplantation to keep the body from rejecting the new organ or tissue. Cushing's syndrome may also develop because the adrenal is simply producing excess cortisol. Pituitary adenomas cause 70 percent of Cushing's syndrome aside from those caused by steroid use. This is then referred to as Cushing's Disease. These adenomas are noncancerous (benign) tumors that stimulate the adrenals through excess secretion of ACTH. Pituitary adenomas are five times more common in women than men and are commonly found around the age of forty.[237] And rarely, Cushing's may be an inherited disease.

There is also a condition known as pseudo-Cushing's syndrome that is commonly found in patients with depression, anxiety, alcoholism, poorly controlled diabetes or obesity. There is still an overproduction of cortisol, but the treatment is more holistic as it relies on correction of the lifestyle or primary disease to be better managed and therefore can rely on less aggressive adrenal repair.[238]

Cushing's is initially considered by a physician based on evaluation of patient concerns, physical examination, and medical history. The diagnosis is then made through a series of tests including blood and urine analysis and often X-rays to detect possible tumors. The three most common lab tests prescribed are salivary cortisol, twenty-four hour urine free cortisol and a dexamethasone suppression test. Cortisol is measured through saliva samples acquired throughout the day. This is the same analysis used in diagnosing and treatment monitoring of adrenal dysfunction and adrenal fatigue. For Cushing's to be diagnosed, it is the late-night levels that are of most value and may often be measured during a hospital stay so as to avoid stress induced false elevation. Urinary free cortisol level measures the amount of cortisol released in the urine over a twenty-four hour period. Elevated levels in an adult of 50-100 micrograms a day would be suggestive of Cushing's. For the low-dose dexamethasone suppression test (LDDST), a person is given a low dose of dexamethasone, a synthetic glucocorticoid, by mouth every six hours for two days. Urine is collected before dexamethasone is administered and several times on each day of the test. A modified LDDST uses a onetime overnight dose. Glucocorticoids inform the pituitary that they do not need to produce as much ACTH so as to not stimulate the adrenals to produce more cortisol. If blood and urine cortisol levels do not drop after the medication is administered, then Cushing's is suspected.

It is important to note that some factors can interfere with accuracy of testing. A false diagnosis can be made in patients with high estrogen levels, acute illness, abnormally high stress, depression or alcoholism. Medications such as phenytoin and phenobarbital (seizure medications) may mask a true Cushing's diagnosis by suppressing cortisol.

If Cushing's is diagnosed then the cause of the syndrome must be determined so as to best treat the condition. Treatment is then based on the cause, severity, and personal preferences of the physician-patient team. The primary factor in determining the best treatment course is identification of the cause of the hypercortisolism. Since tumors tend to be the primary cause of the Cushing's syndrome then surgery is seen as the most effective and common treatment. Surgery may be coupled with radiation, chemotherapy or cortisol-inhibiting medications. In situations where the Cushing's is a result of steroid use to control another disease, then alternate dosing schedules or medications may be considered. [239]

Remember that Cushing's and Addison's are major medical conditions that need to be evaluated and monitored by physicians. However, holistic approaches to any dis-ease can be considered. With the recommendations of your healthcare provider many of the adrenal supportive treatment recommendations that you will learn in this book may be considered as compliments to traditional care.

Chapter 10
Sex Hormone Imbalances: Female Menopause and Male Andropause

Life Stages of Hormonal Balance in Women

The uterus is the most fantastic and awe-inspiring human organ. Medical science merely examines its beautiful mysteries and attempts to make sense of it. I often tell my female patients, "I bow humbly to the mysteries of the uterus…" I explain it this way because the uterus has a mind of its own often, a heart of its own, and trying to control it or figure it out can be challenging for both doctor and patient. I constantly try to better understand these challenging issues and bring light and awareness to all of my female patients.

In Traditional Chinese Medicine (TCM), the uterus is closely related to both the kidneys and the heart. Traditional Chinese medical philosophy sees the kidneys and adrenal glands as storing life energy that would be needed to allow the uterus to function properly. And the heart, with all of its potential for experiencing both joy and pain, may hinder the function of the uterus. Thus, the uterus is seen as "the second heart" and a very special connection exists between these two organs. This is why stress from all sources, related to both the kidneys/adrenals and the heart, can disrupt a woman's cycle, whether causing painful periods, long periods, missed periods, or many other gynecological issues. As women move through the different stages of life, and the clearer this relationship to the emotions and the uterus is understood, the smoother and more meaningful the journey becomes.

Pre-menopause

This stage is essentially defined as the time from beginning menstruation up until the first signs of peri-menopause. However, during this time, women can still have issues related to sex hormone balance. It is important to note that the issues women have with their hormones during this time are not necessarily associated with dysfunctional ovaries as it is related to peri-menopause and menopause. But you will still feel imbalanced at times and gynecological issues can still occur.

Some of the typical reasons why a woman would have issues during this time relate to other organs and conditions separate from the ovarian function, such as:

- Stress: One of the easiest ways to disrupt an otherwise normal monthly menstrual cycle is to go through an excessive amount of psychological, emotional or physical stress. Again, when erratic cycles or PMS occurs, it is assumed that it is an organic problem with the ovaries and their ability to produce hormone, or that it is the balance of the sex hormones that is causing the problem. This is generally not true, in and of itself.

- Poor estrogen metabolism: If your body is not properly breaking down estrogen, then it can lead to many issues and symptoms. Be sure to see the metabolic health protocol section of this book that discusses sex hormone balance and estrogen metabolism.

- Adrenal dysfunction: When the adrenals become weak from chronic stress, the entire body, including the metabolism of estrogen, progesterone, and other sex hormones becomes impaired. Additionally, the adrenals produce a large percentage of the sex hormones in your body and when they are weak, they are not contributing adequately to your sex hormone needs. This topic is also covered in Chapter 9 and in Step 6 of The Metabolic Health Protocol.

- Thyroid dysfunction: This is one of the most underestimated relationships with gynecological issues including erratic periods, uterine conditions, pre-menstrual syndrome and more.

⊘ Organic gynecological issues: At times, women can have direct problems with the ovaries themselves, such as ovarian cysts that can be very painful. There is also a condition known as premature ovarian failure that is a very early menopausal state occurring before the age of thirty. Also, uterine conditions such as cysts and fibroids can occur that will need to be addressed directly.

Lab values during this time tend to be fairly consistent in most cases, even when perceived issues occur, which could be related to other conditions stated above. There is a normal cycle of up and down of estrogen during a typical twenty-eight day menstrual cycle, with estrogen being lowest right before and during menstruation with levels even below 50 pg/mL and levels that can peak as high as 500+pg/mL at ovulation, all of which would be completely normal. During this time the FSH is well below 20 mU/L and more typically below even 10 mU/L most of the month.

One condition worth mentioning here is menstrual migraine. This type of headache will occur right before the menstrual cycle and is typically relieved upon menstruation or soon after. This is a condition related to very low estrogen that occurs right before the time of menstruation. By adding in a small amount of estradiol (estrogen) during this time, menstrual migraines can be relieved in many women.

Peri-menopause

Peri-menopause is the time directly before menopause that is marked by irregular menses and hot flashes and can last up to ten years or longer. For some women, the peri-menopausal transition is very rapid and they just suddenly find themselves in menopause, having a normal period one month and with little warning or transition, they can just stop having periods. This is rarer, but I have seen it many times. Typically, peri-menopause lasts about one year for most women and is accompanied by erratic periods and many of the typical symptoms of menopause, but not in great severity yet.

The peri-menopausal menstrual cycles can be very erratic with a change in flow, either heavier or lessened, a change in timing from more frequent periods to skipping months. During this time, ovarian function is fluctuating with ups and downs as it is moving into full menopausal sleep. In other words, the ovaries can produce adequate amounts of estrogen and progesterone one month and then an inadequate amount the next. Or, adequate amounts one day and inadequate amounts the next. Typically during this time, the majority of symptoms are related to testosterone deficiency and perhaps progesterone deficiency. The FSH (Follicle Stimulating Hormone) reading is often greater than 10 mU/L but still less than 20 mU/L.

> The peri-menopausal menstrual cycles can be very erratic with a change in flow, either heavier or lessened, a change in timing from more frequent periods to skipping months. During this time, ovarian function is fluctuating with ups and downs as it is moving into full menopausal sleep.

The menstrual cycle can be tricky to follow during this transition. And just because a woman has not had a period for a few months or more, it does not mean her ovaries are done producing hormone… yet. Hormone treatments can still be used at this time, but typically, a doctor will wait for complete menopause before hormone treatment will be given. With proper monitoring, hormone replacement can be given during this time to make the transition of change more bearable. Know that providing hormone replacement therapy will not stop the transition into menopause or delay it in any way, but it will make the ride a little smoother.

Menopause and Post-menopause

By the year 2030, the World Health Organization estimates 1.2 billion women will be age fifty or over, more than three times the number in

1990.[240] Menopause is the permanent cessation of menses and fertility. Technically, menopause begins twelve months after the last menstrual cycle. However, the symptoms and conditions can be a problem and may need treatment during the transitional peri-menopausal time. Post-menopause is also a term used to define the time experienced by women once they are in menopause. Essentially, the terms are interrelated.

> By the year 2030, the World Health Organization estimates 1.2 billion women will be age fifty or over, more than three times the number in 1990.

A common misconception related to menopause is that a woman will "go through" menopause. This is only partly true. It is true that a woman transitions into the menopausal state and once she reaches a certain age her menstrual cycles stop. However, once she has walked through the door into menopause, the condition and its various related symptoms are for the most part permanent. So, once you're there, you're there. The misconception comes from the idea that a woman will have a rough time emotionally while she is transitioning, which is true, and that she will have vasomotor symptoms (hot flashes/flushes and night sweats) that eventually go away after a few years. Once these vasomotor symptoms stop, women and their doctors will declare that you went "through menopause" and "it's all over now."

However, I cannot define menopause simply by the presence of vasomotor symptoms. I have treated hundreds of women who have never had a hot flash in their life. I have also treated many women well into their 80s who will still get hot flashes and night sweats. Therefore, we must expand the definition of menopause and redefine it to include the multitudes of symptoms women suffer from, and also understand that menopause is a continuum and permanent state of being. Please understand that I do not believe it means a woman must suffer needlessly if she is permanently in menopause, it simply means that it is a stage of life that needs to be respected and honored for what it permanently is. From this perspective, a woman can more effectively receive the treatment she needs to feel her best.

The Symptoms of Menopause

Hot flashes, hot flushes, cold flashes, heat sensations. Women often have varying body temperature sensations. These vasomotor symptoms are related to the hypothalamic control of blood vessels, which is greatly regulated by proper estrogen balance. When estrogen is low, the blood vessels dilate leading to a sudden inflow of blood, resulting in the flushes response. Women will experience this phenomenon differently and to varying degrees. In my experience, more than two-thirds of the women I treat experience this symptom.

Night Sweats. This type of symptom often accompanies hot flashes and can occur in premenopause, peri-menopause, menopause or post-menopause. Night sweats can also be a basic sign of stress, as well as disturbed sleep and insomnia. Extreme night sweats can even be a sign of cancer. This fact is not to startle anyone who may be experiencing these symptoms, but to make you aware that night sweats can in fact be related to other things. Be sure to check with your physician if you are experiencing night sweats.

Irregular and erratic periods. As stated before, the cycle can start to change during certain times of life, but also for many other reasons. During peri-menopause, the menstrual cycle starts to become erratic. The cycle may not be as timely as it always was. Perhaps the monthly cycle is longer or shorter. The length of the actual menstruation could also be increased or decreased. These types of changes hearken a movement towards menopause. Always check with your healthcare provider if you are having these issues.

Lowered Libido. This is one of the most common complaints that I hear. Libido is defined as the "psychological desire and drive" to want to engage in sexual activity. And, as both estrogen and testosterone begin to decline as peri-menopause and menopause approach, the sense of sexuality can begin to decline. Testosterone is particularly responsible for stimulating libido as well as stimulating the structures of the vulva in terms of vaginal secretion and muscular strengthening of the area. Estrogen helps in this respect also. It is important to mention that testosterone, or any sex hormone, is not the only thing related to poor libido. Other conditions such as hypothyroidism, adrenal dysfunction, depression and stress, psychological issues and even spiritual and moral conflicts, to name a few, can be responsible for altering libido negatively.

Vaginal dryness. As sex hormones diminish, the ability to properly lubricate the structures of the vulva also diminishes. Estrogen is a key hormone responsible for stimulating vaginal secretion. However, it is also testosterone that stimulates an increased blood supply to the vulva that helps to stimulate secretion helping with dryness. Many women experience improved vaginal secretion.

Here are some additional strategies to help with vaginal dryness:

- Increase water. Do not underestimate how helpful this could be. Vaginal secretions come from water, so if you are dehydrated, then it is obvious that producing lubrication would be difficult.
- Increase essential fatty acids. For any type of dryness in the body, such as skin, hair, eye and vaginal dryness, providing essential fatty acids from a source such as fish oil can be very helpful. Skin and its related mucous membranes need the proper essential fatty acids to be healthy. If you are not using a fish oil supplement, consider this today.
- Take your time. As women reach menopause, arousal can take longer. If penetrating sex is rushed, then the vaginal secretions may not have had a chance to respond. This can take up to an hour in some cases, but why rush something worth the wait?
- Use a personal lubricant. Always make sure any personal lubricant is water-based as oil-based can disrupt the vaginal flora (good bacteria) and it also breaks down latex condoms.
- Vagifem® is an estrogen pill that is inserted into the vagina twice weekly and can be effective for some women.
- Estriol creams are topical bioidentical hormone creams.

Mood swings and irritability. Both estrogen and testosterone are responsible for balancing the effects of many neurochemicals or "brain chemicals" including serotonin and dopamine. When these neurochemicals are limited or imbalanced, then emotional instability can result. Additionally, when testosterone declines and your energy lowers, it is harder to cope with stress, which results in irritability. During peri-menopause, the roller coaster effect of good production of estrogen one day and poor estrogen production another can also contribute to mood swings.

Depression and anxiety. Estrogen is highly correlated to depression and anxiety. Estrogen acts in a very similar way to Monoamine Oxidase Inhibitor (MAOI) drugs (such as hydralazine) and the more popular Selective Serotonin Reuptake Inhibitor (SSRI) drugs (Prozac®, Celexa®, Zoloft®, Lexapro®, Paxil®). Estrogen inhibits monoamine oxidases which are enzymes involved in the breakdown of 5-Hydroxytryptophan (5-HTP). 5-HTP is a natural amino acid that is a precursor to serotonin, the neurochemical responsible for mood stability and enhancement. Estrogen also increases serotonin synthesis and the amount of serotonin found in the nerves of the brain. Estrogens also increase the neurochemical norepinephrine that is also responsible for mood stability and alertness.[241] I have seen countless women have dramatic improvement in depression and anxiety when estrogen and testosterone balancing and replacement are employed.

Fatigue. This is one of the most common complaints that I hear on a daily basis. It can result from many different things such as a poor diet and meal schedule to hormonal imbalances. During menopause, stress on the body can be considerable and fatigue can result. Testosterone deficiency is one of the key hormone imbalances that can result in fatigue, and restoring this hormone can work wonders at increasing your energy.

Thinning hair or loss of hair. It is important to stress the basic fact that it is normal to lose up to about one hundred hairs a day that can be seen in your brush, sink or on your pillow. Sometimes patients perceive this hair loss and think there is a problem, when it is not necessarily a problem. If the hair loss starts to seem more excessive than this, then it should be investigated. During menopause, as hormone levels change, hair can start to thin. Estrogen is involved in the basic physiology of the hair cycle. Hair goes through three distinct growth stages:

- ❂ Anagen: The active stage of hair growth
- ❂ Catagen: The brief transition stage
- ❂ Telogen: The resting stage

Hair loss can actually be related to not just the hair coming out, but that the hair follicle has remained dormant in the telogen or resting stage. This is called "telogen effluvium" hair loss. Poor diet and high stress are key reasons why hair would stay in the telogen resting stage. After a shock to the system, up to 70 percent of scalp hairs are shed within two to three months after the shock. This shedding usually slowly decreases over six to eight months once the cause for the hair loss is no longer there. It is extremely important to determine the cause of the hair loss and treat it appropriately.

Common causes of sudden hair loss (telogen effluvium) are:
- ❂ High fevers and illness
- ❂ Childbirth
- ❂ Severe infections
- ❂ Severe chronic illness
- ❂ Severe psychological stress
- ❂ Major surgery or illnesses
- ❂ Hypo-(low) or Hyper-(high) thyroidism
- ❂ Crash diets with inadequate protein and low calories (such as the HCG diet)
- ❂ Certain medications such as retinoids (retin-A), beta blockers, calcium channel blockers, antidepressants, and NSAIDS (including ibuprofen)

Sleeping difficulties. This is one of the most common complaints of both pre- and post-menopausal women. As sex hormones start to decline, the ability of the body to properly regulate and produce melatonin and other important brain neurochemicals also declines. Melatonin and dopamine are important brain chemicals that help to provide restful and uninterrupted sleep. Another common reason for sleep disturbances are hot flashes and night sweats that interrupt the ability to get to sleep and stay asleep. Once sex hormone balance has been achieved, particularly with estrogen replacement, then sleep may normalize and become more productive.

It is important to note here that a key reason for sleep difficulties in many menopausal women is magnesium deficiency. With a magnesium deficiency sleep is characterized as restless, agitated, and wakeful. Estrogen improves the ability of the body to utilize magnesium.[242] As estrogen declines, magnesium absorption and utilization declines, and this contributes to the disrupted and restless sleep experienced in menopause.

Consider adding in magnesium supplementation if your sleep does not improve during menopause or during sex hormone replacement. The best food sources of magnesium are chocolate, nuts, seeds, and dark, leafy greens. The proper magnesium dose is 5 to 10 mg per kilogram of body weight or 2.5 to 4.5 mg per pound of body weight. Look for a form of magnesium that is optimally absorbed. The magnesium sulfate found in Epsom salts has a tendency to bring on loose stools and is rapidly cleared through the body. Magnesium chloride is a gentler form of magnesium and helps to effectively restore magnesium levels. [243, 244]

Be sure to understand that sleep disturbances can be very complex and be for multiple reasons beyond lack of sex hormones while in menopause. Explore carefully other possibilities such as establishing good sleep hygiene which is covered in some detail in the Metabolic Protocol in this book.

Memory and Focus Impairments. When hormones decline, the ability to concentrate declines. We have all had the experience of forgetting simple words, or the name of someone we know, or where we put our car keys. In menopause, these experiences become more prevalent. Estrogen has the function of balancing brain chemistry for sure, but memory and focus is regulated largely by testosterone, one of the key hormones that regulate mental cognition and information recall.

Of course stress plays a key role in our ability to concentrate and remember basic things. In this case, the stress hormone cortisol has the deleterious effect of disrupting memory. The common theme throughout this book will always point towards stress reduction as being a key towards optimizing all menopausal symptoms. Keep this in your... *memory*.

Weight Gain. Obesity is becoming an ever-increasing epidemic in our country. As women enter menopause, the struggle to maintain weight becomes even larger as fat begins to accumulate despite efforts of diet and exercise. Estrogen plays a positive role in maintaining body weight. During menopause women tend to gain body fat. The increase in adiposity is likely due to the decline in estrogen.[245] Animal model studies have shown that estrogens caused significant decreases in body weight and fat content without affecting food intake.[246]

Palpitations. As hormone levels start to fluctuate with both increases and decreases, your heart responds to this stress by increasing heart rate and the force of contractions. Specifically, estradiol (estrogen) has the effect of reducing ischemia, or restrictive tightening, of blood vessels.[247, 248] Although most palpitations are not life threatening, an EKG from your doctor should be done for people who have palpitations associated with syncope (fainting) or with a very rapid pulse approaching one hundred beats per minute. Conditions commonly associated with menopause can also lead to heart palpitations. These include anemia, hypoglycemia (low blood sugar), and hyperthyroidism (high thyroid function).

> Although most palpitations are not life threatening, an EKG from your doctor should be done for people who have palpitations associated with syncope (fainting) or with a very rapid pulse approaching one hundred beats per minute.

Leaking Urine or Incontinence. When the structures and musculature of the pelvis and vulva begin to weaken, particularly the muscles that surround the urethra, urine can leak through. When we place extra pressure in the area with a cough, hard laugh or a sneeze, then it is even easier for the urine to accidentally leak out. Both estrogen and testosterone help to improve this situation. Estrogen keeps the urethra moist. When significant dryness is present, it is harder for the urethra to close properly, which makes it easier for urine to leak out. Testosterone strengthens the muscles of the pelvis and around the vulva, which can further prevent urine from leaking.

Incontinence can be more serious, with a constant sensation of having to urinate and even to the point of having no sensation that you have to urinate at all. These are more complicated issues. Sex hormones may not have much to do with this type of incontinence and your healthcare provider should be alerted if your incontinence presents like this.

Bloating. During menopause, it is very common for women to experience overall gastrointestinal distress that leads to bloating and irritable bowel syndrome. It is uncertain if this is directly or indirectly related to the decline in sex hormones.[249] Either way, menopausal women experience this often and most of my patients express this to me. This common complaint can be related to gastrointestinal issues such as poor digestion and underlying food allergies. This should not be underestimated if you have constant bloating and difficulty with digestion. Be sure to consider seeking out the advice of a healthcare professional that can help with improving digestion and enhancing diet choices.

Allergies and Asthma. Currently there is some medical research that suggests a correlation with sex hormones such as estrogen and progesterone, and asthma and allergic responses.[250, 251] As hormone levels decline, allergic reactions can set in. Sex hormones can have the effect of helping with allergic responses and asthma, and I have witnessed this clinically many times. However, asthma and allergies are very complex and can be due to many other reasons.

Headaches. As estrogen lowers before the menstrual cycle, some women can have a "menstrual migraine" that can be relieved by low amounts of estrogen supplementation. For others, it can be during any hormonal shift within the menstrual cycle, such as at ovulation, when hormone levels are peaking. During peri-menopause, this could be the time of the largest swings in ovarian production of sex hormones and headaches could result. The fluctuations in estrogen levels associated with headaches produce changes in inflammatory producing substances called prostaglandins as well as changes in opiod receptors that are part of the pain process.[252] In menopause, both estrogen and particularly testosterone deficiency are related to headaches. Headaches are often a sign of fatigue, poor metabolism, sugar regulation, and lack of sleep. Once energy, insulin regulation, and normal sleeping patterns return, headaches can be helped in many people. However, headaches are complex in their origin and are not always helped by balancing and replacing sex hormones. Be sure to check with your doctor if you have chronic headaches.

Muscle and joint aches and pains. As hormone levels decline, the overall metabolic rate slows which can lead to body aches and pains. Specifically, testosterone can help heal the tissue around bone joints, improving perceived pain. Estrogen has also been shown to play a significant role in stimulating muscle repair and regeneration.[253] However, hormone deficiency also leads to other psychological disturbances such as depression that has been associated with muscle aches and joint pain.

Breast pain. For younger women, the most common reason for breast pain or mastalgia is "cyclical mastalgia" referring to the breast pain experienced around the menstrual cycle. During peri-menopause, the breasts will swell

> One hormonal abnormality frequently detected in mastalgia (breast pain) is increased prolactin levels that are due to increased TSH levels that occur in hypothyroidism.

and become painful in response to fluctuating estrogen and progesterone levels. Research on hormonal fluctuation reasons for breast pain is actually unclear, relating it to both excess and deficient estrogen or progesterone.[254] However, one hormonal abnormality frequently detected in mastalgia (breast pain) is increased prolactin levels that are due to increased TSH levels that occur in hypothyroidism.[255, 256, 257, 258] When women go into menopause, low thyroid function is very common. Hypothyroidism leads to increased levels of TSH that can stimulate the pituitary to increase another hormone called prolactin, which in turn stimulates breast tissue leading to pain.

One common reason for breast pain can be from fibrocystic breast changes, which is becoming more and more prevalent. The relationship of iodine deficiency, thyroid disease, and fibrocystic breast changes is starting to be revealed by research. I encourage any woman experiencing menopausal breast pain to consider if iodine could help. I have had women drastically improve their fibrocystic breast changes and related pain simply by adding iodine to their supplement regimen. I have also had women experience improvements in their mammogram demonstrating less fibrocystic breast changes, even after having it for years. If you are experiencing breast pain that is constant, very severe, and particularly one sided, then consult your healthcare provider right away, as this type of pain is more often associated with breast cancer.

Medications Associated With Breast Pain in Women

There are many medications associated with breast pain.[259] Of course, minimizing or eliminating these medications can be an excellent start at helping with breast pain. Explore these lists and then consult with your healthcare provider.

Hormonal medications: oral contraceptives, menopausal hormonal therapy, clomiphene (Clomid®, an infertility medication).

Antidepressant and antianxiety medications: Sertraline (Zoloft®) and other serotonin reuptake inhibitors (i.e. Prozac®, Wellbutrin®, Paxil®, Celexa®); Mirtazapine (Remeron®); Chlordiazepoxide (Librium®);

Amitriptyline (Elavil®); Doxepin (Silenor®); Haloperidol (Haldol®) and other antipsychotic agents.

Antihypertensive and cardiac medications: Spironolactone (Aldactone®); Methyldopa (Aldomet®); Minoxidil; Digoxin (Lanoxin®); Reserpine.

Antimicrobials: Ketoconazole; Metronidazol (Flagyl®).

Miscellaneous drugs: Cimetidine, Cyclosporine, Penicillamine.

Strategies to help with breast pain

Consider hormone replacement therapy. I have seen menopausal women have relief from breast pain when hormone replacement therapy was employed. I have also seen the opposite. It is not uncommon to see a postmenopausal woman have breast pain within a few weeks after natural estrogen replacement therapy. This is a transient symptom that tends to resolve itself quickly. Be sure to let your healthcare provider know about any changes.

Get fitted for a proper brassiere. An estimated 70 percent of women wear an improperly fitted brassiere,[260] and this should not be underestimated in trying to help with breast pain. Most major department stores have specialists on staff who do this, but the skill level of the salesperson is unpredictable. Certain lingerie boutique stores specialize in properly fitting a woman in an appropriate brassiere. Also, be sure to wear a properly supportive sports bra when exercising.

Reduce excessive caffeine intake. Research in this area is not consistent and overall it appears that restricting caffeine in women with breast pain does not lead to improvement. However, in women who consume excessive amounts of caffeine, such as several cups of coffee daily, there could be some improvement if this amount is reduced.

Use Evening Primrose Oil (EPO). This oil has been used extensively over the years for the effective treatment of breast pain for women.[261] It is an essential fatty acid oil known as gamma linolenic acid which has been found to be an effective anti-inflammatory in the body and specifically for breast tissue. Women can get immediate relief within days, but for many it may take months. Keep the EPO dose at around 3,000 mg per day to be effective, which is 240 mg of gamma linolenic acid.

The Health Benefits of Estrogen

Brain effects and neurochemicals.[262] Estrogen affects a multitude of brain chemicals such as endorphins, helping with mood stability and memory. Particularly, estrogen has multiple effects on the mood stabilizing chemical serotonin and even blood levels of the amino acid tryptophan where serotonin is synthesized. Estrogen also helps to increase "brain derived neurotrophic factor," a protein that helps to preserve and protect brain cells and improve brain cell circuitry. Estrogen has primary target receptors in the brain and therefore estrogen will have a positive effect on brain tissue at any age.[263]

> Estrogen also helps to increase "brain derived neurotrophic factor," a protein that helps to preserve and protect brain cells and improve brain cell circuitry.

Cardiovascular benefits. In general, women have a lower risk for cardiovascular disease as compared to men. However, following menopause, women show an increased risk of heart disease to a level equal that of men. Research continues to support the idea that estrogen replacement is cardioprotective if initiated around menopause. It appears that estrogen reduces the progression of atherosclerotic plaque that leads to narrowed_arteries and increased risk of heart attack and stroke.[264, 265] Estrogen increases high density lipoprotein (HDL, the good cholesterol), decreases low density lipoprotein (LDL, the bad cholesterol),[266, 267] and lowers a substance called fibrinogen, which contributes to improving the lowering of plaque in the arteries. Estrogen helps blood vessels to heal when damaged,[268] and increases nitric oxide (NO) that dilates blood vessels and lowers blood pressure.[269]

Bone health. Bone loss and increased fracture risk is a major concern among post-menopausal women. For the year 2000, there were an estimated nine million new osteoporotic fractures. One in three women over fifty will experience osteoporotic fractures, as will one in five men. Between 1990 and 2000, there was nearly a 25 percent increase in hip fractures worldwide. The peak number of hip fractures occurred at seventy-five to seventy-nine years of age for both men and women, and for all other fractures, the peak number occurred at fifty to fifty-nine years.[270] Estrogen has a positive affect on bone health, helping to decrease the degradation of bone over time. Low estrogen represents the main cause of bone loss and osteoporosis.[271] Most of this bone loss occurs within the first five to ten years following menopause, making early intervention critical.

Estrogen acts on bone in two ways: 1) directly on the bone cells called osteoclasts (cells that naturally break bone down, liberating needed minerals), and osteoblasts (cells that build bone and store minerals), and 2) indirectly through promoting calcium metabolism in the intestine, kidneys, and parathyroid glands. In estrogen deficiency, the osteoclasts are uncontrolled and break down too much bone and the osteoblast builders actually get destroyed. Also, calcium has difficulty in being digested and absorbed when estrogen is low.

The bone loss issue is further complicated by another important function of estrogen. Estrogen inhibits and controls a hormone called parathyroid hormone (PTH), that is secreted by the parathyroid glands located within the thyroid gland. PTH normally takes some calcium and other bone minerals out of the bones to be used by the body. However, when PTH is in excess because of estrogen deficiency, it extracts too much calcium and minerals, and the bones become brittle leading to osteopenia (partial bone loss) and osteoporosis (severe bone loss).

Bone Health and Calcium

Magnesium is an important mineral for bone health that becomes deficient during menopause because estrogen increases bone magnesium uptake.[272, 273] Magnesium supplementation in postmenopausal women prone to osteoporosis has shown improvements in bone density.[274] In particular, a large Swedish study found that calcium alone did not protect against hip fracture as well as did adding magnesium, iron, and vitamin C.[275] Also, the mineral boron and vitamin K are essential in bone formation as well as magnesium.[276, 277]

> Magnesium supplementation in postmenopausal women prone to osteoporosis has shown improvements in bone density. In particular, a large Swedish study found that calcium alone did not protect against hip fracture as well as did adding magnesium, iron, and vitamin C.

Calcium is of course needed for bone health, but the over-focus on this mineral and the lack of focus on magnesium presents some risks:

- Calcium in excess is "pro-thrombotic" or promotes clotting.
- Magnesium has the natural tendency towards being "anti-thrombotic" or unclotting the blood.
- Magnesium also focuses on building the flexible bone "matrix" which is the protein and collagen containing portion of bone.
- Calcium promotes the hardening of bones. Yet too much makes the bones thicker, but more brittle and prone to fracture.
- Remember: alcohol depletes magnesium levels.

Be sure to explore the section on vitamin D and the sun in this book. As a reminder, vitamin D is essential for bone health and a multitude of other health benefits. Be sure to balance your vitamin D supplementation with magnesium, zinc, boron, vitamin K2, and a small amount of vitamin A.[278]

The Health Benefits of Testosterone for Women

Testosterone is not just for men! More women are beginning to understand this, but testosterone still remains an elusive topic in female hormone replacement therapy. Testosterone provides many benefits for women including improvements in bone density, brain health, mood stabilization, energy, sexual enhancement, and libido.

Some Technical Information About Testosterone

- When you add up all the sex hormones in a woman's body, she actually secretes greater amounts of androgens (that include testosterone) than of estrogen![279] And just like men, women produce all of the other androgens that are related to testosterone.
- The major circulating androgens include DHEA-S, DHEA, androstenedione, testosterone, and dihydrotestosterone or DHT, in descending order of blood concentration, though only testosterone and DHT significantly bind to the androgen receptor on the cell to produce all of the wonderful benefits.
- The daily production rate of testosterone in women is about 0.1–0.4 mg.[280] Most of the testosterone is being produced primarily through the conversion of these other androgens, such as DHEA, into testosterone.
- Androstenedione contributes 50 percent of the total testosterone production through conversion with the remainder of testosterone production concentrated in the ovary (25 percent) and adrenal (25 percent).[281]

Testosterone and Bone Health

Testosterone is very important for bone health in women and studies support this.[282, 283, 284] The presupposition is that estrogen is all that is needed for bone health for postmenopausal women, but estrogen is only half the battle. Testosterone is stimulating the important osteoblast cells within bone that actually build up bone tissue and make it stronger and denser.

Testosterone and Sexual Desire

Lowered libido is the most common complaint that women express during peri-menopause and postmenopause. Libido is a complicated issue and there are some common issues that are associated that include:

- ❧ Pain with sexual activity
- ❧ Emotional distress
- ❧ Life stress
- ❧ Relationship conflicts
- ❧ Lowered testosterone

The low testosterone was placed at the bottom of the list to emphasize the importance of the other factors. I have seen testosterone therapy be able to completely change the sexual lives of countless women and men to the point of them saying to me, "It saved our marriage." And it is true that large randomized controlled trial studies using testosterone replacement therapy show benefits on sexual desire, arousal, orgasm, pleasure, and satisfaction.[285] But I have also seen the other factors greatly influence libido despite adequate testosterone levels. Do not underestimate the other factors and consider lowering stress and enhancing coping mechanisms and explore relationship counseling when appropriate.

Testosterone and Mental Enhancement

There have been studies demonstrating improvement in overall well-being[286] and enhanced memory in testosterone replacement therapy.[287] Keep in mind that in these studies they were able to demonstrate improvement even when using synthetic forms of testosterone and estrogen. Utilizing bioidentical testosterone, particularly in a subcutaneous pellet form, can yield continuous improvements for women in sexual libido, memory and focus, and overall sense of well-being. Testosterone also works on recall of information and the ability to retain it.[288]

A Word on Testosterone
Replacement Therapy for Women

The use of testosterone therapy in women is controversial in mainstream medicine. This is the main reason most conventional doctors simply do not prescribe it, wanting to avoid the controversies. However, in 2007 in the *Journal of Sexual Medicine*, a review commentary was published supporting the clinical use of testosterone for women.[289]

It has been suggested in the literature that to be effective, testosterone levels for women must be increased above the current normal ranges.[290] Clinically, this has been my experience and the ranges our practice employs is higher than what is typically used. The testosterone ranges seen, depending on the lab, will be from as low as 2 ng/dL up to 82 ng/dL. For most women, symptomatic and clinical relief will not occur until serum blood levels of approximately 60 ng/dL to 180 ng/dL are achieved.

Finally, if women are using estrogen replacement therapy, then levels of Sex Hormone Binding Globulin (SHBG) are increased. SHBG is a protein that binds testosterone making it unavailable and inactive. Therefore, it is reasonable to utilize testosterone replacement while estrogen is being used.

The Health Benefits of Progesterone

Progesterone is a hormone produced primarily by the ovaries and adrenal glands. It affects the function of the reproductive system, the nervous system, the cardiovascular system, and the skeletal system.

The main reason progesterone is used in hormone replacement therapy is to protect the uterine lining from developing endometrial hyperplasia, or thickening. A thickened lining increases a woman's risk for developing endometrial (uterine lining) cancer.[291] Estrogen thickens the lining of the uterus while progesterone thins it and keeps it intact.

For uterine lining protection, I recommend oral micronized progesterone which can be obtained by prescription under the trade name Prometrium® or compounded more cost effectively at a compounding pharmacy. Micronized progesterone is natural progesterone, whose average particle size has been reduced or "micronized," leading to decreased destruction in the gastrointestinal tract, a longer half-life, and enhanced absorption and bioavailability.

Problems with Progesterone

The clinical use of progesterone, mostly with topical creams, was popularized by Dr. John Lee and he has written about it extensively. My personal experience has been that most menopausal women do not benefit greatly from progesterone therapy, beyond the normal application of giving it to protect the uterine lining. The symptoms of menopause still often persist. This is largely because the body still wants and needs the more potent and effective estradiol. Once estradiol is given, then the menopausal symptoms will be eliminated. Some of the direct problems with progesterone include:

- Many women are sensitive to progesterone and will suffer from the typical side effects of extreme fatigue and drowsiness, nausea and irritability. In my practice, when giving progesterone to protect the uterine lining, I make sure to have them take it before bed. It can in fact help with sleep. However, women have mistakenly taken it in the morning, and for some, the result can be a drowsiness not unlike being drunk. In fact, progesterone is similar in action to benzodiazapine drugs.[292]

- Progesterone is a very warming hormone, and for some this could be a good thing, for others it could not. It could potentially lead to worsening hot flashes and night sweats and the overall sensation of feeling warm.

- Progesterone is related to water retention. Progesterone is the likely culprit for women who get very bloated right before their menstrual cycle. It is progesterone that is highest at that time and estrogen is low. The bloating is often relieved as soon as the period comes as progesterone is now lowered and estrogen is rising. Remember, estrogen is a diuretic!

❋ Excessive progesterone may increase urinary incontinence and counteract the beneficial effects of estrogen in maintaining urinary control.[293, 294]

❋ Excessive amounts may decrease libido due to an anti-estrogen and anti-testosterone effect.[295]

❋ Excessive levels are related to depression.[296]

❋ Progesterone is related to insulin resistance[297] that leads to poor blood sugar control, diabetes, and weight gain. (Estrogen does the complete opposite, helping you to lose fat!)

❋ Both synthetic and natural progesterone has been associated with the increased risk of diabetes.[298, 299, 300]

❋ The normal amount of progesterone produced by women in the second half of their menstrual cycle (the luteal phase) has been associated with inducing insulin resistance in certain women.[301]

Progesterone Benefits Worth Considering

In general, I have not seen much benefit from women taking progesterone, particularly progesterone creams. However, some of my patients absolutely swear by its affects. Progesterone will have its greatest benefits in peri-menopausal women, who have not really experienced low estrogen and its many symptoms.

If progesterone is to be used, I recommend oral micronized progesterone. It may be worth considering the following benefits of progesterone in certain clinical situations:

❋ Insomnia. Because of the powerful sedative affects of progesterone, some women can benefit from adding in progesterone to aid in sleep.

❋ Anxiety. Just as with insomnia, the sedating affects of progesterone can be helpful for some women.

❋ Osteopenia/Osteoporosis. This is a consideration for a woman who has already been diagnosed with bone loss. Be sure to keep in mind that both estrogen, and particularly testosterone, stimulate bone growth very effectively, and should be the mainstay of any hormone replacement regimen if bone loss has occurred. However, progesterone also has stimulating effects on bone building cells called osteoblasts,[302, 303] as well as an increased secretion of IGF-1 and other growth factors by the bone cells[304, 305] all resulting in increased bone building activity.

A word of caution: For any woman who has a uterus, adding in progesterone to a hormone replacement regimen can lead to breakthrough uterine bleeding and spotting. A woman's cycle is a potentially delicate balance, and adding in progesterone can lead to bleeding difficulties in some women. For those women who have had a hysterectomy or a uterine ablation procedure, bleeding would obviously not at all be a concern, and it would be easier to employ progesterone.

Estrogen and Testosterone for Fat Loss

This book focuses around the concept of metabolism and its relationship to health. Obesity is an epidemic problem in our country and as we age and hormone levels decline, weight management becomes more challenging, contributing to this epidemic. Sex hormones play an integral role in enhancing fat loss and increasing lean muscle. There is hope…

Testosterone for Fat Loss

In a previous chapter, lipoprotein lipase (LPL) and its role in weight management was covered. As a review, LPL is an enzyme that breaks down triglycerides into their fatty acid components for transport and use inside cells. An increase in LPL activity means an increase in the flow of fatty acids into the cell. An increase in LPL activity in muscle cells means they will use more fat and less sugar for energy, which enhances muscle strength and size. However, an increase in LPL activity in fat cells leads to an increase in stored fat.

Testosterone blocks lipoprotein lipase particularly in subcutaneous fat, or fat under the skin on the body.[306, 307] This helps prevent fatty acids from being stored into fat cells in this area, keeping you lean.

Estrogen for Fat Loss

One of the largest misconceptions is that estrogen makes a woman gain weight. If fact, when properly balanced, estrogen does the complete opposite. Specifically, estrogen maintains and evenly distributes the subcutaneous fat content of the body. This thin layer of skin fat maintains a feminine and youthful appearance to skin and the body, characteristic of pre-menopausal women. Pre-menopausal estrogen levels also keep fat from accumulating around the stomach. As women go through menopause and estrogen levels decline, a fat content shift occurs from under the skin around the body to the abdomen, leading to sagging skin and abdominal obesity.[308]

Just like testosterone, estrogen reduces lipoprotein lipase[309, 310] lowering the uptake of fatty acids in fat cells and making them decrease in size. Estrogen also reduces appetite by regulating melanin-concentrating hormone (MCH),[311] which is a brain protein associated with controlling the hunger mechanism.

> One of the largest misconceptions is that estrogen makes a woman gain weight. If fact, when properly balanced, estrogen does the complete opposite.

Making Sense of Menopause: A New Beginning

Menopause is not a disease. Menopause is a stage of life. Menopause is no more a disease process than puberty. We view puberty as a time of blossoming and beginning, and the related difficulties of the time period are accepted because we perceive that we are coming of age and transitioning into a time where the best is yet to come. Why is it that menopause is not viewed in the same way? This is a time

> Menopause is not a disease. Menopause is a stage of life. Menopause is no more a disease process than puberty.

when most women have the opportunity to truly begin to know who they are and what they really want, and menopause harkens this transition. As most journeys are wrought with peril, the journey of menopause is no different. But there are tools that you can carry with you along the way to aid and assist, making the journey possible, a little more manageable, and even enlightening. This book intends to provide you with some of those tools.

Some of the psychological issues that women experience during this time largely surround the idea of fertility and the ability to conceive. As most women have revealed to me, conception is a centralized theme in a woman's life. I have spoken to women who have absolutely never wanted to conceive and had no children of their own, but upon entering the permanency of menopause, mourned the passing of this rite of womanhood. But, the best is yet to come, if you know how to find it. The idea of conception is not just limited to conceiving a child. It is also about conceiving ideas, embracing new projects, and finding deeper truths about yourself and others. Women possess a unique perspective and ability in this regard.

Nurturing the Nurturer

Women inherently are caretakers. My own mother was and is spectacular in this regard. She sacrificed much for me along my own journey, as so many mothers and women do for their children and loved ones. I have spoken with so many women who are absolutely devoted to their families, putting all aside for them. Sometimes this devotion is to an extreme, where a woman will even neglect herself during the process of taking care of others, often to the detriment of her health. And that is the irony. If the caretaker does not take care of herself, she will ultimately not be the best caretaker for those who need her. Be good to yourself. Now is the time.

As a woman enters into this new stage in her life, she may find that her role as caregiver is not the same. Children grow up and leave the home to create new lives for themselves.

This creates a natural space for a woman to explore herself and the things she has always wanted to do, to fill that space with lifelong dreams. Now is a time to be alive in a different way. Your creative force is now even more powerful, if you allow it to flourish.

- Travel the world, or at least in your own back yard with a good book.
- Be philanthropic on your own terms, giving when and how you choose.
- Go back to school and learn for the sake of learning.
- Create your own business, or offer your gifts to the workforce.
- Focus on your own spiritual path, join and contribute to a church or faith group.

Most of all, menopause can be a time of releasing old fears and wounds to the spirit. It can be a time of resolve, when a woman can experience more freedom and wisdom than ever before in her life. I encourage all women patients to celebrate where they are in life and to *ask for help* if they feel they need it, whether it be medical help or more support from partners, children, friends, and their community.

Chiron Returns: Healing the Wounded

"You shall count seven weeks of years, seven times seven years, so that the time of the seven weeks of years shall give you forty-nine years. On the Day of Atonement you shall sound the trumpet throughout all your land... And you shall consecrate the fiftieth year, and proclaim liberty throughout the land to all its inhabitants... That fiftieth year shall be a jubilee for you... It shall be holy to you." Leviticus 25:8-11

In Greek mythology, Chiron the centaur, a half man and half horse, was revered as a teacher, philosopher, astrologer, and great healer. His own tragedy befell him when he was wounded in the leg, but being immortal, was destined to continue to have the wound and seek out his own healing. Chiron later arranged to give up his immortality and his suffering by exchanging it for Prometheus to be set free. Prometheus had stolen fire from the gods and given it as a gift to humanity, leading to an eternal punishment of having his liver pecked out daily by a griffon. When Prometheus was released, Chiron died and was freed from his suffering. The gift of fire is symbolic of the gift of consciousness and deeper understandings. Chiron helped to see this concept fully realized with his own sacrifice that led to his own personal understanding about his healing journey.

Astrologically, Chiron is a comet that orbits in close proximity to Saturn and Uranus. It makes a full cycle every forty-nine, fifty, or fifty-one years, back to the original place it started in relationship to a person's birth. The return of Chiron is the time when most women enter into menopause. The average menopausal age is in fact fifty-one. And this is the average age that both women and men initially come to see me, seeking help and understanding about the new challenges they face. This is a time when a lot of changes are occurring and this is the time that people start to instinctually seek to "heal the wounded." This is a special and important transition into a time where real understandings can be realized. And as the passage from Leviticus explains, *"It shall be a jubilee for you."* It also explains that at this pivotal time, it is a Day of Atonement, implying forgiveness, healing, and reckoning for yourself and others.

At this time of life, we are given an opportunity for growth—to delve into ourselves and understand a deeper meaning about the pain and suffering that we are experiencing. This is a time to address unresolved issues and pain completely and for the last time. It is only when we address and face these wounds and issues can we make room for our truest purpose.

It is this concept of the "wound" that we should actually embrace in order to learn from it. Or, we can continue to avoid it, mask it, and deny it, which is often the case. This is part of the quick fix, take-a-pill mentality that occurs in our society which leads to missing the opportunity for growth. This time in your life, with

> This time in your life, with all of its difficulties, is a gift. And your very essence and being is poised to make changes and realizations more than at any other time in your life.

all of its difficulties, is a gift. And your very essence and being is poised to make changes and realizations more than at any other time in your life. The more we see menopause (and male andropause) as an opportunity for growth, the more we will embrace and learn from it. If we seek to just fix it without any other regard for it, then the opportunity is missed, and our "wound" will never really heal. Full healing is always possible, but not from avoiding what the condition really is and what it likely represents. We must embrace it to understand its true nature, leading toward better solutions such as the things offered in this book, and much more.

Andropause: The Male Menopause

Amid the crowded sports bars, men are gathering and whispering about things never before discussed. At gyms and social clubs, in locker rooms and boardrooms, men are starting to discuss how things… maybe, just maybe, are changing for them. Yes, men have hormones too. And men are figuring out that these hormones have a powerful impact on how they feel and perform… and they want to keep them. But, where do you go? Who do you talk to? Will your doctor understand?

Fortunately, the practice of men's health has begun to emerge as a prominent medical and social phenomena where previously little was known, or at least appreciated, about the specific health concerns of men. This historically occurred for a few reasons. One, gender specific concerns were largely related to women and the multiple concerns that they can potentially have from a gynecological perspective. Two, men tend to avoid going to the doctor and presenting their complaints and concerns due to perceived social pressures and concepts of the male role as one of invincibility and non-complaining. This of course is very often to the detriment of the health of men, often waiting to go to a healthcare professional only when their health is seriously impaired far beyond the preventative stage. Finally, the practice of urology is only recently starting to consider the significant impact of sex hormone imbalances in men, particularly as they age. Additional specialties such as anti-aging organizations are taking a closer look at the specific health needs of men, focusing on the hormonal impact of conditions such as cardiovascular disease, osteoporosis, insulin resistance and diabetes, mental health and sexual function.

What is Andropause?

Andropause is defined as the gradual decline of androgens, mainly testosterone, in the aging male leading to various related health concerns, conditions and symptoms such as fatigue, memory loss and difficulty concentrating, weight gain and abdominal obesity, joint pain and loss of muscle mass, emotional instabilities including irritability and depression. Other terms such as "ADAM" and "PADAM" are more technical terms accepted and used by many researchers. A.D.A.M. stands for Androgen (Testosterone) Deficiency/Decline in the Aging Male. P.A.D.A.M. stands for Partial Androgen (Testosterone) Deficiency/Decline in the Aging Male.

> Andropause is defined as the gradual decline of androgens, mainly testosterone, in the aging male leading to various related health concerns, conditions and symptoms such as fatigue, memory loss and difficulty concentrating, weight gain and abdominal obesity, joint pain and loss of muscle mass, emotional instabilities including irritability and depression.

How Do I Know if I am in the Midst of Andropause?

The first place to start is determining some of the basic symptoms of andropause. Then you should look into the sections that discuss even more symptoms and conditions and see how you may relate. From there, you should seek medical advice from a healthcare provider that specializes in andropause and hormone replacement and have your "total" and "free" testosterone levels checked with a simple blood test.

The following is a basic screening questionnaire to give you an idea of the symptoms and it provides an opportunity to score yourself to see if you should pursue further medical evaluation.

ADAM Screening Questionnaire

(You can find a complete andropause questionnaire in the Appendix)

1. Do you have a decrease in libido (sex drive)?
2. Do you have a lack of energy?
3. Do you have a decrease in strength and/or endurance?
4. Have you lost weight?
5. Have you noticed a decreased enjoyment of life?
6. Are you sad and/or grumpy?
7. Are your erections less strong?
8. Have you noted a recent deterioration in your ability to play sports?
9. Do you fall asleep after dinner?
10. Has there been a recent deterioration in your work performance?

Scoring and Interpretation

You may be in andropause if: You answered "yes" to question one or question seven, or you answered "yes" to any three questions.

Another consideration as to the entrance into andropause is age. After the age of thirty-nine, total testosterone decreases by about 0.4 percent per year. Sex Hormone Binding Globulin (SHBG) increases by 1.2 percent per year leading to free testosterone levels also declining by 1.2 percent per year.[312] The magic number that I tend to see in practice where both the symptoms and the actual testosterone number seem to be an issue is right around fifty years old. Testosterone can be low at any age, but many men even in their forties can still have adequate testosterone even though they have many testosterone deficiency related symptoms. In this situation, other aspects of the metabolism need to be explored.

The Symptoms of Andropause and
Low Testosterone: You're Not Alone

All patients can feel alone when experiencing new symptoms and conditions. However, men can feel particularly isolated when they are moving through andropause. Men all too often do not know how to share personal feelings and troubles, particularly with other men. And men also have the problem of limiting their resources of confidants. The issues, conditions, and symptoms listed here are experienced by millions of men every day. You are not alone and there is hope.

Depression and Irritability. As testosterone levels decline as men age and enter andropause, the ability to cope with things mentally and emotionally declines. Testosterone has the function of balancing and optimizing various brain chemicals, including serotonin.

Poor concentration and memory. Testosterone helps to improve your ability to recall information and focus on tasks.

Sweating and hot flashes. We typically think this is something only women will go through during menopause, but men can experience this also. For women, it tends to be more focused around estrogen deficiency, although testosterone deficiency can be the reason in some cases for women. In men, excessive sweating and hot flashes results from low testosterone.

Decreased libido, erectile dysfunction, testicular shrinkage, and delayed ejaculation with decreased volume. Testosterone stimulates the mental drive to want to have sex. It increases blood supply to the penis, assisting in obtaining and maintaining erections. When testosterone deficiency is very low and chronic, the testicles shrink and the volume of the ejaculate diminishes with lessened force.

Loss of facial and body hair. When testosterone levels are very chronically low, then hair will start to thin on the face, armpits, pubic area, and legs. A typical sign is hair loss on the lower legs.

Fatigue. Testosterone stimulates the metabolism and helps to improve energy.

Insomnia. Testosterone is a metabolic fuel for your body's furnace. As explained before, it helps to enhance your energy. And, paradoxically, we need energy to sleep and maintain sleep. Testosterone also helps directly with calming the nervous system and helping to balance brain chemistry to aid in sleep.

Body fat gain, particularly abdominal weight gain, and decreased muscle mass. When testosterone declines, muscle mass is lost and fat is gained.

Aches and pains. Lack of testosterone can lead to increased body aches and joint pain.

Anemia. As stated before, testosterone stimulates tissues to grow. Blood is a tissue, composed of cells that need proper nourishment and stimulation to remain vital and fulfill the job of circulating and carrying oxygen. When testosterone lowers, red blood cells can shrink, leading to anemia.

Osteoporosis. Testosterone is a key anabolic hormone which means it is responsible for the growth of body tissues, including bone. As men age, the risk for osteoporosis increases. Testosterone enhancement and therapy can improve osteoporosis outcomes, and I have seen this many times in clinical practice.

Diabetes. There is a direct correlation with diabetes and low testosterone in men. I cannot think of one time seeing a diabetic patient who had optimal levels of testosterone.

The Health Benefits of Testosterone

Here are some of the most common health benefits of testosterone in more detail.

On the issue of cardiovascular disease, men have over twice the risk of dying from coronary (blood vessel) disease than women.[313] When testosterone is low, the risk factors associated with cardiovascular disease are increased, such as elevated cholesterol, insulin resistance that leads to abdominal weight gain, obesity, and increased blood clotting.[314] When testosterone levels are restored and consistently maintained, these associated risk factors are reversed. Additionally, testosterone is an effective coronary blood vessel vasodilator, having the ability to relax and open blood vessels and therefore decrease chest pain and angina.[315, 316]

It is often assumed by doctors unaware of current research, that testosterone causes an increase in cardiovascular disease. This stems from bodybuilders using very high "supraphysiologic" doses of testosterone who experience a higher risk for cardiovascular disease.[317] This does not occur with normal dosing of testosterone or optimizing your own body's ability to produce testosterone.

> It is often assumed by doctors unaware of current research, that testosterone causes an increase in cardiovascular disease. This stems from bodybuilders using very high "supraphysiologic" doses of testosterone who experience a higher risk for cardiovascular disease. This does not occur with normal dosing of testosterone or optimizing your own body's ability to produce testosterone.

Diabetes and Insulin Resistance

There is a clear association with diabetes and low testosterone in men. After consulting with hundreds of men with diabetes, I have never seen testosterone levels in the optimal range. In fact, the testosterone levels for these men are very low. Diabetes and insulin resistance are an epidemic in this country. The National Health and Nutrition Examination Surveys (NHANES) predicts that by 2021, approximately thirty-three million people will have diabetes in the United States or about 13.5 percent of the population.[318] Testosterone optimization is one important piece of the puzzle to medically helping this crisis.

When the hormone insulin can no longer effectively and efficiently recognize the body cells, we call this "insulin resistance." This leads to excessive levels of glucose (sugar) being left in the blood. Testosterone has the ability to help insulin perform its job of bringing glucose (sugar) from the blood and shuttling it into the cell. Testosterone replacement has been shown to improve outcomes for diabetic and insulin resistant patients including lowered inflammation, improved insulin function, lowered cholesterol, and decreased abdominal fat.[319, 320]

Low testosterone levels can even predict the development of Non Insulin Dependent Diabetes Mellitus (NIDDM) or type II diabetes. A large nutritional survey study called the National Health and Nutrition Examination Survey (NHANES III survey), found that men with the lowest free testosterone levels were four times as likely to have diabetes as those with the highest free testosterone levels.[321]

Osteoporosis in Men

The problem of osteoporosis is often overlooked with men, as most of the concentration of diagnosis and concern has been with women. But in fact, 10-20 percent of people with osteoporosis over the age of fifty in the U.S. are men.[322] Low testosterone levels in men are associated with decreased Bone Mineral Density (BMD) and osteoporosis. Testosterone replacement therapy has been shown to increase bone density.[323]

> **10-20 percent of people with osteoporosis over the age of fifty in the U.S. are men.**

Mortality

The facts are in. Low testosterone is directly associated with a shorter life in men.[324, 325, 326] In fact, the EPIC-Norfolk study[327] found that for every 172 ng/dL (6 nmol/L) reduction in serum testosterone, all-cause mortality and cardiovascular disease were increased. So, as testosterone levels decrease, risk for death and disease increases. The good news is: testosterone therapy can improve this situation.

Erectile Function

Erectile dysfunction or ED, affects millions of men and has a large impact on quality of life. Lowered testosterone leads to various sexual symptoms such as lowered libido, complete or partial erectile dysfunction, difficulty achieving orgasm, and diminished sexual sensation.

There is a wealth of studies using animal models showing that testosterone directly affects erectile function. Clinically, the correlation is also established showing that one-third of men with ED have low testosterone levels.[328] And as men age, they require higher levels of circulating testosterone for libido and erectile function compared to younger men.[329] However, it is not just a direct association that exists with testosterone deficiency and ED. Other key factors in ED such as hardening of the arteries (atherosclerotic disease), elevated blood pressure, diabetes, and the pre-diabetic condition called the metabolic syndrome, all correlate strongly with low testosterone.[330] It is well established that erectile dysfunction is very common in diabetic men, with prevalence reports of between 30 and 90 percent.[331]

When testosterone levels are improved, then ED is affected directly by the testosterone molecule, but also indirectly by helping to treat and lower the risk for other ED related diseases.

Brain Function, Mood Regulation, and Quality of Life

As we age, one of the most common and frustrating problems encountered is memory problems. Forgetting simple words or why you walked in a room can become commonplace. When testosterone levels decline, visual and verbal memory decline,[332] contributing to these problems. When testosterone levels are optimized evidence shows that cognitive performance such as spatial abilities and mathematical reasoning are also improved.[333] And men with a higher amount of testosterone have a lowered risk for Alzheimer's disease.[334]

The benefits do not stop with cognitive function, but also help with mood. Testosterone has been found to improve overall well/good feelings, friendliness, and lowered anger, nervousness, and irritability.[335] Interestingly, when men are irritable, it is assumed that they have too much testosterone, when in fact it is typically because they do not have enough.

> Interestingly, when men are irritable, it is assumed that they have too much testosterone, when in fact it is typically because they do not have enough.

Metabolism, Muscular Strength, and Muscle Mass

Testosterone is one of the best metabolism boosting substances, unlocking the restraints on energy production in a multitude of body areas and tissues. Testosterone legendarily improves strength and muscle mass, and most people are aware of this. Particularly, it will improve body composition by increasing muscle mass and lowering fat mass.[336]

Biochemical Laboratory Analysis

If it is suspected that you have low testosterone levels, then your doctor should run a simple blood test. This blood test should include:

Total Testosterone. This is the total amount of testosterone present in the blood at any one time. Typically in the U.S., the value will be in ng/dL. Sometimes, even in the U.S., but particularly in Canada and Europe, the value will be in nmol/L.

❧ Optimal Range: 700 – 1100 ng/dL or 24.29 – 38.17 nmol/L

Free Testosterone. Testosterone in your blood travels either bound to a carrier protein called Sex Hormone Binding Globulin (SHBG) or it can travel in the blood unbound, or free. Unbound free testosterone is actually the active form of testosterone that has the direct potential to get into the cells of the body to do work. This is a smaller relative portion, but it is the significant portion. Your total testosterone levels can be optimal, but the free testosterone could be very low.

❷ Optimal Range: > 25 pg/mL

Here are three reasons why it is important to lower SHBG to increase free testosterone:

❷ Obesity, particularly a high hip to waist ratio, produces more estrogen and more SHBG in men.

❷ High protein and adequate fat intake keep SHBG down and increase total and free testosterone.[337]

❷ Keep alcohol intake to a minimum to prevent burdening the liver, which will lead to increased liver production of SHBG.

The Optimal Range of Testosterone

When interpreting blood levels of testosterone, it is important to utilize an average range that attempts to reflect an optimal physiological situation. You and your doctor should strive for the high end of the range in most cases. Typically, the higher end of the range of testosterone reflects a more youthful count of testosterone and would therefore, if achieved, have more potential at making you feel your best. For example, total testosterone has a range anywhere from 200 ng/dL to 1100 ng/dL. These ranges are considered "population" ranges that include all men of all ages, including the very elderly. Some doctors will observe a 201 ng/dL testosterone level and note that, "It's on the low end of the range, but it is still *normal*." Many other doctors, including myself, would observe that number to be woefully low. And if the patient had many symptoms and clinical indicators of low testosterone,

> Typically, the higher end of the range of testosterone reflects a more youthful count of testosterone and would therefore, if achieved, have more potential at making you feel your best.

then every attempt would be made to optimize the testosterone levels into more youthful levels.

Estrogen in Men

For men, it is important to keep estrogen relatively low, particularly to help protect the prostate gland from developing cancer. Most of the research focus has been on testosterone and its possible relationship to increasing the activity of prostate cancer once present in the body. More recently, research attention has been brought to the relationship between prostate cancer development and estrogen.[338]

Excessive estrogen levels are also associated with gynecomastia, or enlargement of breast tissue. This is seen particularly in men who use testosterone replacement. The nipples can even become sensitive or sore when estrogen levels elevate. Estrogen levels should be maintained at less than 30 ng/mL or about 3-5 percent of the total testosterone level.

> **For men, it is important to keep estrogen relatively low, particularly to help protect the prostate gland from developing cancer.**

Making Sense of Andropause: A Rite of Passage

Yield and overcome;
Bend and be straight;
Empty and be full;
Wear out and be new;
Have little and gain;
Have much and be confused.

—From the *Tao Te Ching* by Lao Tzu

Here you are, in the midst of this thing we are calling andropause. You now have an opportunity to place a unique perspective on understanding this truly powerful transition.

The first step is to embrace this time of your life. Learn the art of letting go. Let go of the old mythologies and assumptions about yourself. Don't fight it, try to beat it, avoid it, or deny it. As men, we are very good at doing this. Instead, accept. To accept means to "receive something that is offered." This

> To accept means to "receive something that is offered." This time, right now, is a gift, an opportunity, an offering.

time, right now, is a gift, an opportunity, an offering. Embrace it so you can find the deeper understanding about what it means, and then cash in on the truths it reveals. This entire book is about making the transition of aging not just smoother, but about finding deeper personal understandings and reaching dream fulfillments.

"When I was a child, I spoke as a child, I understood as a child, I thought as a child; but when I became a man I put away childish things." —1 Corinthians 13:11

Now is the time to:

- **Re-prioritize what is truly important.** Spend your precious energies carefully. Get to know yourself so you can take care of yourself. Now is the time, and the opportunity, to work on your soul and less on your career.

- **Joseph Campbell reminded us to "Follow your bliss and the universe will open doors for you where there were only walls."** Your bliss is not hedonistic. Your bliss is now about, as it always was, your true purpose, the art of letting go and Lao Tzu's idea of "Empty and be full." Realize your true purpose. This a common theme in this book. At this time of life, it becomes even easier to find out this secret, as you learn to let go of old patterns that are not needed anymore.

- **Learn to see the sexual act as a potential for true connection with yourself and your partner.** Sex is about a connection with ecstasy and the true imaginative and creative force. Focus on quality and not quantity. In youth, men can miss the point of this powerful act. The transition of aging provides an opportunity to see that sex is not always about the sexual act.

- **Embrace your role as an Elder Statesman**. Think of this time as an opportunity to bring your wisdom and experience forward for the benefit of your family, your community, your country, and the world. The world needs Statesmen. The world needs integrated men.
- **Find a male mentor**. See other men, both young and mature, as part of a brotherhood and as men who can and will help you if you desire it. Now is the time to understand that men are actually "with you" and "for you" and "not against you."
- **Mentor younger men**. Teaching helps you understand more about yourself. "Empty and be full." Let others benefit from your wisdom.

Section 5
The Metabolic Health Protocol:
Seven Steps to The Hormone Zone

Introduction

This is the actual protocol for increasing and enhancing your metabolic health, improving the effectiveness of your thyroid gland and other hormone endocrine organs, and optimizing the effectiveness of any possible prescription thyroid hormone or other metabolic enhancing medications or supplements you have been prescribed or are using as over-the-counter. It is divided into seven sections, or steps: assessment of your health, building a foundation to support good health, supplements, sex hormone optimization, thyroid treatment, adrenal hormone balance, prescription medications, and your metabolism. Each step is part of the pathway that leads to building health into your body and keeping your health status in great working order.

Step 1: The Metabolic Assessment. This section is about getting a diagnosis and an understanding of your condition, which includes education on endocrine disorders such as thyroid disease, thyroid hormone resistance, fibromyalgia and hypometabolism, sex hormone imbalances and deficiencies, insulin resistance, diabetes, adrenal insufficiency and adrenal/ chronic fatigue. This guide is intended for education only and does not intend to diagnose any condition. It will help you ask the right questions or to talk about what you are feeling in order to guide your healthcare provider towards a better understanding of your overall health. It will give you the power to work well with your healthcare provider so that you both may enjoy great results on your behalf.

Step 2: The Metabolic Health Foundation. If you do not already have a good foundation upon which your health is built, there is a way to work toward getting onto a better platform. This is the largest section and should be given a lot of attention. There are five key pillars in establishing metabolic health. These include following a metabolic diet, engaging in metabolic exercise, making metabolic lifestyle changes, managing your mental health, and addressing your spirituality.

Step 3: Metabolic Supplements. In Section 1 of this book you were given basic information on how nutritional and herbal supplements can enhance your health. In this section, specific metabolic nutritional supplements and herbal preparations are listed to help you match your symptoms with helpful supplements.

Step 4: Sex Hormones. A thorough explanation of both male and female sex hormones will be offered with strategies to optimize and balance them.

Step 5: Thyroid Hormone Treatment. A highly detailed explanation of differing thyroid hormone treatments is provided, including the natural alternatives that I recommend for my patients.

Step 6: Adrenals. This section provides an explanation of the often-missed diagnosis and treatment of a common condition known as adrenal fatigue. Properly functioning adrenals are vital towards achieving your metabolic health.

Step 7: Prescription Medications. This section discusses some of the commonly prescribed medications given for symptoms of what is actually an undertreated low metabolic state. Many prescription medications interfere with achieving the health and wellness most patients desire. A discussion of how to decide if weaning off these medications is possible, while under the care and guidance of your healthcare provider.

The Many Levels of your Metabolism

Your metabolism could be only slightly affected due to a simple lack of exercise. Perhaps your metabolism is off due to B vitamin deficiency. It could also be much more complex, such as a result of a sex hormone imbalance or low thyroid gland function that necessitates thyroid hormone replacement. If there are certain unresolved mental and emotional stresses, your health is compromised. Your health imbalance could be all of these things and more. The important thing to understand about your metabolic health and this protocol, is that you must explore the entire array of your metabolism and health to ensure you achieve the complete health and healing you are seeking. You may start to move through the protocol and notice that once you are exercising properly, that was all that was necessary for you to enhance your metabolic health and achieve balance. But you may find that you will need to move through each step before you achieve what you are looking for.

Start at the Beginning

It doesn't matter which step you take first, but YOU MUST MOVE THROUGH EACH STEP! You must also continue to examine how well you have completed each step, all the time, every day, every month, every year, while moving through your health journey. When you hit a roadblock along the way of improving and enhancing your metabolism and health, you must reexamine each step carefully, completely, and without reservation. If any one step is missing or if any one step is not being taken seriously, then it often explains why a patient is not improving.

> It doesn't matter which step you take first, but YOU MUST MOVE THROUGH EACH STEP!

Remember:

- Regaining and enhancing your metabolism is a process just as health is a process.
- Ultimately, your success is largely up to you and your level of commitment.
- Your healthcare practitioner should be helping to guide you along the way.

The Follow Up Routine

If you are beginning treatment for a slow metabolism such as hypothyroidism, the key to your success is to follow up with your healthcare provider consistently. I map out a specific format for all patients to follow up with their treatment on a monthly basis to monitor their progress. This is accomplished by monitoring your body's response to treatment based on your existing symptoms and signs as they relate to your lowered metabolism.

Based on this clinical assessment, the treatment plan may be altered slightly or even significantly to meet your changing needs on a monthly basis. Often, if thyroid hormone has been prescribed, the dose is changed monthly or every other month, depending on your progress. In the beginning stages of treatment, thyroid hormone will be increased more frequently, often on a monthly basis. As a patient improves, normally within a few months or even sooner, the dose will be changed less frequently and monitoring can be extended to every two to three months.

For sex hormone balance, adrenal dysfunction, and weight loss, monitoring your symptoms and signs and making adjustments will also be important to complete on a monthly basis or even more frequently. Keeping a journal is a great idea. Writing daily observations of both your symptoms and good health provides your healthcare provider with a great tool when working with you.

Metabolic Health Protocol: A Layered Process

Keeping in mind that you are required to complete each step of the protocol, you can work on several layers of each step at the same time. But again, *you will have to complete each step*. Health, as a process, is always being enhanced and altered. It is constantly ebbing and flowing, evolving and devolving. So feel free to move and flow through each step and even skip around to see what works for you. But, I will stress again, you will need to go through each step eventually, and eventually you will need to go into each step with some depth, depending on your personal condition and how bad things are for you. Some patients can skim the surface of each step and achieve amazing results for their health and metabolism. But others will need to probe deeply to achieve what they are looking for. This is true of any process in life.

It is possible for you to achieve success without the direct guidance of a healthcare provider versed in supporting your metabolic health. However, in many cases, professional guidance and support will be necessary and I encourage you to seek this kind of advice before embarking on any health journey. Be sure to follow up with your healthcare provider on a routine basis to have their assistance in your progress and to gain encouragement.

So, good luck and know that you are supported as you follow this protocol. Know that you can find the professional support you will need while going through this process. If you are not working directly with me, know that practitioners are out there who understand what you are trying to achieve. This book provides resources to find these practitioners.

Step 1: Analysis of Your Metabolism, Body Composition, Hormonal Status, and Progress Monitoring

This is one of the most important steps to go through. As explained in the introduction to this section, you must go through each step continuously to determine your current metabolic health status. Reassessment and revisiting your current health situation is the only way to know if you are progressing or not and if you are following the correct diagnosis. Determining if your metabolic health is low and/or out of balance is your first important step. Here are some important points about Step 1:

- ❦ It should be gone through *at least one time completely*, answering all of the questionnaires found in Appendix 6.
- ❦ If you have a particular condition, such as sex hormone imbalances or adrenal dysfunction, be sure to focus on that section continuously, rechecking your status at least monthly and communicating this progress with your healthcare provider.
- ❦ If you are hypothyroid and/or on thyroid hormone medication and/or are trying to optimize your thyroid function, then monthly monitoring of signs and symptoms is imperative to determine whether you are over-stimulated by your thyroid hormone medication dose.

Use the Questionnaires

These Specific Condition Questionnaires are in Appendix 6. Hypothyroid/Thyroid Hormone Resistance Symptoms:

- ❦ Adrenal Insufficiency
- ❦ Menopause
- ❦ Andropause
- ❦ Hypoglycemia
- ❦ Metabolic Syndrome

When you have filled out all applicable questionnaires and significant symptoms exist, then it means that either you've just been diagnosed by a healthcare provider and are still not feeling well or you need to take them with you to an appointment with a health care provider.

With the help of this book and the questionnaires, you can work with your healthcare professional to make clinical adjustments in medications, supplements, and lifestyle adjustments to improve your situation. No matter which professional you choose to help guide you to optimal health, you will need to continue to move through all the Seven Steps to Success.

Laboratory Assessment

Your healthcare provider will lead you through the following kinds of lab work for both diagnosis and periodic monitoring:

- Complete Thyroid Panel
- CBC (Complete Blood Count)
- CMP (Comprehensive Metabolic Panel)
- Sex Hormone Panel
- Adrenal Panel
- Fasting Insulin
- Oral Glucose Tolerance Test
- Ferritin
- Prolactin

Clinical Assessment

The following items are clinical as well as self-assessment tools and procedures that are convenient and accurate, when employed in concert, at assessing metabolic health.

- **Resting Metabolic Rate Testing (ReeVue®).** This is a specialized test that measures oxygen that the body consumes and then calculates the number of calories an individual burns at rest in a day. This is a direct measurement of metabolism and can be used to diagnose and monitor low metabolic conditions such as hypothyroidism and fibromyalgia.
  - This test works best when performed as a baseline before thyroid hormone therapy or weight loss therapy begins. It should then be used as a monitoring device at three to six month intervals.

- **ECG (Electrocardiogram).** Another very simple test that measures the electric conduction of the heart muscle. There are several non-specific changes that occur in low and high thyroid function. An EKG can be used both diagnostically and for close monitoring while on thyroid hormone. The following information of ECG is more specific for the physician.
    - In hypothyroidism, the EKG may reflect either low voltage (voltage of an entire QRS complex in all limb leads ≤ 5mm) or bradycardia (slow heart rate, < 50 beats per minute).
    - In hyperthyroidism, the EKG may reflect sinus tachycardia (fast heart beat > 100), shortened QT interval, PR interval prolongation, and continuous atrial fibrillation.
- **Basal Body temperature.** This measurement is correlated with a person's resting metabolic rate. The test is convenient using a simple thermometer that is typically placed in the armpit early in the morning before rising, over at least three days to determine normality. Normal axillary (armpit) temperature is 97.8 F to 98.2 F. Measurements lower than that are *suggestive* of low metabolism and *possibly* mean an inadequate amount of thyroid hormone and/or low adrenal function.
    - Measurements of three days in a row should be reported monthly.
- **Blood Pressure.** A simple test that can produce accurate monitoring of body changes. Obtain a basic digital blood pressure cuff from a drug store. The blood pressure monitor will also be able to provide an accurate digital readout of your heart rate. Blood pressure should be no higher than 120/80 mm mercury. Often, hypothyroid and hypometabolic patients will have very low blood pressure readings, such as a typical 90/60, without the physical fitness to warrant it.
    - An early morning blood pressure reading over the course of three days should be provided on a monthly basis.
- **Heart Rate.** To measure your heart rate, either utilize the convenience of a blood pressure cuff that provides the number automatically, or you can do this easily on your own. Place two fingers over your radial

pulse point located just past your wrist crease on your arm on the thumb side. You can also find your carotid pulse which is done by using two fingers placed on the side of your neck just in front of the large neck muscle but to the side of your throat. While watching the second hand of a clock for sixty seconds, count the number of pulses for your score. An average heart rate is about seventy-two beats per minute. Many patients with low metabolisms will have a heart rate in the low sixties or even lower. If your heart rate starts to elevate into the nineties, and you are taking thyroid medication, your dose could be too high.

- Provide an early morning resting heart rate for three mornings in a row or any additional measurement when you believe your heart is racing or having any perceived irregularity.

- **Achilles tendon reflex.** This is a very simple test that can be performed by your healthcare provider with a reflex hammer. The Achilles tendon is struck and the relaxation portion of the reflex is observed. A relaxation time that is very slow is suggestive of a hypometabolic state that is often consistent with hypothyroidism or low thyroid function. Hyper-reflexive responses can be suggestive of hypermetabolic states including excessive thyroid hormone stimulation.

- **Body weight.** Changes in overall body weight can be used to determine improvement, particularly if the patient is overweight. Rapid reductions in weight can be suggestive of excessive thyroid hormone or a hypermetabolic state.

  - Avoid weighing yourself often. Monthly is adequate. Checking too often can be discouraging as body weight can fluctuate daily.

- **Body fat percentage.** Body fat percentage is a far more accurate measurement of weight loss goals. Utilizing a bioelectrical impedance analysis (BIA) body fat analysis machine that can easily be purchased at a drug store can help to monitor body change progress more accurately.

● Body Composition Index (BCI): This is a different measurement for considering fat loss. The BCI is the net result of scoring losses of fat and gains in lean as positive, and gains in fat and losses in lean as negative. In other words, there is more emphasis on the net result of gaining lean muscle while losing fat, versus simply looking at the overall *weight* loss as is considered in the Body Mass Index (BMI). You could lose only one pound of weight after a month of altering your diet, but have actually lost 10 pounds of fat and gained 9 pounds of muscle. This would be better than losing 10 pounds of weight where much of it was muscle and only a little of that was fat.

● Checking your body fat percentage should only be done every two to four weeks—not daily.

● Optimal body fat percentages vary based on age and gender. In general, women should seek to keep their body fat percentage from 25-30% or lower. Men should optimally range from 20-25% bodyfat or less.

● **Waist-to-Hip ratio.** This ratio helps determine your level of health and fitness. It is also a predictor of disease, particularly diabetes. The waist is measured usually with a tape measure, in inches, at the smallest circumference of the natural waist, usually just above the navel, and the hip circumference may likewise be measured at its widest part of the buttocks or hip. To calculate your ratio, divide waist inch count by your hip inch size.

● A waist-to-hip ratio of 0.7 for women and 0.9 for men have been shown to correlate strongly with general health and decreased tendency towards metabolic syndrome and diabetes. The normal waist-to-hip ratio for women is 0.7 to .08 and 0.9 to 0.99 for men.

Over-stimulation from Thyroid Hormone

The common signs and symptoms of taking excessive amounts of thyroid hormone medication are an elevated heart rate, shaking and tremors, anxiety, excessive sweating, and even unexplained diarrhea. These signs and symptoms should be watched for on a daily basis while on thyroid hormone to help to determine if an individual dose is too much. Be sure to monitor this situation more closely using the Questionnaire in Appendix 6.

Common reasons for over-stimulation from thyroid hormone include:

- Poor cardiovascular conditioning, being out of shape.
  - Remedy: Exercise and follow Step 2 of the Metabolic Health Protocol.
- Poor nutrition, particularly a lack of B vitamins.
  - Remedy: Take nutritional supplements and follow Step 2 and Step 3 of The Metabolic Health Protocol.
- Increasing the thyroid hormone dose too rapidly, or not giving the body time to adjust to an increased dose.
  - Remedy: Decrease the dose, take more time adjusting the dose, and discuss with your healthcare provider.
- Increased anxiety due to life stressors (this situation can mimic over-stimulation).
  - Remedy: Understand the stress, discuss it with your healthcare provider to determine how to minimize or avoid it, or cope with it more effectively.
- Adrenal fatigue that has been confirmed through testing and clinical determination.
  - Remedy: Treat the adrenals, see Step 6 of the Metabolic Health Protocol..
- Low ferritin (the storage form of iron).
  - Remedy: Take additional iron and maintain a ferritin level at least above 50 ng/mL.
- Hypoglycemia (low blood sugar) due to inadequate protein intake, skipping meals, poorly treated diabetes (causes or mimics over-stimulation).
  - Remedy: Avoid it in the first place.

Avoid Hypoglycemia

Hypoglycemia is a condition that is due to low blood sugar. Many of the symptoms that patients present with are due to temporary and often long drops in blood sugar. Be sure to complete the Hypoglycemia Questionnaire both initially and if you ever become overstimulated on thyroid hormone, because hypoglycemia and excessive thyroid hormone can symptomatically present similarly.

Some of the symptoms of hypoglycemia are:

- Constant hunger
- Dizziness
- Fatigue
- Excessive sweating
- Inability to sleep and stay asleep
- Tremors
- Anxiety and nervousness

Note: Many of the signs and symptoms of hypoglycemia are similar to the signs and symptoms of overstimulation of thyroid hormone. There are times when patients believe that they are over stimulated on thyroid hormone, when in fact they are having signs and symptoms of hypoglycemia. Interestingly, thyroid hormone can exacerbate an already existing condition of hypoglycemia because thyroid hormone increases the metabolic rate and therefore the clearance of glucose (sugar) and the need for glucose to maintain the increased cellular reactions.

Here is a suggested diet for hypoglycemia:

- Focus on lean sources of protein, vegetables, and minimal fruit
- Eat protein at every meal, no matter what
- Avoid processed foods, particularly sugar
- Eat every two to three hours
- Never skip meals
- Consider eating a small meal before bed

Talk with your healthcare provider about a diet if you have been diagnosed with hypoglycemia, especially if you have food allergies or other special dietary concerns.

Determining Clinical Thyrotoxicosis
(Thyroid Hormone Overstimulation)

This section is more technical, but can be a valuable tool for you and your healthcare practitioner to determine if you are actually overstimulated from thyroid hormone versus simply relying upon thyroid laboratory values.

- Laboratory Result Interpretations
  - Chemistry Panel
  - Alkaline Phosphatase: increased due to increased bone turnover.
  - Calcium: increased due to increased bone turnover.
  - Phophorus: increased due to increased bone turnover.
  - Creatinine: decreased due to increased glomerular filtration, or possibly due to low physical conditioning.
  - BUN: increased due to increased muscle mass turnover.
  - BUN/Creatinine ratio: increased due to increased muscle mass turnover.
- Thyroid labs
  - TSH: if suppressed it DOES NOT indicate thyrotoxicosis but may lead to determining the possibility.
  - Total T4/T3, and Free T4/T3: if elevated it does not indicate thyrotoxicosis but may lead to determining the possibility.
- N telo-peptide: an increased value can suggest increased bone turnover.
- Physical Signs and Symptoms
  - Hyperactivity
  - Hyperreflexia: particularly at the Achilles tendon
  - Muscle weakness
  - Stare, and eyelid retraction
  - Systolic hypertension
  - Tachycardia or arrhythmia
  - Tremor
  - Warm, moist skin
  - Widened pulse pressure

- Hyperdynamic precordium
- Shortness of breath on exertion
- Nonspecific EKG changes:
    i. Complete or third degree right bundle block
    ii. Increased U wave amplitude
    iii. Persistent atrial fibrillation
    iv. PR interval prolongation
    v. Right axis deviation with atrial fibrillation
    vi. Shortened QT interval
    vii. Sinus tachycardia
    viii. ST segment elevation
    ix. Wolff-Parkinson-White syndrome
- Symptoms
    - Appetite change (usually an increase)
    - Fatigue and muscle weakness
    - Heat intolerance
    - Hyperactivity
    - Tremors
    - Increased perspiration
    - Menstrual disturbances
    - Nervousness
    - Palpitations
    - Weight change (usually a decrease)
    - Dry, itchy skin

NOTE: A cold hand, moist or dry, virtually excludes thyrotoxicosis. A warm, moist hand is very indicative of thyrotoxicosis.[339] This is a very useful clinical sign and I have used it many times before with very accurate success.

Step 1: Analysis

The Importance of Your Symptoms

In the practice of holistic health, we consider the totality of the individual and the individual's personal experience. In 1810, the German physician Samuel Hahnemann wrote the seminal work of what is known today as *The Organon of Medicine*. In it he lays the foundation of a philosophical and scientific approach to medicine known as homeopathy. The text was just as relevant then as it is today as he reveals a holistic and comprehensive examination of viewing a patient and their illness. Specifically for this section and discussion on symptoms, he explains:

> **In the practice of holistic health, we consider the totality of the individual and the individual's personal experience.**

> The unprejudiced observer realizes the futility of metaphysical speculations that cannot be verified by experiment, and no matter how clever he is, he sees in any given case of disease only the disturbances of body and soul which are perceptible to the senses: subjective symptoms, incidental symptoms, i.e., deviations from the former healthy condition of the individual now sick which the patient personally feels, which people around him notice, which the physician sees in him. *As far as the physician is concerned, is not that which reveals itself to the senses in symptoms the very disease itself?* [Emphasis added.]

Here Hahnemann is leading us to a rational approach to medicine and imploring the physician to focus on a holistic view of what is presented to the senses with utterly no need to find the mystical "thing" lurking deep within the recesses of the blood. For medical doctors who practice conventional, or evidence-based medicine, the cause of disease is somewhere on a blood test. And if the blood test does not reveal a supposed abnormality or "definition of disease," then there is thought to be no disease, even though the patient and the dis-ease expression is still sitting right in front of him or her in the suffering of it.

This section of the book was written to help you understand your own symptomatic picture and how that can lead you towards understanding what you are dealing with. Follow your symptoms carefully and report them regularly to your healthcare provider.

You may ask, "Why doesn't the doctor want to assess my clinical signs and symptoms? Why does my doctor only look at the lab values?" The answer to this question began to be answered in the previous section. The philosophical belief of conventionally trained doctors is at least part of the reason they place so much emphasis on lab results. But there are other reasons, too.

As a scientific and medical culture, we are in the "age of the laboratory." There has been an ongoing push in medicine towards an attempt to simplify the consult by reducing and eliminating any subjectiveness in diagnosis and treatment. Patients are left with the supposed objective measurement of laboratory values. Where there have been undoubted advances in medicine due to laboratory tools, this approach has also proven disastrous in thyroid hormone diagnosis and treatment specifically and general medicine as a whole.

This medical model has been named different things. The term "reductionistic" is often used, implying everything can be reduced to the "sum of its parts," and even biological systems such as human beings, are nothing more than a complex machine. This is also known as the Cartesian philosophy, formulated by the seventeenth century philosopher Renè Descartes. Interestingly, even by the 1950s, the Newtonian Law of Conservation (stating that matter is neither gained nor lost) was used explicitly to disprove this perspective in relation to biological systems, but we still see this philosophy firmly entrenched in current conventional medical thought.[340]

Another term for this medical philosophical approach is "technocratic medicine." Dr. John C. Lowe defines the term eloquently as:

> Medical technocracy is advocacy of reforming medical practice so that it is conducted according to the reported findings of technologists. In this form of practice, diagnostic and treatment decisions are based solely on the outcome of objective tests. Typically, the practitioner of

technocratic medicine disavows the methods of clinical medicine. *He tends to devalue the patient's symptoms and signs and communication with the patient.* [Emphasis added.] Commonly, the practitioner has an extremist faith in the outcome of objective measures peculiar to his specialty. Patients and medical generalists typically do not have the background education to comprehend some of the measures and the rationale for their use. The technocratic practitioner's specialized knowledge tends to give rise of a sense of superiority that alienates both patients and practitioners of clinical medicine.[341]

The opposite philosophical view to the Cartesian reductionist and technocratic approach in medicine is holism. With holism, one can see that indeed the human body, the human condition in relationship to its environment, is much more than simple parts. In reductionism, 1 + 1 always equals 2. In holism, particularly as the human body is concerned, 1 + 1 often equals 3, with the extra amount being that ineffable and unknowable essence that makes us complex humans. When it comes to considering the disease process of a patient in a holistic medical practice, the entire individual is considered in order to approach and restore health.

Step 2: The Five Pillars of Metabolic Health
in Your Hormone Zone:
Diet, Exercise, Lifestyle, Mental Health, and Spirituality

If your goal is thyroid health, sex hormone balance, adrenal health, fat loss, physical conditioning, mental health and well-being, then this step contains what is necessary for those things to be realized. Within this step are the Five Pillars of Optimal Integrated Health. These concepts are the core of any "house" a patient wants to build for themselves and their health, no matter what the diagnosis or goal.

The Five Pillars of Optimal Integrated Health:

- The daily habits of a proper diet, normal body composition, sunlight, fresh air, proper breathing, and restful sleep.
- Exercise performed in the most efficient manner.
- Lifestyle attention and awareness in order to minimize stress and using periodic dietary cleansing as a process.
- Appropriate behavior toward others, balanced motivations and intellectual stimulation and growth.
- A spiritual belief system and practice.

Pillar 1: Diet, Body Composition,
Sunlight, Breathing, and Sleep

Diet and Metabolic Nutrition

Diet is probably one of the largest four letter words in the English language. It means so much to people. It has cultural, social, and religious meanings. Diet affects us physically and drives our mental and emotional being, inducing sensations and beliefs of joy, celebration, devotion, familiarity, and love. But for many, the idea of diet is the unknowable, uncertain and unconquerable thing, leading to frustration, disconnection from the process of food, and ultimately poor food choices.

The chapter on metabolic nutrition laid out an argument for a particular type of eating that can help with many things including weight loss and overall health improvement. And if you are empowered to follow that particular nutritional lifestyle, many good things can come of it. I happen to believe that the concepts presented in that chapter are based on sound reasoning and a historical track record of success, particularly for fat loss. But truly, there is more to it.

Metabolic nutrition is a "nuts and bolts" and academic perspective that explores the "why" of proper diet. Here, I offer a comprehensive approach to nutrition and eating that encompasses multiple levels of insight towards its accomplishment that also explores both the "who" and the "when" of dieting. It is yet another layer to understanding food as a lifestyle that provides deeper insight into the mental, emotional and even spiritual aspects of food.

An Integral Nutritional Approach

The Integral Theory offered by contemporary philosopher and theorist Ken Wilber has offered an "integrated" theory that holistically incorporates a world view based on the perspective of:

- The IT: The item studied.
- The I: The experience of the individual.
- The WE: The rationale of the interior collective.
- The ITS: The exterior global collective.

Integral Theory answers to the collective of human experience including the physical, mental, emotional and spiritual all from a globally constituted amalgam of personal, cultural and religious experiences. Using this theory, which is completely in line with the naturopathic medical paradigm, we can view nutrition comprehensively leading to a more purposeful food experience and lifelong "lifestyle" approach and commitment to the food experience.

Optimal Eating: The IT

This can be summarized conveniently: Eat as close to nature as possible, eat organic, and eat a variety of foods. It probably sounds too simple. But this strategy covers largely, but not completely, the gamut of nutritional health in terms of "what" to eat. Let's examine each portion of this profoundly simply sentence:

"Eat as close to nature as possible."

This means avoid processed foods. Almost all food, to some degree, has been "processed." This means that if you cut an apple in half to eat it, you "processed" it. If you squeezed the juice out of it, that is even more processing. If you squeezed the juice out of it and then heated it, you processed it even more. If you did all of that and then added sugar and artificial flavors and preservatives to it, you processed it even more. The less processing the better and this leads to "Eating as close to nature as possible." Choose foods that are whole and involve minimal cooking and preparation when possible. This also means "eat for quality."

"Eat organic."

The news is out… organic is better. It tastes better and the organic farming practices have a lower impact on the environment and raises healthier animals. Organically grown food has a lower pesticide load, and is devoid of the most dangerous chemical used in farming known as organophosphates which have been linked with conditions such as cancer, lowered male fertility, fetal abnormalities, chronic fatigue syndrome in children, and Parkinson's disease.[342, 343] The U.S. Government ranked pesticides among the top three environmental cancer risks.[344] Organic food appears to clearly have a higher nutritional content than conventionally grown foods, although this is controversial to some extent. The basic farming practices of organically grown food helps to replenish mineral content within the soil. The Soil Association in the U.K. found that on average organic food contains higher levels of vitamin C and essential

> **The less processing the better and this leads to "Eating as close to nature as possible."**

minerals such as calcium, magnesium, iron, and chromium.[345] Additional reviews of the evidence found that organic foods had significantly higher levels of all twenty-one nutrients analyzed compared with conventional produce including 27 percent higher vitamin C, 29 percent more magnesium, 21 percent more iron, and 14 percent more phosphorous.[346]

Most supermarkets have at least some organic food choices and these should be considered whenever possible. Also, when possible, seek out locally and organically grown produce at farmers' markets. Shopping at them helps the local economy you live in and the produce is even fresher and better for you.

Do you know the Dirty Dozen and the Clean Fifteen? The Environmental Working Group (www.ewg.org) has found twelve food items to have the highest pesticide load when grown conventionally, listed in order of highest level of pesticide load. Your "organic dollar" should go towards choosing organic for these fruits and vegetables whenever possible.

- Peaches
- Apples
- Bell peppers
- Celery
- Nectarines
- Strawberries
- Cherries
- Kale
- Lettuce
- Imported grapes
- Carrots
- Pears

All conventionally grown fruits and vegetables are also not all bad. The Clean Fifteen have the lowest pesticide load and you can choose to not spend your "organic dollar" with these foods.

- Onions
- Avocados
- Sweet corn
- Pineapples
- Mangoes
- Asparagus
- Sweet peas
- Kiwis
- Cabbages
- Eggplants
- Papayas
- Watermelons
- Broccoli
- Tomatoes
- Sweet potato

"Eat a Variety of Foods."

Your body craves variety. Different organs in your body need different arrays of vitamins, minerals, and other various meat and plant based chemicals. Particularly, it is important to eat a large variety of fruits and vegetables, so experiment whenever you can. The more you experiment, the more you keep the concept of fresh foods alive and well within your daily habit, and you will be healthier for it.

> The U.S. Government ranked pesticides among the top three environmental cancer risks.

Mindful Eating: The I

Mindful eating means you are connecting with your food experience. This is a purposeful and intentional experience versus the often disconnected and rushed eating experience most people engage in.

Do you actually take time to relax when you eat? One of the best metabolic boosters is to simply relax, particularly while you eat. Slowing down actually increases your metabolism. The metabolic burden of stress increases your "sympathetic nervous system" or "fight-or-flight" response. During an increased sympathetic response, your digestion decreases and nutrient excretion increases. Additionally, cortisol increases and insulin becomes resistant, both of which can lead to increased fat deposition, particularly around the midsection.

> Mindful eating means you are connecting with your food experience. This is a purposeful and intentional experience versus the often disconnected and rushed eating experience most people engage in.

Ask yourself, do I:

- ❦ Eat with intention of conscious choice, aware of my body and environment while eating?
- ❦ Listen to my body while eating and heed its responses to the eating experience?
- ❦ Create a space of thankfulness before and during eating?
- ❦ Take at least ten to fifteen minutes for breakfast? Thirty minutes for lunch? Thirty to sixty or more minutes for dinner?
- ❦ Breathe deeply, relax, and SMILE during eating?
- ❦ AVOID FEAR, worry, guilt, and judgment of yourself and food choices and ultimately, trust your inner guidance and accept your body as it is?

Meaningful Eating: The WE

The social aspect regarding food includes a meaningful experience with others as well as a conscious connection with your immediate community. The "we" of eating includes the process of growing and preparing food locally, which includes the local farmer and the local "mom and pop" restaurant. This helps our eating experience to stay connected with our larger but immediate community. There are multiple occasions for social eating within the community, but one of the most important social eating events is a meal with family.

Even though family dinner time was on the decline for years, recently it has been on the rise and the benefits for the family are numerous. W.J. Doherty has written a book entitled *Putting Family First: Successful Strategies for Reclaiming Family Life in A Hurry Up World* where he explains, "For young children, meal time at home is a stronger predictor of academic achievement and psychological adjustment than time spent in any of the following activities: school, studying, sports, church/religious activities, or art activities. For teens, having regular dinners with parents is a strong predictor of academic success, psychological adjustment, and lower rates of alcohol use, drug use, early sexual behavior, eating disorders, and risk for suicide."

The benefits expand to the parents also, lowering stress and creating a stronger family bond. Make dinnertime a fun and sacred space so that all can benefit and enjoy. Avoid stressful conversations or involved reprimands, which can wait until later. This ensures not just proper digestion, but a space where all family members will want to continually and happily return.

Ask yourself, do I:
- Support local farming and food sources?
- Eat with others whom I want to share time with?
- Get involved in the preparation of food for the sake of others?
- Have at least five family dinners weekly? Or, do I at least eat socially with friends with this frequency?

Eat Sustainably: The ITS

This refers to the global eating experience. The world itself is getting smaller as we are continually connected by technology and global social awareness. This inevitably includes food and the eating experience. When you eat there are larger implications for the world at large and this understanding expands your global perspective that helps everyone involved, including yourself.

Some foods have more impact on the environment and may be produced in a way that is not fully conscious. The more we understand this, the more our eating experience will be complete.

Ask yourself, do I:
- Include seasonal foods to honor the earthly cycles and rhythms?
- Understand where my food came from and do I ethically, morally, politically, socially and even religiously support this?
- Do you know how your food is grown and by whom?

There was a time when families grew their own food together, worked the fields, hunted and gathered food, harvested based on the rhythmic seasons, prepared for future months and even future years, prepared food with purpose, reverence and joy, and consistently feasted socially with family, friends and community for celebratory and religious reasons. It was a complete, comprehensive, and holistic process from beginning to end. Having this complete type of experience may not be possible in our modern world. However, we can learn from this model and incorporate as many aspects of this as possible, if we try.

Body Composition

I specifically use the technical phrase "body composition" versus "body weight." When you focus on the actual composition of your entire body mass veruss how much you weigh, health status is seen more clearly and accurately. You could weight 150 pounds and be very healthy or very unhealthy, depending on how much total body fat you hold and where you hold it. Body composition refers to the actual amount of fat under your skin, over your abdomen, and around your internal organs, in relationship to the amount of muscle and bone mass you possess. In general, the more muscle and bone you have the better. Body fat should be kept low in relationship to muscle and bone mass. Stay away from focusing on your actual body weight and keep your focus on body fat percentage. There are commercial scales available that measure body fat through bioelectric impedance, simply by stepping on the scale barefoot. Step 1 of the Metabolic Health Protocol discusses how to monitor your body fat percentage.

> **When you focus on the actual composition of your entire body mass veruss how much you weigh, health status is seen more clearly and accurately.**

Sunlight

Sunlight is good for you. Since the dawn of time, the earth and its inhabitants have been dependent upon the rays from the sun. We have developed as human beings, generation after generation, with the benefits of the sun. All the food that we eat, in any form, is essentially captured sunlight, synthesized in higher and higher forms. Recently, we have now been made to believe that the sun is some kind of enemy, particularly to our skin, whether it is wrinkles or cancer. This fear of the sun has led people to avoid the sun like a plague. From a practical health standpoint, this strategy has been detrimental at the least and even deadly at its worst.

The benefits of sunlight:

- Provides a healthy looking complexion.
- Moderate tanning will make your skin more resistant to infections and sunburns than if your skin is not tanned.
- Ultraviolet rays act as a natural antiseptic that kills viruses, bacteria, molds, yeasts, fungi and mites in air, water and on different surfaces including your skin.
- Improves skin conditions such as acne, athlete's foot, psoriasis and eczema.
- Sunlight stimulates your appetite and enhances digestion, intestinal motility and overall metabolism.
- Sunlight improves circulation and enhances red and white blood cell production.
- Sunlight increases endorphins and serotonin enhancing mood and improving depression.
- Sun exposure helps to regulate proper circadian rhythms because it increases melatonin production at night to improve sleep.
- And, sunlight produces vitamin D!

Step 2: The 5 Pillars

Vitamin D Deficiency

The Centers for Disease Control and Prevention estimates that more than 180 million Americans, or 60 percent of the population, are vitamin D deficient. Getting enough vitamin D is as easy as either getting out in the sun or taking a supplement when sun exposure is not possible. But, fear of malignant melanoma, the fatal form of skin cancer, keeps most people out of the sun and away from the amazing benefits of vitamin D. The truth is that the incidence of melanoma continues to *increase* dramatically although many people have been completely avoiding the sun for years.[347] Not wearing sunscreen, too much sun exposure, and getting sunburn is always a bad idea. However, safe sun exposure allows you to make vitamin D properly at the skin level and ultimately optimizes your health.

> The truth is that the incidence of melanoma continues to *increase* dramatically although many people have been completely avoiding the sun for years.

A recent study in the *Journal of the National Cancer Institute*[348] actually showed a correlation with increased sun exposure to *lowered* death rates in people diagnosed with the skin cancer melanoma. The authors proposed two possible hypotheses as to why this may be:

1. Sun exposure creates vitamin D which has properties that prevent cancer cells from proliferating and also leads to their destruction, called apoptosis.

2. Sun exposure increases the amount of melanin or pigment in the skin which increases DNA repair capacity. This reduces the amount of mutational and cancerous changes within a melanoma.

I want people to know that the sun is good for you! I truly believe this is an obvious, natural statement. Simply being outside in the shade has its calming and warming benefits. We are meant to be outside!

Benefits of Vitamin D

- Maintains your calcium balance.
- Prevents osteoporosis.[349]
- Potent immune system modulator.[350]
- Has a role in insulin secretion under conditions of increased insulin demand.[351]
- Blood Pressure Regulation[352]

The Vitamin D Council available at www.vitamindcouncil.org lists the following conditions that have been found to be correlated with Vitamin D deficiency:[353]

- Addison's Disease
- Allergic Hypersensitivity
- Alzheimer's Disease
- Ankylosing Spondylitis
- Asthma
- Autism
- Autoimmune Illness
- Benign Prostatic Hyperplasia
- Bladder Cancer
- Brain Cancer
- Breast Cancer
- Celiac Disease
- Cerebral Palsy
- Chronic Obstructive Pulmonary Disease (COPD)
- Chronic Pain
- Cognitive Function Difficulty
- Colon and Rectal Cancer
- Cystic Fibrosis
- Depression and Seasonal Affective Disorder
- Diabetes
- Endometrial Cancer
- Epilepsy
- Eye Cancer
- Gaucher's and Fabry's Disease
- Graves' Disease
- Hashimoto's Thyroiditis
- Heart Disease
- HIV and AIDS
- Hypertension
- Inflammatory Bowel Disease
- Influenza
- Innate and Adaptive Immunity
- Liver Cancer
- Liver Function
- Lung Cancer
- *Lymphoma, myeloma,* and *leukemia*
- Melanoma
- Mental Illness
- Mineral metabolism condition such as calcium, phosphate and magnesium
- Mortality
- Multiple Sclerosis
- Muscular Weakness and Falls
- Obesity
- Osteoarthritis
- Osteomalacia, Osteopenia, and Osteoporosis
- Otosclerotic hearing impairment
- Ovarian Cancer
- Pancreatic Cancer
- Parathyroid Function
- Parkinson's Disease
- Postmenopause weight gain and bone loss
- Pregnancy and Lactation
- Premenstrual Syndrome
- Prostate Cancer
- Renal Function
- Rickets
- Sarcoidosis
- Sickle Cell Disease
- Skin Cancer

❧ Stroke   ❧ Tuberculosis
❧ Toxin and Radiation Exposure   ❧ Turner's Syndrome
   Treatment

How Much Sun Exposure is Good?

Dr. Michael F. Holick of Boston University School of Medicine and other experts recommend figuring out how long it takes your skin to get pink, then expose ¼ of your skin (face, arms, legs) for ¼ of that amount of time during the hours of 11:00 a.m. to 3:00 p.m. So, most Caucasian people will only need five to ten minutes per day during that time. Darker pigmented Caucasians and darker pigmented people such as those of East Indian or African descent will need up to an hour in the sun to achieve the same results. Within thirty minutes of full body exposure to the sun most people will make at least 10,000 units of vitamin D.[354]

Testing Vitamin D Levels and Vitamin D Toxicity

For basic health reasons and to optimize your health, you should have your vitamin D levels checked. The best test to determine this is the vitamin D that is ready to convert into the active form called 1,25 hydroxy vitamin D. Some doctors are still using the outdated 1,25 hydroxy (OH) vitamin D test that is essentially useless.

❧ Optimal levels should be between 50 ng/mL and 80 ng/mL.
❧ Remember: Some labs, including Sonora Quest, currently use the mass spectrometry test which makes the results come back too high. If the lab uses mass spectrometry be sure your healthcare provider knows to multiply the 25(OH)D3 value by 0.6 to yield the correct value.
❧ Lab Corp uses the Diasorin test which is more accurate.

Supplementing with Vitamin D:
How Much Vitamin D Should I Take?

If you do not get much sun daily, make sure you supplement in pill form with vitamin D3 or cholecalciferol. Avoid products that have vitamin D2 which is not as effective as D3. Here are the basic guidelines for Vitamin D3 dosing:

- ❦ Healthy children under the age of two years: 1,000 IU daily
- ❦ Children over the age of two: 2,000 IU daily
- ❦ Adolescents and adults: 5,000 – 10,000 IU daily
- ❦ And here are a few cautions:
- ❦ Remember to monitor your vitamin D levels using the 25 OH Vitamin D blood test after about three months from starting the vitamin D supplementation.
- ❦ The following medications increase the way vitamin D is metabolized and may decrease serum D levels:
    - ❦ Phenytoin (Dilantin), fosphenytoin (Cerebyx), phenobarbital (Luminal), carbamazepine (Tegretol), and rifampin (Rimactane).
- ❦ The following medications should not be taken at the same time as vitamin D because they can decrease the intestinal absorption of vitamin D:
    - ❦ Cholestyramine (Questran), colestipol (Colestid), orlistat (Xenical), mineral oil, the fat substitute Olestra, and ketoconazole.

There are some important minerals and one other vitamin that improve vitamin D utilization[355] you should know about:

- ❦ Magnesium is one of the most commonly deficient nutrients and is needed to make vitamin D work. Eat plenty of nuts, particularly sunflower seeds or pumpkin seeds. Consider adding 400 mg of magnesium in a supplement form.
- ❦ Zinc is an essential part of the vitamin D receptor. Consider oysters and lobster or 30 mg of zinc with about 2 mg of copper. Always take copper with zinc.
- ❦ Vitamin K2 improves bone health and assists the calcification process of vitamin D. Consider 500 to 1,000 mcg daily.
- ❦ Boron assists vitamin D at the cell membrane. About 3 mg daily is adequate.

Step 2: The 5 Pillars

❧ A limited amount of vitamin A. It is another underrated fat soluble vitamin that works synergistically with vitamin D; 1,000 IU per day is normally adequate.

In fact, there are now supplements on the market that contain all the co-factors vitamin D needs to work properly including magnesium, zinc (the vitamin D receptor contains a zinc molecule), vitamin K2 (vitamin K helps direct vitamin D to calcify the proper organs and prevents calcification of improper organs), boron (boron is involved in vitamin D action on the cell wall), and a tiny amount of vitamin A.

Food Sources of Vitamin D

It is always good to get additional vitamin D from food sources, particularly in the winter when sun exposure is seasonally limited in North America. Fish liver oils, such as cod liver oil, provides an easy, inexpensive, whole food option to obtaining vitamin D. One tablespoon or 15 mL provides about 1,360 IU of vitamin D. Be sure that you are using a reputable brand of oil such as Nordic Naturals® or Carlson's®, among others. Cod liver oil should not be "fishy" and most reputable brands are actually very tasty. Caution: Do not take in excessive amounts of cod liver oil. Keep the dose at no more than one to two tablespoons daily. The vitamin A content of cod liver oil is variable and can become toxic in large amounts.

Fatty fish species, such as herring, provide about 1,383 IU of vitamin D for every three ounces of fish. Salmon and tuna also provide vitamin D, but the amounts are much lower.

Breathing

Breathing is the obvious essential act that most take for granted. We assume that if we are upright then we must be breathing. But there is a difference between adequate breathing to keep you alive and optimal breathing to keep you healthy. Breathing has been studied for many, many years by several disciplines including science and it has led to understanding the breath and its use in optimizing health, well-being and even spirituality.

While enduring the stresses of life, people train their bodies to restrict breathing. They become "chest breathers" instead of "abdomen breathers." Chest breathing, or shallow, rapid breathing is a sign of stress and limits the exchange of air in your lungs. Most exchange of oxygen occurs in your lower lungs. This is best achieved by deep and slow abdominal breathing or what is called "diaphragmatic breathing."

> **Most exchange of oxygen occurs in your lower lungs. This is best achieved by deep and slow abdominal breathing or what is called "diaphragmatic breathing."**

A simple test of your own breath pattern is to place one hand on your chest and one on your abdomen and breathe as you normally do. If the hand on your chest rises higher than the hand on your abdomen, you are a chest breather.

There are many breathing techniques that you can employ for better breathing. Qigong and yogic pranayama breathing techniques are the most common, but a detailed explanation of those two practices is beyond the scope of this book. I encourage you to explore these methods as they can lead to an understanding of how to control your breath which will optimize your metabolic health. At the very least, you should focus on making sure you breathe with your diaphragm and with your abdomen, not your chest.

Deep, abdominal and slow breathing can help with:
- Increased energy
- Lowered anxiety
- Weight loss
- Memory and focus
- Enhanced immunity
- Improved digestion and elimination
- And much more... like opening the mind to the present moment

Step 2: The 5 Pillars

Here is a list of the most important things to always keep in mind regarding your breathing:

- When at rest, breathe through your nose. Avoid mouth breathing.
- Breathe through the abdomen and not the chest.
- Your exhalation should be twice as long as the inhalation. This should slow down your exhalation considerably.

Here is a great technique to show you how to train yourself to become a diaphragmatic breather:

- Keep one hand on your abdomen and one hand on your chest to monitor your ability to make the abdomen rise highest when breathing.
- Breathe in through your nose for four to seven seconds and breathe out of your mouth for eight to ten seconds.
- When you exhale, attempt to gently force all the air out of your lungs by contracting your abdominal muscles.
- Repeat this cycle for at least a total of five deep breaths.
- When you are ready, incorporate words into the exhalation such as "relax," "calm." or any other positive word that is important to you.
- Practice at least twice a day. This can be done once in the morning and again before bed, taking very little time. Practice this technique when you are under stress or experiencing pain.

Doing diaphragmatic breathing is the first step in understanding your breathing. The technique is largely for relaxation and instruction on basic proper breathing. Here are more techniques to add to your breathing practice.

The Cleansing Breath

For a great start to your day, try this:

- Start by breathing normally.
- Next, forcefully exhale through your nose as fast as you can. Contract your abdominal muscles to help the exhalation.
- Relax your abdominal muscles and the air will come back in automatically through your nose.

- The more complete the exhalation, the more cleansing and rhythmic the breathing process will be.
- Repeat this for about five cycles.

The Stimulating Breath

For an energy boost at any time, try this:

- This is done by rapidly breathing in and out through the nose as fast as possible.
- Start by breathing in and out once every second, build up speed and go for an in and out cycle of three per second. It is difficult at first, but you will get used to it. Just do this slowly and steadily.
- Again, make sure you use your diaphragm and abdomen to do the breathing and not your chest.
- To avoid getting light-headed, do not breathe this way for more than —ten to fifteen seconds initially. You will be able to add more time as you practice.

An excellent resource for optimizing your breathing can be found online at www.authentic-breathing.com.

The Great Outdoors

"Go get some fresh air!" is the advice parents often give children who have been indoors too long. Well, they're right. So now I'm advising you to go outside, go to the mountains, get out of the city, go to a park, just get outside and breathe. As polluted as outdoor air can be, indoor air is actually far more polluted, particularly in large buildings. Consider using an indoor air filter both at work and at home.

Limited access to nature can cause a sense of internal loss that leads to a host of behavioral problems. Richard Louv coined the term Nature Deficit Disorder in his 2005 book *Last Child in the Woods* which references the trend of

> Limited access to nature can cause a sense of internal loss that leads to a host of behavioral problems.

children spending less time outdoors. In fact, both children and adults are spending less time in nature as seen by a decline in the number of visitors to national parks in the U.S.[356]

Your very soul needs the outdoors; it needs to commune with nature. And it's right out there, just beyond your door, just beyond the movie screen, just beyond the shopping mall. Go and see....

Sleep

Humans spend over a third of their lives sleeping. But how do you prepare for this long event every night? Most people view sleeping as an inactive process that should just automatically happen. But sleeping is actually an active process that should be prepared for every night.

Here is some advice on making your night as restful as possible:

- Set your going to bed routine so that you get in bed at the same time each night, say 10:00 p.m. Then set your routine for getting up at the same time each morning, say 6:00 a.m. You should get up and out of bed at the same time each day, even if you did not sleep well the night before. Also, get up at the same time even on the weekends.
- Get seven to nine hours of sleep regularly, based on your needs.
- Exercise daily, but avoid exercise later at night, which can be over-stimulating.
- Get daily sun exposure.
- Limit liquid intake right before bed to avoid awakening due to the urge to urinate.
- Avoid caffeine past 6:00 p.m.; drink decaffeinated herbal teas instead.
- Avoid or keep alcohol consumption low (one drink) before sleep. Alcohol in moderation (two drinks) and in large quantity (three drinks or more) actually disrupts sleep in the second half of the sleep cycle.[357]
- Avoid nicotine at least three to four hours before bed.
- If you cannot get to sleep within twenty minutes, get out of bed, leave the room and read or do something relaxing until you are ready to go back to your bed and sleep again.

- The process of going to sleep should be at least thirty to sixty minutes before you are actually ready for sleep.

- Get to bed as early as possible to mimic normal circadian rhythms.

- Avoid overly stimulating activities during pre-bedtime such as exercise, intense reading or study, and complicated conversations.

- Eat a small amount of protein thirty to sixty minutes before bed. This helps to regulate blood sugar and avoids sleep disruption. A handful of almonds or a small amount of yogurt can be good choices.

- Take a warm bath or shower nightly within an hour before bed. This can also eliminate daily allergy-causing substances that accumulate in the hair and on the body. Allergic reactions can also interfere with sleep.

- Epsom bath salts contain magnesium sulfate which relaxes muscles and softens the skin. No need to rinse after this excellent bath!

- Meditate and breathe deeply for at least five to ten minutes before going to sleep. Use a CD meant for relaxation or meditation, then turn off the electronic device and put it away from your bedside.

- Journal about your day and any stressful previous dreams.

- The bedroom should be for sleep and sex only. Do not work or read in bed.

- Maintain the temperature constant and slightly cool, no warmer than 70° F.

- Keep the bedroom quiet, which means no television or radios. Using earplugs to completely drown out sound might be necessary for a truly restful sleep, especially if you share the bed with someone who snores.

- Complete darkness is imperative to maintain serotonin levels. Use blackout drapes or an eye mask.

- Keep your alarm clock at least three feet from your bed. It emits a small electromagnetic frequency which may cause subtle sleep interference.

- If you suffer poor circulation, wear socks to keep your feet warm.

Step 2: The 5 Pillars

❧ When you wake in the morning, open all the blinds and turn on as many lights as possible.

Natural Sleep Aids

If you must use an aid to sleep that is ingested, be sure to start with the least potent form in order to assess if the simplest measures help. From there, add additional supplements as needed. This list is by no means exhaustive, but provides a good place to start with the most noted effectiveness.

First Choice:

❧ Chamomile Tea or capsules of extract. Chamomile is a slightly bitter herb that soothes nerves and settles the stomach promoting digestion as well as sleep. As a tea, it can be very calming for children and it may even improve menstrual cramps. It is also a mild diuretic. Drink one to four cups of tea, sufficiently steeped for at least five minutes. Time it so that not too much liquid is taken before bedtime. Another option is to purchase an extract in capsule form that is standardized to at least 1.2 percent apigenin, the active ingredient of the herb.

Second Choice:

❧ 5-HTP (5-hydroxytryptophan). This amino acid is a direct precursor to the production of the brain chemical serotonin which is responsible for mood and sleep regulation. The doses can range from 100 mg to up to 300 mg or more right before bed. Be careful that you do not take too much as some people can become tired the next morning, but this is rare. Also, do not take 5-HTP if you are taking any kind of medication for depression such as an SSRI like Prozac®, Celexa®, Lexapro®, Paxil®, Zoloft®, etc.

❧ Magnesium. Consider 250 mg of this mineral, which helps to induce sleep

❧ Vitamin B6. 100 to 150 mg of this vital B vitamin can assist in sleep and the production of serotonin.

❧ Here's a recipe for an effective nightcap: magnesium, B6, about 50 mg of non-flush niacin or B3, and a small amount of juice all with the 5 HTP which assists with the conversion of 5-HTP into serotonin.

Third Choice:

❧ Melatonin. This is a hormone produced by the pineal gland in the brain and it promotes healthy sleep patterns. In the human light-dark cycle, melatonin peaks every twenty-four hours, between 2 and 3:00 a.m. This assumes that sleep is done is complete darkness, which is why the overall sleep hygiene section is so important to follow for optimal sleep. The trick with taking melatonin for enhanced sleep is getting the dose correct. For some people 1-3 mg is sufficient for sleep, and in some can even cause sluggishness the next morning. However, many people take the recommended dose of melatonin then stay at the 1-3 mg dose and never achieve any results. For some, they need to increase the dose to upwards of 25 mg or more before it is effective. These doses are in fact safe as melatonin has been used as a powerful antioxidant in cancer patients safely at doses up to 40 mg daily. The U.S. National Institutes of Health came out with a statement: "Available trials report that overall adverse effects are not significantly more common with melatonin than placebo. And a very large clinical trial in the Netherlands had 1,400 women taking 75 mg of melatonin with no negative effects."[358] As for dosing, when I prescribe this hormone, start with 1 mg at night, possibly with the other supplement suggestions in this section, and then increase each night by 1 mg until sleep has been achieved WITHOUT having sluggishness the next morning. If you become sluggish at a particular dose, then lower by 1 mg or more until the sluggishness has resolved. Remember that your physician can have the melatonin compounded for you into one pill if your dose becomes high and you are taking multiple 1 mg pills. (Special thanks to my good friend and colleague Nael Dagstani, N.M.D., for this melatonin protocol.)

Step 2: The 5 Pillars

Pillar 2: Exercise

An entire chapter has been devoted to this pillar because its relevance for overall health and well-being cannot be overstated. The bottom line is… move. Move with purpose. Move with fervor. Move for fun. Move for your life. Move for your metabolic health.

As a review, be sure to consider the high intensity, short duration exercise as an easy way to stimulate your metabolism, balance your hormones, and get physically fit. The higher the intensity while exercising, the more fruitful your exercise.

Here again are the basics to get you started in the right direction. You can utilize different movements that you find interesting and fun. Almost any movement can be done with high intensity. Remember that *intensity* of the movement is the key. For example:

- Sprinting/Walking
- Stationary bike
- Jumping Jacks
- Jumping rope
- Weight training

With weight training, use compound movements that utilize as many joints in the exercise as possible, such as squats or overhead presses. Then, you can also incorporate hybrid movements by combining traditional exercise movements into one exercise, such as a squat combined with arm curls. This also has the added benefit of taking old movements and giving them a fresh and fun makeover.

To keep the intensity up, alternate between all out exertion of your chosen exercise and then recovery. Here's how:

- Beginners: (new to this type of exercise) Exert yourself for 30 seconds in your exercise of choice, then recover for 120 seconds. Repeat this six to eight times.
- Intermediate: (training for about one month) Exert for 30 seconds, then recover for 90 seconds. Repeat this eight to ten times.
- Advanced: (training for over three months) Exert for 30 seconds, then recover for 60 to 90 seconds. Repeat this eight to ten times.

Keep your exercise time to forty minutes or less. In fact, when you first start utilizing high intensity exercise, ten to twenty minutes can be extremely beneficial. Remember to warm up and cool down before and after your exercise, and include light stretching once you are warmed up and at the end of the routine. You only need to exercise two to four times per week. Be aware that the increased metabolic rate is lasting well past your time spent exercising.

Pillar 3: Lifestyle Changes and Cleansing as Process

I define lifestyle change as avoiding stressful situations, or even more accurately, moving towards non-stressful moments. Stress comes in many forms. Typically, stress is perceived as something that affects us mentally and perhaps emotionally. But usually we do not consider the other types of stress, such as spiritual and physical/chemical stress. Spiritual stress comes from many things, but is most often related to a lack of connection with your true self and fundamental purpose.

Most often, when I explain to patients that they need to avoid stressful situations, they smile, roll their eyes, and lament that they are in situations that they cannot avoid. Because that reaction is so common, a further definition of lifestyle change is learning how to cope with those situations that you cannot avoid.

> I define lifestyle change as avoiding stressful situations, or even more accurately, moving towards non-stressful moments.

How Do You Truly Make a Lifestyle Change?

The easy answer is to avoid the stress in the first place! You do not have to run away from it, simply move towards something else that is fulfilling. Do you see the difference? We often believe that we will have success from running away, quitting or avoiding. This strategy usually leaves us vacant and unsatisfied and we go back to what was known, even if it is unhealthy for us. The trick is to find the things that are fulfilling on all levels and then move towards those things. Once that is done, there will be no room or need for the other stressful situations, and they will, by necessity, just go away. This may be a simplification, but in most circumstances, it is true. For example, patients say to me that they want to quit smoking. Quitting anything can be difficult because your brain does not want to give up almost anything, even if it is bad. A better strategy is to

> We often believe that we will have success from running away, quitting or avoiding. This strategy usually leaves us vacant and unsatisfied and we go back to what was known, even if it is unhealthy for us. The trick is to find the things that are fulfilling on all levels and then move towards those things.

become a non-smoker. This means thinking, acting, breathing, becoming, and living like a non-smoker. Once that focus has been established and practiced, the act of smoking, by necessity, just goes away. It is not part of the "computer program in your brain" anymore and just slips away as your focus on the new way of being. A further key example is losing weight. Another way of looking at this process is by telling yourself to become a physically fit person free from the constraints of negative attitudes and food choices. One of the reasons that many diets do not work is because the dieter does not set up any type of permanent lifestyle change, or a pattern of events that can be built upon and individualized along the path and journey of health. Diets focus on the things that you can't have only until you lose the weight. Many diets do not focus enough on teaching you to explore the wonderful and new things that you can enjoy.

Learning How to Cope: Mental Health

As we all know and understand, we cannot always move away from stress. People get themselves in situations that for one reason or another, necessitates them to engage directly and face the problems directly. Actually, these moments of stress are gifts, as they provide unique opportunities to make change, grow, and learn.

Consider this advice when you find yourself in a stressful situation:

- Learn to let go. Sometimes, just say no. Eliminate things from your to-do list and learn to delegate. Simplify your life. Being busy does not necessarily increase your worth as a person, as so many people believe. Give yourself permission to just be.
- Forgive. Forgive yourself. Forgive others. Let go of your pain and judgment.
- Find balance. Express your emotions, but learn to be silent. Assert yourself and your sense of will, but allow others around you to do the same. Discipline yourself, but do not raise the bar too high. Let go. Expend your energy for others, give to others, but draw the line at giving too much. Learn to give from the space of your own fulfillment so that you are not giving in order to receive.
- Be good to yourself. Know your boundaries and stick to them. Communicate your needs and strive for understanding in all relationships.
- Be positive. Perspective is a choice. Attitude is a choice. Use positive words; think positive thoughts. Fill your mind with the positive thoughts of those who think and speak positively.
- Have fun. Laugh with others, laugh at others when appropriate; laugh at yourself. One of the greatest secrets is the power of mirth. Do not take life too seriously.
- Remember, bondage is an illusion… only you have the power to control an outcome.
- Know that your perception of a problem is your perception. You have a problem because of your ignorance, or lack of understanding. Your lack of understanding is born out of accepting some appearance at

face value. And as your problem worsens, your word choices express poor observation.

Cleansing for Your Metabolic Health

Cleansing is the ultimate process of moving towards something while letting go of other things. The process of cleansing helps to discipline you towards exploring what is important and can teach you to accept your true self. There are all kinds of ways to cleanse, ranging from food related dietary cleanses to eliminating old ways of being, thinking, and old habits. Cleansing has spiritual and religious implications and has been used since time immemorial to help prepare someone for higher echelons of being. Within the rich history of naturopathic medicine and the spas and sanitariums from the late eighteenth century into the early nineteenth century, cleansing was at the very core of the medical prescription. The particular physical benefits are many and should be part of a basic yearly process for anyone looking to optimize their metabolic health.

Eliminating and Avoiding "Endocrine Disruptor Chemicals"

Your endocrine system is extremely sensitive to foreign chemicals, particularly manmade chemicals. These chemicals have been linked to a multitude of endocrine disorders such as diabetes, cardiovascular disease, thyroid disorders, sex hormone imbalances and gynecological issues, endocrine cancers, and even obesity. The chemicals that are related to obesity have been dubbed "obesogens" and are being studied as key endocrine disruptor chemicals that are contributing to the obesity epidemic. The top three obesogens are:

- Bisphenol-a (BPA), found in plastics with recycling codes 3 and 7 and in the linings of cans of canned food products.
- Organotins, which are biocides found in conventionally grown produce.
- Phthalates are found in plastics and personal care products like nail polish, shampoo, lotions, and perfumes.

To avoid obesogens and other endocrine disruptor chemicals, follow this advice:

- Chose organic foods when possible to avoid pesticides. (See The Dirty Dozen and The Clean Fifteen in Step 2 of The Metabolic Health Protocol.)
- Buy canned foods in BPA-free cans. Vital Choice and Eden Foods produce canned goods with BPA free liners.
- Drink spring water in safe BPA-free bottles or filter your water using reverse osmosis and store it in glass containers.
- Store your food in glass containers. Never heat your food in plastic containers in the microwave because it leaches phthalates directly into your food.
- Use organic personal care products when possible. Whole Foods, Trader Joe's, Sprouts, and many local health food stores have excellent choices.
- Avoid plastics. The "new car smell" indicates phthalates are present.
- Cleanse on a regular basis.

A Simple Cleanse

This is an introduction to cleansing. If you are curious about more in-depth cleansing, then consult a qualified healthcare professional. But this first step can be very profound. There are many cleanses out on the market and you should absolutely be sure to consult your healthcare provider before embarking on any cleanse. Before you buy any cleanse product, follow the protocol below for a simple cleanse.

- This is a simple week long cleanse. It is an elimination process that slowly adds foods back into the daily diet. For the first three days eat organic fruits and vegetables, light organic vegetable broths, and herbal teas. Avoid animal flesh, dairy, grains, and legumes such as beans and nuts on the first three days. On the fourth day you can add in protein sources such as organic raw nuts and sprouted grains. On the fifth day, add fish. On the sixth and seventh day, you can add in poultry and regular grains if desired. However, you could continue on fish as the only animal protein, with all the nuts and legumes you would like. That's it. Nothing fancy in terms of ways of eating and specific supplements. This strategy alone helps to improve digestion and eliminate unwanted fat stores in a slow, gentle, and safe manner.

Key Considerations While on the Simple Cleanse

These considerations are sometimes more important than what you should eat or what supplements to take. When you cleanse, you take the opportunity to cleanse from everything that comes into your system, not just food and drink.

Rest

- This is a time to rest and reflect.
- Avoid as many stressful situations as you can by putting off appointments or any situation that you absolutely do not need to deal with for the week.
- Get that extra hour or two of sleep during this week by simply going to bed a little earlier.
- Do not watch the news. Take a break from the excitement of our times, just for the week.
- Eliminate smoking, alcohol, and caffeine during this time.

Water

- Drink 1/2 ounce of water per pound of body weight. This is similar to the advice you may have heard about drinking eight cups of water per day. This is very important during this time.
- Add a small amount of Celtic Sea Salt to your water to help with electrolyte balance.

Daily Practices

- Dry brush your skin with a dry loofa. This increases circulation and assists the elimination process. Always brush towards the heart.
- Cleanse the sinuses with a Neti Pot using a sea salt solution using distilled bottled water. Avoid tap water when using a Neti Pot as the contaminants in tap water could potentially be harmful to the sinus

cavity. You can find a Neti Pot at drug stores and health food stores. Do this in the morning when rising and then right before bed.

- When taking a shower, run hot water for thirty seconds then cold water for thirty seconds. Repeat this seven times to create a cleansing hydrotherapy effect.
- Minimize use of chemical-based household products and choose all-natural personal healthcare products.
- Breathe deeply to get oxygen circulating.
- Meditate, think, reflect, write about your cleanse experience in a journal.
- Sit in a dry sauna to sweat in order to eliminate waste. Start slowly for about ten to twenty minutes.
- Keep exercise to a minimum during this time, but do not avoid it all together. Take a thirty minute walk in the morning for exercise. This helps to kick start the digestion and elimination processes and keeps the mind aware. Add a few days of light yoga.
- Have at least one colonic during this time to encourage bowel elimination and toxin removal. Colonics are gentle and safe and not to be feared.

Pillar 4: Mental Health

This book has provided some suggestions for helping with your mental well-being. And these suggestions are by no means exhaustive so I encourage you to explore more avenues specific to your own personality and life path. Books can be an excellent source of inspiration and thought-provoking ideas that have the ability to lead you to a moment of change. Seminars of all types are also available that can bring a more interactive component to the equation. Sometimes people need more, such as a direct level of care, the advice and guidance of a professional. Do not be shy if you think you may need to be in the care of a psychiatrist, psychologist or counselor.

Here is a simplified list of these types of mental healthcare activities, therapies, and professionals.

Mental Activity: Keep the Mind Sharp

Learning is a lifelong process and layers of thought and understanding must be laid down continuously. When your true purpose is understood, you can more easily make your way through the efforts of thought and learning to fulfill your mission. The newest understandings of neurology and the study of the brain shows that it is very plastic and capable of learning new things, despite age and even brain damage. One of the best ways to keep the mind sharp throughout life is to simply keep learning new things. Challenge yourself to do crossword and number puzzles. Make a practice of reading books. Take a class in a topic that interests you. Use your leisure time to engage in activities you enjoy instead of just watching television.

> **When your true purpose is understood, you can more easily make your way through the efforts of thought and learning to fulfill your mission.**

Prayer and Meditation

This activity has some definite overlap with both mental and spiritual aspects. If there is any one thing that you take from this book and incorporate in your daily life, this would be it. Meditate, think, pray to a higher source, reflect, be thankful, release, contact yourself internally and recognize how you are intertwined with your personal concept of God. This ancient science has proven effective over and over again throughout the ages by scientific method, religious and spiritual testament, and even by agnostic medical pragmatists. Meditation is simply mental concentration on a particular thought, object or on nothing particular except relaxation and attention to your breath. Meditation is natural. And when we meditate, our true desire naturally expresses itself. You do not need to learn *how* to meditate. What you need to learn is what you've been doing or not doing *with* your powers of meditation all along. A good example of this is that when you drive, your mind is on getting to where you are going.

This attention to task is a form of meditation! When you are cooking something and following a recipe and process, this attention is a form of meditation! If you are walking and thinking, you are actually doing a meditation. A great way to calm your mind is to close your eyes, take two deep breaths and then place your index finger in the middle of your forehead. The sensation of touch will focus your

> Meditate, think, pray to a higher source, reflect, be thankful, release, contact yourself internally and recognize how you are intertwined with your personal concept of God.

Step 2: The 5 Pillars

thoughts forward to the feeling and bring you a momentary bit of peace which will lead you to better direct your next thought.

Meditation teaches you how to be in the moment and fully present by focusing your mind and attention. But the purpose of this ability to focus while meditating is to solve a problem. That's it. Yes, it is relaxing, or at least can be relaxing. Yes, it helps you to breathe. And yes, it helps you to focus. But, focus on what? Meditation helps you to focus your intention to discover the *solution* to a problem. Even your deepest desires, something that you would like to move toward, can be framed into the context of a problem. And then focused meditation can help to release the answers you have within you. Simply focus on the problem and wait for the answers to reveal themselves.

If you do not already meditate, start. If you already meditate or pray, do not assume that you are doing it enough or even correctly. I am not offering the right way at all. I am offering, however, that you must continue, at all levels, to explore. Any of the past spiritual masters could tell you that they continually worked on their meditation skills. It was never over, even for them. I have many patients, when the concept of spirituality is brought up, who assume that because they go to church every Sunday, they have and do incorporate spirituality enough for them. The frequency may or may not be enough. The connection may still need enhancement. Keep working on this.

Be sure to find out exactly what you want, your true purpose, and move towards that. Move towards the way you envision your lifestyle would be. Decide. Truly decide. Words seem inadequate to explain this fully. Work to create a vision for your life. See what you could be capable of and send yourself to that kind of a future by using your mind

> **Be sure to find out exactly what you want, your true purpose, and move towards that. Move towards the way you envision your lifestyle would be. Decide. Truly decide.**

and the power of your imagination. And let your healthcare provider in on what you are doing to create the lifestyle you desire. He or she will be a willing participant in helping you reach your goal.

Bodywork and Massage Therapy

This is one of the most profound things you can do for your mental healthcare. Of course, it helps with your body also. I have a personal vestment in this advice due to my previous career as a massage therapist for over fourteen years and had the wonderful opportunity to work with many people helping them in body, mind, and soul with this simple art and science. Utilizing the methods of massage and bodywork can help to unwind the mental turmoil of the day and even the emotional anguish of years of pain. Massage therapy truly is medicine as it has the dramatic potential of providing lasting healing and profound understandings about yourself, if you let it. Establishing a relationship with a good therapist over time can guide you to new levels of health. Of course, beyond the mental and emotional benefits there are direct physiological benefits that can change posture, eliminate pain, free restricted joints, improve circulation and health to organs and enhance your metabolism. Do not underestimate its potential for healing and change.

Books and Seminars

Countless examples and resources are at your disposal. Read and engage your mind and power of reason towards discovering the various truths about the soul that exist. The trick about the books that people read and the seminars they attend is actually following through with the message and incorporating the change that is recommended. Be sure to follow through and take action. Personally, Anthony Robbins has been an inspiration for me over the years, being influenced by his work early at the age of eighteen, contributing to my later personal successes. His true gift is his ability to inspire people to actually take action on the information that he is providing. A physician can suggest many amazing things for your health, but if you do not take action and follow through, it means very little. And of course, taking action is the whole point of this book you are reading right now. Take action!

Support Groups

Some people need the one-on-one setting when it comes to finding others to help them find their way. Others naturally seek out the validation and support of a group of like-minded individuals who truly have had similar experiences and who enjoy sharing the lessons learned. Explore these options for yourself, based on your personality. One of the key human experiences is to feel validated by at least one other human being, particularly about a problem or a painful experience. Validation lets you know that you are alive. By being in the company of loving witnesses, you then become a loving witness yourself.

Counseling/Life Coaching/Psychotherapy/Psychiatry

Many of my patients do not necessarily need to advance to this level of mental healthcare. Some of them do, and I do not hesitate to direct them to resources. When the decision is made to explore this level of involvement, it can be profoundly life-altering and beneficial. If either you or your healthcare provider believes you need to explore this option, do not fear it. You will learn the lessons of self in a most profound way when you align yourself with a professional who can guide you, and possibly even prescribe a medication if what you are suffering is due to a chemical imbalance.

Pillar 5: Spirituality

"Truth is that which is; there can not be that which is not. Therefore, that which is, or truth, must be all there is."

George Burnell

Spirituality is an internal and external exploration of the question, "Why am I here?" It is one of the most profound questions you can ask. Spirituality is a connection with the "Other," the "Source," the "Primal Will," with whatever you perceive to be God. Spirituality, and its internal exploration, is practiced in many ways, including through participation in an organized religion, prayer, meditation, study, and self-contemplation. To be the healthiest you can be, to have the personal freedom that you desire, a sense of spirituality is necessary. The majority of scientific studies agree that people who have a sense of spirituality and who have an active spiritual practice, such as a being a member of a religious group or spiritual community, live longer and are healthier.

I have found that patients do in fact wish to discuss with me their spirituality or a spiritual crisis that they are experiencing. I have also found that, all too often, patients forget that their lack of spiritual connection and practice could be leading, or at least contributing, to their physical ailments. This is a repeated theme throughout this book: our physical makeup is influenced directly and indirectly by the other facets of our being,

> **The majority of scientific studies agree that people who have a sense of spirituality and who have an active spiritual practice, such as a being a member of a religious group or spiritual community, live longer and are healthier.**

which is who we are and how we operate on mental, emotional, and spiritual levels.

Often, our spirit calls out for a connection with the present moment, but we overlook it in order to review the burdensome past or skip into the unpredictable future. Spiritual stress can come in the form of lacking a connection with a fundamental source of life, however you may define that. Or spiritual stress can be with the innermost being of yourself. When you question the source, when you question why you are here, you may get a sense that you are not here under your own power. You may get a sense of something larger and outside of the human being you think you are. Sometimes people realize that there really are no answers to their personal questions and that moving forward is a matter of trust and faith. It is in those times that one really learns of their power to love, learn, and grow.

Spiritual Unfoldment:
Answering Questions, Solving Problems

Here is a way to utilize different spiritual aspects to find peace and a connection with your higher self. I am describing here the stages of spiritual growth, common to most religions. These stages can also be viewed as steps towards analyzing and moving through a problem. As you read through each step, you will be asked different questions about your practices, or beliefs about the concept that is presented. Take some time to think about your answers and consider writing your answers in a journal.

Step 1: Bondage is an illusion and there is more to life than what the five senses may indicate. Do not take any situation at face value. Realize that your problem as it appears on the surface, is the illusion of suffering and difficulty. Suffering comes from only looking at things instead of looking into them. So, look deeper. Also, stand back and take a different view of the bondage that you feel holds you. See it in your imagination as an illusion and figure out the way you would

Bondage is an illusion.

act if it were invisible. Learn to laugh at the absurdity of your problem. Remember the power of mirth. Ask yourself:

- Do I judge a problem at its face value without looking past the absurdity?
- Where and why do I feel trapped?
- Have I blamed my shortcomings on others?
- Will I be able to face my dark side?
- Is this problem smaller or larger than I imagine it to be?

Step 2: Enter an awakening from the nightmare and the flawed structure that you self-created. Position and allow yourself to be shocked out of your own erroneous structure. Problems often continue even when we think we solved them, because our ego structure is still the same. Pain is the resistance to change. You are only in pain when you resist. Allow the change that is necessary. Free yourself from judgment and do not expect a certain outcome. Realize that only you are in this process—no one else can read your mind or swoop in with a miracle to take care of you. But know that you have all the power you need on your own to understand your problem and see a way around it or out of it. Ask yourself:

> **Position and allow yourself to be shocked out of your own erroneous structure.**

- What deep-seated belief or fear needs to be uprooted?
- What am I holding on to? Why am I holding so tight?
- What unpleasant realization or truth must I now confront?
- What lesson am I in the process of learning?

Step 3: After you have opened your mind, revelation, clear thought, and of true purpose, is open to arise and make itself known. This is all about understanding the need for brotherly and sisterly love, experiencing relief and tolerance and seeing a truth beyond yourself. This comes from meditation and focus of attention. Ask yourself:

- What truth do I wish to know, no matter what it reveals?

- Why do I avoid the internal reflection of prayer and meditation?
- What is my Purpose?
- Am I afraid to focus on the things I desire?

Step 4: Once you have gotten clarity, organization of thought and imagination within, your *body* will lead you towards your true purpose. You must align your body to incorporate your new thought patterns towards your problem. This entire book reflects this need. Go back and review the Health Affirmation Statement you took time to write when you saw it introduced at the beginning of this book. It helps to cement new thought patterns by exploring the specific effect of each of your thoughts on the body make up.

Ask yourself:

- What memories haunt me? If you experienced abuse or other kinds of negativity as a child, take a look at www.acestudy.org for a way to help your healthcare professional assess the effects of any adverse childhood experiences you may be carrying. Healing is possible.
- What hidden thoughts and feelings am I not expressing?
- What does my purpose look and feel like?
- Is my body ready and willing to change along with my new thought pattern?

Step 5: After you face your innermost questions with honesty, regeneration of your mind and body begins to occur. Your purpose in life and lessons to learn will become clear. Regeneration is also a stage of conscious self-identification with God. You begin to change as a person

> After you have opened your mind, revelation, clear thought, and of true purpose, is open to arise and make itself known.

> After you face your innermost questions with honesty, regeneration of your mind and body begins to occur.

Step 2: The 5 Pillars

and you will begin to live life at a different level than in the past. Ask yourself:

- How can I bring my personal revelations and purpose to the world?
- How can I create an enjoyable life?
- In what ways can I serve others or my community?

Step 6: Realization and knowing the world as it truly exists begins to bubble up into your new mind. This will help you get past a problem and on towards a larger perspective. This is an understanding that we are all interconnected as one, even the people that we believe are diametrically opposed to us and who create problems for us. At this level, you will begin to view even strangers as part of your personal existence and see them as part of the mass consciousness in which you exist. Ask yourself:

- Is the judgment of myself and others harmful?
- What is the effect of judgment by others on me?
- What new realization with regard to being one part of the whole am I open to experiencing?

Step 7: After doing all the work involved in these steps, you begin to be aware of the cosmic consciousness and you may even have a personal experience with God. This is the ineffable thing. You must figure this out for yourself. But the more you strive for connection on this level, the more your problems will gain perspective and therefore be easier to handle and solve. Strive for self-mastery to overcome the mundane.

> Strive for self-mastery to overcome the mundane.

Ask yourself:

- Where have I achieved mastery?
- What does it feel like?
- Am I connected to God or Spirit? How?

Facing the Shadow

"Everyone carries a shadow, and the less it is embodied in the individual's conscious life, the blacker and denser it is. At all counts, it forms an unconscious snag, thwarting our most well-meant intentions."   —Dr. Carl G. Jung

The shadow is our hidden, suppressed, and often directly rejected feelings that typically manifest themselves in negative reactions towards ourselves and particularly others. I have placed this concept in this section because the shadow can be defined to have mental and emotional difficulties, as well as spiritual and moral conflicts.

When we repress any experience it typically will find a way to manifest itself. This is a basic law of nature and is an integral part of the naturopathic philosophy. Nature will find a way to express itself, and negatively if necessary. This negative expression or "voice of the body" is called a symptom. These symptoms can be physical as well as mental and emotional. But here, we are exploring the mental and emotional manifestation of suppressed shadow aspects. For example, when we always feel rejected by others, it could be that the hidden shadow form is that you yourself reject others. Or your sense of self-consciousness stems from the shadow form of placing a constant outward focus on others. When you are sad, it is because you have repressed being angry, or when you always say "I can't" it is really because you are afraid to say the truth of, "I won't."

The shadow is created when we suppress our true feelings and this creates behavioral patterns of symptomatic expression that continue to block our route to happiness.

Why is Facing the Shadow Important?

Facing your shadow side takes work. But shadow work frees up wasted energy. It increases your metabolism. Keeping your true emotions suppressed while maintaining the structure of a shadow form takes energy, and a lot of it. This type of work also creates a sense

> **Shadow work frees up wasted energy. It increases your metabolism.**

of compassion, forgiveness, and empathy towards others, particularly those who are in your life to bother you, stir your emotions, and to help you learn the lessons you need to learn to be a happier, healthier, better person.

People instinctually fear this process. People do not want to face these hidden aspects of themselves. Nor do they want to accept that they are carrying around such debilitating beliefs. But the longer you wait, the worse it gets. And this ultimately affects your health on all levels. It is these types of issues that are dictating so many of the physical symptoms that patients present with to me on a daily basis. Either you will decide to own your shadow, or it will continue to own you.

The 3 – 2 – 1 Shadow Process

Psychotherapy is a process that can help you to delve into your shadow self, at significant cost and time. It can be very beneficial and is often necessary. Psychologists and psychiatrists are trained to help you make changes at the core of your being. However, there are options and ways to work on your shadow without working directly with a psychotherapist. There are many options available. Ken Wilber and The Integral Institute have developed one particular simplified process that shows you how to delve into shadow work on your own. Here is a summary of this 3 – 2 – 1 process adapted from Ken Wilber's book *Integral Life Practice*.[359]

Choose an experience in your life that you want to work with. Choose a person with whom you have difficulty who may irritate, disturb, annoy or upset you. Or a person you feel attracted to, obsessed with, infatuated with or possessive about. Just choose someone with whom you have a strong emotional charge, whether positive or negative.

3 – Face It: Describe the qualities about this person that most upset you, or the characteristics that you are most attracted to using third-person language (he, she). Talk about them out loud or write it down in a journal. Take this opportunity to let out all the emotions you feel. Don't try to be skillful or say the right thing. The person you are describing will never hear or see this.

2 – Talk to It: Begin an imaginary dialogue with this person. Speak in second person to this person (using "you" and "me"). Talk directly to this person as if he or she were actually there in the room with you. Tell them what bothers you about them. Ask them questions such as "Why are you doing this to me?" "What do you want from me?" "What are you trying to show me?" "What do you have to teach me?" Imagine their response to these questions. Speak that imaginary response out loud. Record the conversation in your journal if you like.

1 – Be It: Become this person. Take on the qualities that either annoy or fascinate you. Embody the traits you described in "Face It." Use first-person language (I, me, mine). This may feel awkward, and it should. The traits you are taking on are the exact traits that you have been denying in yourself. Use statements such as "I am angry," "I am jealous," "I am radiant." Fill in the blank with whatever qualities you are working with: "I am_____." To complete the process, notice these disowned qualities in yourself. Experience the part of you that *is* this very trait. Avoid making the process abstract or conceptual: just BE it. Now you can re-own and integrate this trait in yourself. Facing your shadow is a life-long process. This should not be a fear, but a relief that nothing is perfect and we can function very well even when we have some shadows lurking. But we still need to face them to optimize our health. Shadows come and shadows go. Just as health has been described in this book as a dynamic process of ever-flowing change, so too does this apply to your psychological and spiritual well-being.

Step 3:
Nutritional and Herbal Supplements for Metabolism and Body Composition Management
Introduction

You may think you can have optimal health without help. But let's start with the basic supplements that I believe everyone should know about. After those, you'll read about metabolic supplementation. Here are the four most important things to consider adding to your diet:

❷ Multivitamin

❷ Essential Fatty Acids (Fish Oil)

❷ Vitamin B Complex containing a complete array of B vitamins

❷ Vitamin D

When I was in naturopathic medical school, one of my nutrition professors put it plainly when describing the need for basic nutritional supplements. She said, "If you are alive and breathing, you should at least be on a multivitamin and fish oil!"

Due to depleted vitamin and mineral contents of our soil, even organically grown fruits and vegetables are lacking in proper nutrition. This makes basic nutritional fortification essential. Additionally, due to the overabundance of omega 6 fatty acids in our diets coming from corn, sunflower, and safflower oils, our need for a proper ratio of omega 3 essential fatty acids from sources such as fish oil is critical. I also recommend a B complex formula and vitamin D as additional basic foundational vitamins. The B vitamins are imperative for proper cellular metabolism and the benefits of vitamin D are innumerable and have been mentioned elsewhere in this book. If most people regularly took these four vitamin supplements, many health issues would and could be avoided and improved.

To avoid stomach irritation from your supplements:

❷ Unless specifically noted, take supplement pills with food.

❷ Do not lie down immediately after taking your supplements.

❷ To increase the likelihood that you will take your supplements:

> - Keep supplements in view as much as possible such as on a counter in the kitchen or bathroom.
> - Take most of your supplements with breakfast or dinner—the two times of the day that most people experience some routine. Taking supplements in the middle of the day, unless you have some consistent pattern well established for lunchtime, is more difficult.

Multivitamins

Patients often inquire about which type or brand of multivitamin to take. There are many on the market. The easiest way to ensure you are procuring the best possible quality and efficacious supplement, be sure to choose something your healthcare provider suggests for you. Usually, a healthcare provider is familiar with higher quality supplements from reputable companies that maintain excellent standards. This helps to eliminate much of the guessing.

In general, your multivitamin should be complete in its array of nutrients, but at the same time have adequate amounts of the things offered. This needs to be balanced. Most people do not have degrees in chemistry and need help to determine what the right amount of a certain mineral will be for them. Sometimes, a multivitamin will have many different things in it, but without the potency of each thing to make it effective. On the other hand, it could have a smaller array of potent factors in the formula, but not offer a large enough array of what the body needs. Again, check with your healthcare provider.

Essential Fatty Acids (Fish Oil and Flax Seed Oil)

One of the most common problems in our diets today is the lack of "good" fats. Key essential fatty acids are the omega 3s. There are two, with names you need to know: eicosapentaenoic acid (EPA) and docosahexaenoic acid (DHA). Both of these essential fatty acids have been linked to lowered cholesterol and triglycerides, improved heart health, decreased joint pain, and lowered inflammation. When inflammation is high in the body, diseases of all types can occur. Essential fatty acids keep inflammation to a minimum.

Fish Oil

Patients are very concerned about the taste and quality of fish oil. When fish oil has been manufactured poorly with little concern for quality and purity, then the potential for a rancid, fishy odor and taste is high. Be sure to choose a high quality fish oil that is free from odor. In fact, when the quality is high, fish oil can have a very pleasant taste.

Flax Seed Oil

This option is for anyone who is a strict vegan and wants to avoid animal sources for their supplements. I mention it here because it is a popular oil. Flax seed oil provides mostly omega 6 essential fatty acids and less omega 3. A large portion of the omega 6 fatty acids in the flax seed oil can be converted into a substance known as arachidonic acid which is a known pro-inflammatory substance. Also, the omega 3 fatty acids in the flax seed oil have a difficulty in being broken down chemically into EPA and DHA, as mentioned above. In general, I do not recommend this vegan source for essential fatty acids, but prefer chia seeds.

Vitamin B Complex

A vitamin B complex supplement should contain a complete array of the B vitamins: B1, B2, B3, B5, B6, B12, biotin, and folate (folic acid). These vitamins are absolutely imperative for energy production in the cell and this formula should not be underestimated in its ability to help improve energy levels in general. When cells are being driven by stimulants such as thyroid hormone, caffeine, and others, the demand for B vitamins increases to make the chemical reactions occur, and ultimately you feel your best.

There are a few potential problems with the B complex formula. Nausea, flushing, and anxious energy are the three most reported symptoms. The best strategy to alleviate these problems is to take the recommended amount in divided doses such as two or three times per day versus once daily and/or lower the overall amount of the dose. Taking a lowered tolerable amount is better than taking nothing at all.

Vitamin D

The benefits of this pro-hormone are numerous and they were covered in Step 2 of The Metabolic Health Protocol. This is a key metabolic supplement and its vast role in enhancing human health should not be underestimated. Be sure to take a liquid form of this vitamin as it is the most absorbable and therefore efficient way of optimizing vitamin D levels in the blood.

Metabolic Supplements

The first section focused on the basic supplements that are important for everyone who is trying to achieve optimal health in general. Now we can focus on additional supplements that can help to take your metabolic health to the next level. There are so many nutritional supplements and medicinal herbal medicines available for optimized health, increased metabolism, and weight loss. This list is not exhaustive, but rather focused on the main elements that reflect sound research and my personal clinical experience.

Use the outline below to customize what supplements you might consider based on your individual needs and goals. Refer back to this chart to ensure you are getting the basics in place as you move along on your health journey. There is overlap of some of the supplements based on the category. The specific explanations and dosage recommendations of each supplement are provided below in alphabetical order. Some of the supplements have been discussed in previous chapters and sections.

- ❧ Weight Loss
  - ❧ Cleansing and Detox
    - ❧ Metabolic spices
    - ❧ Milk Thistle (*Silybum marianum*)
    - ❧ Fiber (Salba [chia] seed: *Salvia hispanica L*)

- Appetite control
  - Fiber (Salba [chia] seed: *Salvia hispanica* L)
  - Metabolic Spices
  - Bitter Orange (*Citrus aurantium*) (Synephrine)
  - Yerba mate *(Ilex paraguayensis)*
  - Gudmar (*Gymnema sylvestre*)
- Mood Enhancement
  - Cocoa (*Theobroma cacao*) (Theobromine)
  - 5-hydroxytryptophan (5-HTP)
- Blood sugar and insulin management
  - Metabolic spices
  - Chromium picolinate
  - Bitter melon *(Momordica charantia)*
  - Fenugreek (*Trigonella foenum-graecum*)
  - Gudmar (*Gymnema sylvestre*)
  - Goat's rue (*Galega officinalis*)
  - Fiber (Salba seed: *Salvia hispanica* L)
- Metabolism boosting and Energy
  - Metabolic spices
  - Green tea and Green tea extract (EGCG)
  - Bitter orange (*Citrus aurantium*) (Synephrine)
  - Coleus (*Coleus forskohlii*) (Forskolin)
  - Citrulline malate
  - Calcium pyruvate
- Exercise Support
  - Protein Supplements
  - Creatine monohydrate
  - Citrulline malate
- IV (Intravenous) and IM (Intramuscular) Nutrient Therapy
- Thyroid Support
  - Bladderwrack (*Fucus vesiculosis*)
  - Iodine
  - Coconut Oil

- Zinc with copper
- Selenium
- Tyrosine
- Iron
- Guggul (*Commiphora mukul*)
- Blue flag (*Iris versicolor*)
- Dietary desiccated thyroid powder
- Adrenal Support
  - Vitamin C
  - Magnesium
  - Zinc
  - Selenium
  - Pantothenic acid (B5)
  - Phosphatidyl serine
  - Licorice (*Glycyrrhiza glabra*)
  - Ashwagandha (*Withania somnifera*)
  - Dietary desiccated adrenal glandular
- Sex Hormone Support
  - For Women
    - DIM (di-indoyl methane)
    - Calcium and magnesium
    - Black cohosh *(Cimcifuga racemosa)*
    - Maca (*Lepidium meyenii*)
  - For Men
    - Zinc
    - DIM (di-indoyl methane)
    - Longjack (*Tongkat ali*)
    - Puncture vine (*Tribulus terrestris*)
    - Maca (*Lepidum meyenii*)

5-HTP (5-Hydroxytryptophan)

5-HTP is an amino acid derived directly from the amino acid l-tryptophan, and is used in the production of the brain chemical serotonin.

Serotonin is responsible for regulating mood and normal sleep patterns and has been highly associated with helping with depression. Other brain chemicals such as melatonin, dopamine, norepinephrine, and endorphins have also been shown to increase when using 5-HTP.[360, 361]

The use of 5-HTP has also been associated with improving headaches, pain associated with fibromyalgia, and even weight loss. Regarding weight loss, 5-HTP acts mostly as an appetite modulator. When calories are initially lowered along with carbohydrate restriction, serotonin levels drop.[362] These low serotonin levels lead to carbohydrate cravings and binge eating. Using 5-HTP can be helpful to control this.[363, 364]

Caution! It is possible that 5-HTP could interfere with SSRI drugs such as Prozac®, Zoloft®, Wellbutrin® and others, although there are no published reports to my knowledge and I have never seen this before. However, if 5-HTP is to be used while on one of these medications, close monitoring by your healthcare provider is recommended.

The initial dosage for 5-HTP is usually 50 mg three times per day with meals and may be increased to 100 mg three times per day, depending on need. When helping with depression, the dose often needs to be at least 300 mg total for the day, and even more. Some studies have used up to 3,000 mg daily. I would not recommend that at all, but the point is that to be effective for some people, the dose may need to exceed 300 mg daily. Always consult with your healthcare provider.

Bitter melon *(Momordica charantia)*

Bitter melon has been shown to aid in weight loss in studies with both animals[365] and humans.[366] Interestingly, bitter melon has been shown to increase the actual size of the insulin producing β cells in the pancreas that also led to increased insulin production.[367, 368] This is important in both the treatment and prevention of insulin-dependent or type I diabetes. All too often, poorly monitored and treated patients with non-insulin dependent diabetes worsen to eventually need insulin. Bitter melon has effectively and consistently demonstrated to be effective in the management of diabetes and/or metabolic syndromes for years.[369]

When bitter melon is used with other supplements, such as the ones listed in this section, a synergistic effect is created leading to an enhanced additive benefit for lowering and controlling blood sugar.[370]

> **All too often, poorly monitored and treated patients with non-insulin dependent diabetes worsen to eventually need insulin.**

Reported adverse effects of bitter melon include hypoglycemic coma, convulsions in children, reduced fertility in mice, a fauvism-like syndrome, increased enzyme activities of γ-glutamyl transferase, alkaline phosphatase in animals, and headaches in humans.

For dried bitter melon, effective doses range from 3-15 grams. For a standardized extract pill, use 100-200 mg three times daily. Bitter melon tinctures are condensed liquid herbal preparations that can also be used at about one teaspoon (5 ml) two to three times per day. As a "power food," a small melon can be eaten daily. You can also drink the fresh juice, about two ounces (60 ml) daily. Always avoid eating or juicing the seeds as they are potentially toxic in large amounts.

Bitter orange (*Citrus aurantium*) (Synephrine)

Citrus aurantium, or bitter orange, comes from a flowering, citrus fruit-bearing evergreen tree native to tropical Asia, but is now widely cultivated in the Mediterranean region and elsewhere. It has been shown to provide excellent results at stimulating metabolism, increasing fat loss, facilitating uptake of amino acids into muscles, and mildly suppressing appetite.

There have been over two dozen research articles published on the safety and efficacy of *Citrus aurantium* since 1997.[371] The specific controversial concern has been on the active ingredient synephrine and its supposed negative effect of increasing blood pressure and heart rate. It is true that a particular molecular isomer of synephrine or the m-synephrine isomer is used to increase blood pressure in emergency medical situations.

However, the form of synephrine occurring naturally in extracts of *Citrus aurantium* is the p-synephrine isomer. This is an important distinction, not just for understanding the misunderstood claims about this herb in regards to heart rate and blood pressure, but realizing its potential for weight loss and metabolism enhancement. Heart rate and blood pressure will increase if alpha-receptors are stimulated. Metabolism and fat breakdown (lypolysis) will increase if beta-2 and beta-3 receptors are activated. This is important because alpha-receptors bind with the m-synephrine, increasing heart rate, while the beta-receptors, found in *Citrus aurantium*, bind with p-synephrine, and aid in fat loss.

Avoid bitter orange completely during pregnancy and take extreme caution if you have any history of heart disease. Be sure to consult with your healthcare provider before you start any new supplement.

A standardized extract should be considered that ranges from 5 to 30 percent p-synephrine. The dose of actual p-synehprine, which will be different depending on the strength of the extract, should be from 100 to 120 mg total daily, divided into two to three doses.

Calcium pyruvate

Our bodies make pyruvate daily during the metabolism of sugars and it is utilized in the energy producing reactions in the cell called the Krebs cycle. In short, pyruvate is associated with increasing cellular respiration, which is the basis for increased metabolism. There are many substances that achieve this including thyroid hormone, most of the supplements mentioned in this chapter, and calcium pyruvate.

Pyruvate use is associated with weight loss.[372] One controlled trial study found that pyruvate supplements enhanced weight loss and resulted in a greater reduction of body fat in overweight adults consuming a low-fat diet, but the doses were from 22 to 44 grams daily.[373] Other studies using more reasonable doses of 6 to 10 grams per day of pyruvate combined with an exercise program reported greater effects on weight loss and body fat than that seen with a placebo plus the exercise program.[374, 375]

I have seen patients have good success with this supplement, but I would not rank it as one of the best. I add it here because it is commonly discussed, it possesses the strong theoretic basis of increasing cellular respiration, and some individuals have good results. Calcium pyruvate may cause gas, bloating or diarrhea in sensitive individuals. Keep the dose at least near 6 grams per day to be effective.

> The study on chromium found a significant change in "body composition index" which is an index measuring the sum of the loss in body fat plus the gain in muscle mass. The BCI is a much more accurate gauge of weight management progress than using total body weight or BMI (body mass index).

Chromium picolinate

This is a nutritional trace element responsible for stimulating insulin to utilize glucose (sugar) more effectively in skeletal muscle and fat tissue.[376] This is an important distinction. Chromium does not stimulate more insulin to be produced, it helps insulin to do its job more efficiently. This is very important to help treat and prevent insulin resistance, the precursor to diabetes and one of the largest reasons people are overweight and obese.

The picolinate version of chromium is the most bioavailable or absorbable version of this trace element. Chromium has been shown to possess a positive effect on weight loss in a recent meta-analysis study, which pooled multiple studies and analyzed the effectiveness of chromium on weight loss.[377] A specific double-blind placebo controlled study[378] examined average Americans in Texas given between 200 mcg to 1,000 mcg per day of chromium picolinate with no special instructions in diet or exercise. The study on chromium found a significant change in "body composition index" which is an index measuring the sum of the loss in body fat plus the gain in muscle mass. The BCI is a much more accurate gauge of weight management progress than using total body weight or BMI (body mass index).

The use of chromium should be considered for its blood sugar balancing effects and its ability to assist in changing body composition versus *direct* fat loss effects. If blood sugar is properly regulated, it is easier to lose body fat, gain muscle, and maintain weight, and chromium is very well known for its blood sugar balancing effects.[379] Additionally, clinical research clearly supports the use of chromium to lower cholesterol and manage blood sugar in actual diabetics.[380] If you are diabetic and on specific diabetic medications, particularly insulin, be sure to let your doctor know before you start chromium.

A proper dose is from 200 mcg to 1,000 mcg or more daily. The higher doses should be monitored by a healthcare practitioner.

Citrulline malate

This simple amino acid is derived from the rind of watermelon and has been used for years as a medication in Europe called Stimol® to treat asthenia, or weakness and loss of strength[381] as well as weakness from psychological difficulties.[382] Citrulline can help with improving energy and an overall sense of mental and emotional well-being. Citrulline can also improve exercise performance. One study with forty-one men used 8 grams of citrulline and found that both strength and stamina improved during high intensity resistance exercise.[383] Cirtrulline appears to help with endurance. One study demonstrated that when cyclists took 6 grams of citrulline before a long bike ride they had a measurable increase in amino acid utilization and growth hormone production.[384]

Citrulline is responsible for optimizing blood levels of the amino acid arginine. Arginine is related to increasing nitric oxide (NO), which is a blood vessel dilator that helps achieve and maintain erections. However, arginine is poorly absorbed due to intestinal enzymes, such as arginase, that break it down before it gets into the circulation.[385] Citrulline, in doses as low as 1.5 grams daily, have been shown to improve mild to moderate erectile dysfunction.[386] By adding in oral citrulline daily it has been found to greatly increase the absorption of arginine, increasing NO.[387, 388]

People with a cardiac history and who are on high blood pressure medications, medications for angina (chest pain), or who have a history of very low blood pressure should consult with their physician before considering this supplement. Some people may have gastric upset using the higher-end doses. Start low with the dosing to determine your personal tolerance.

The dose ranges from 4-10 grams daily of citrulline malate. Start low at about 1-2 grams and then build up the dose to tolerance and effectiveness.

- To improve your overall energy, metabolism, and sense of well-being, doses as low as 3-4 grams may be sufficient.
- If you are using it before a workout, then take it at least an hour before and with a meal.
- For erectile dysfunction, use the citrulline with up to 2,000 mg of arginine. Start low with the arginine dose, building it up steadily over time.

Cocoa (*Theobroma cacao*) (**Theobromine**)

In the chapter on metabolic nutrition, cocoa was mentioned and promoted. I will cover it again here because it's always worth mentioning *Theobroma*, or the "food of the gods." One key active ingredient in cocoa is theobromine and this is directly related to mood enhancement, which can aid in any weight loss program.

> One key active ingredient in cocoa is theobromine and this is directly related to mood enhancement, which can aid in any weight loss program.

Often, theobromine is touted as a direct weight loss agent in terms of stimulating fat loss, but this is actually a relatively weak effect when compared to caffeine.[389, 390] However, it still has the basic stimulant, fat burning, and diuretic (water loss) effects as caffeine, but with a much more mild effect. This makes the theobromine found in chocolate an alternative to caffeine to those who are sensitive.

> **Cocao helps control appetite by providing a sense of mental and emotional well-being, and prevents the need to eat more to find that sensation.**

Cacao also affects mood versus its direct effect on fat loss. Additionally, cacao functions as a reward food and keeps you on track with making other positive changes in your nutritional lifestyle. Raw cacao contains some key elements including very high levels of magnesium, which is the most common mineral deficiency, also PEA or phenylethylamine which is related to increased mental focus and connectedness towards others, and anandamide, or the "bliss" chemical. The important take-home message is that cocao helps control appetite by providing a sense of mental and emotional well-being, and prevents the need to eat more to find that sensation.

When choosing a cacao or chocolate source, the best forms available are raw cacao nibs and raw cacao powder. Raw cacao nibs are pieces of the inner portion of cacao beans that have been roasted and hulled. Cacao powder is simply the cacao bean, that through cold-pressing, has had the fat (cacao butter) removed. As far as choosing a bar of chocolate, always be sure to stay with dark chocolate that is at least 70 percent dark chocolate. This lowers the overall sugar content and makes the bar much more healthy. Raw cacao nibs and roasted cacao cocoa powder contain the highest antioxidant content of any food ever tested, more than green tea, acai berries, and red wine combined. Raw cacao ranks the highest of any food on the Oxygen Radical Absorbance Capacity scale that measures the ability of antioxidants to absorb cancer-promoting free radicals. Raw cacao powder has an ORAC Score of 95,500. As a comparison, blueberries, which are very good for you, have an ORAC score of 2,400.

Step 3: Supplements

Some sensitive people may experience insomnia, anxiety, tremor, nervousness, palpitations, gastric upset, and withdrawal headaches. Always be aware of how any food or nutritional supplement affects you and your unique physiology. Everyone is different. There are some people who are very sensitive to cacao.

Dose at one or two teaspoons of raw cacao powder or raw cacao nibs daily. Keep 70 percent dark chocolate bars to a minimum, perhaps a few squares daily. There is still a sugar content with these bars. Dark chocolate is much more satisfying than milk chocolate which has a very high sugar load.

Coleus (*Coleus forskohlii*) (Forskolin)

The root of the Coleus botanical herb has been used classically in Hindu and Ayurvedic traditional medicine for centuries to treat hypertension, congestive heart failure, eczema, and respiratory disorders. The active ingredient is forskolin and this has been found to increase lipolysis (fat breakdown) in fat cells[391, 392, 393] via activation of the enzyme adenylate cyclase which increases levels of the cellular metabolism boosting substance known as "cyclic AMP." Forskolin has also been shown to stimulate thyroid hormone release and increase thyroid hormone production[394, 395] which further demonstrates improvement for your metabolic health.

Research has demonstrated that forskolin can increase the rate and strength of heart contractions [396] and lowers blood pressure.[397] Forskolin is also associated with increases in lean body mass and muscle[398] and increased testosterone production.[399] This is particularly important for anyone on a weight loss program, as preserving muscle mass can be a challenge when reducing body fat. And muscle mass is directly related to an increased metabolic rate.

Contact your healthcare provider if you have any of the following conditions before starting forskolin: low blood pressure, if you are taking medications for high blood pressure, bleeding disorders (due to forskolin's ability to decrease platelet aggregation), or if you take blood-thinning medication. Do not use if pregnant.

To achieve the potent metabolism and weight loss effects, the extract of Coleus must be standardized to at least 10 percent diterpene forskolin. Then the typical dose would be 250 mg twice daily of a 10 percent forskolin extract or 50 mg total forskolin once daily.

Creatine monohydrate

One of the most extensively researched supplements for muscle maintenance is creatine. This supplement not only aids in muscle growth, but helps to keep muscle around, even when dieting and in aging. One of the key factors in longevity is maintaining muscle mass and tone, and this is just as important for women as it is for men.

Creatine is very safe and when used in appropriate doses, there are no reports of adverse effects, such as the popularly touted kidney failure. Keeping the dose from 2-5 grams per day is both effective and safe.[400, 401] However, since there is limited long-term data, cycling off for one month and then back on for one month is a reasonable precaution.

Fenugreek seed (*Trigonella foenum-graecum*)

The extract of fenugreek seed yields high concentrations of a unique amino acid called 4-hydroxyisoleucine. This extract has been studied and was found to have the effect of lowering insulin, balancing blood sugar,[402] and improving insulin resistance and the metabolic syndrome.[403] It has also been found to lower cholesterol and triglyceride levels in the blood.[404, 405] The longer blood sugar remains in the circulation, the easier it is to store that sugar as fat. The stimulating effects of 4-hydroxyisoleucine on the pancreas to secrete insulin limits the time blood glucose (sugar) remains in circulation, thereby helping to reduce body fat production.

In general, fenugreek has a long history of use in India and is considered generally safe. There have not been any reported issues with the proper use of fenugreek. If you are diabetic and on diabetic medications, always consult with your healthcare provider before starting fenugreek.

As for any medicinal substance employed by a healthcare practitioner for his or her patient, the dose is the most important aspect. This is particularly true of nutritional and botanical substances where low dose, poor quality and manufacturing practices, and overall weak concentrations of herbal active constituents yield poor clinical results. When these factors are not considered, the clinician, the research scientist, and particularly the unsuspecting patient all believe that the substance did not work as promised. The following studies regarding fenugreek demonstrate this point.

As for any medicinal substance employed by a healthcare practitioner for his or her patient, the dose is the most important aspect. This is particularly true of nutritional and botanical substances where low dose, poor quality and manufacturing practices, and overall weak concentrations of herbal active constituents yield poor clinical results.

In three small short-term random control trials, fenugreek seed powder and its effect on fasting blood sugar was evaluated in patients with type II diabetes. In one trial, twenty-five patients took 1 gram of seed extract or placebo for two months with no change in FBG levels.[406] In another study, ten patients added 25 grams of defatted seed powder to one meal or ate the meal without the powder for fifteen days that also yielded poor results.[407] One study using 15 grams of powdered fenugreek seed soaked in water lowered blood sugar significantly.[408] However, a third study used a higher dose of 100 grams of defatted seed powder in fifteen patients for ten days did report improvements in fasting blood sugar values.[409]

❷ As a general rule, about ½ of a gram of the defatted seed per pound of body weight is a good starting dose and then increase gradually from there based on results.

❷ A water/alcohol extract of fenugreek is available which greatly lowers the amount you have to ingest in order to achieve results. The extract standardizes the content of the active ingredient 4-hydroxyisoleucine. This should be 500 mg one to two times per day (up to 1,000 mg daily).[410]

Fiber as Chia/Salba seed (*Salvia hispanica L*)

Adding fiber to the diet has many benefits to your health. Fiber provides a sense of fullness leading to appetite control. It traps and therefore lowers cholesterol, and it slows the digestion of sugar, keeping blood sugar smoothly regulated and controlled. Fiber influences the good bacteria in your colon that in turn assists the immune system to fight infections. Fiber helps to keep your bowel movements regular. There are many different sources of fiber including oats, fruits, and vegetables. But here's a focus on a unique source of fiber that has many other wonderful benefits for your health.

The South American seed known as chia gained some popularity when people started planting them on little clay animals. "Chuh chuh chuh Chia"…remember the advertisement? This seed has far more potential as a nutritional powerhouse than as a vegetative animal *for* your house and is one of the best things you can add to your diet, whether for general nutritional support, weight loss or optimizing your metabolic health. I am always looking for nutrient-packed foods for family, patients, and myself. Foods that offer the highest density of nutrients relative to their caloric content tend to be the best for our health and longevity. Other foods fitting this profile are seaweed and coconut oil discussed in the chapter on thyroid treatment. As explained throughout this book, humans should always eat as close to nature as possible when trying to optimize health and chia leads the way.

Chia seed has the following nutritional profile:

- It is high in soluble fiber. This is extremely important for digestion, fighting hunger cravings and blood sugar control. Soluble fiber helps to slow digestion, particularly the conversion of carbohydrates into sugar, thus controlling blood sugar spikes.
  - When water is added, chia seed will turn into a gelatin after about ten minutes. This is due to the high "soluble" fiber content. This gel can easily be added to most recipes.
- Chia is very high in omega-3 essential fatty acids. This is truly a remarkable content. In only two tablespoons of chia seeds you receive over 5 grams of omega-3 (equivalent to five fish oil gel caps) and 1.7 grams of omega-6 fatty acids.
- It is an excellent source of calcium. Two tablespoons provide over 200 milligrams of calcium.
- Chia boasts abundant mineral and antioxidant content.
- Among grains or seeds, chia seeds have the highest protein content by weight. Two tablespoons provide 4 grams of highly digestible protein.

There have been two significant studies on the particular seed hybrid *Salvia hispanica L.* demonstrating improvement in blood sugar control and cardiovascular outcomes in diabetics.[411, 412] The combination of nutrients found in this wonderful seed all directly and synergistically assist in helping the diabetic.

Debate exists regarding the differences between chia seeds and salba seeds. The producers of the patent-pending brand Salba claim that their specific seeds are more nutrient dense than regular chia. Perhaps this is true. But the difference here is really between the white and black chia. Salvia hispanica is considered the black chia seed. *Salvia hispanica L.* is the white chia, a.k.a "salba." They are just two different species of the same plant. I have done my best to explore the differences to see which one would be better, and it seems about the same… other than the price. Salba or the white chia is much more expensive and this should be considered when making a choice for yourself.

There really are no major cautions with this wonderful seed. Always consult with your doctor about any kind of new food, particularly if you have gastrointestinal issues. Be sure to find a trusted source of chia that grows the plant ethically and organically. The great news is that adding pesticides to the plant is unnecessary because insects avoid the plant completely.

Use about two to four teaspoons daily. Chia seeds can be eaten raw, sprouted, ground, cooked or as a gel. Chia has a neutral taste and therefore a mostly neutral affect to most recipes, making it easy to add in to many of your favorites. They add easily to cereals, yogurt, soups, smoothies, or salads and can be eaten as a snack. Ground chia mixes very well in baking. A popular Mexican drink called chia fresca has two teaspoons of the seeds mixed in a glass of water with added lime, lemon or honey.

Goat's rue (*Galega officinalis*)

Galega officinalis is a very effective herb with a wide variety of uses. Traditionally, it is used to lower blood sugar levels and treat the excessive urination that accompanies diabetes. It has been used to reduce fevers and has effective sweat inducing (diaphoretic) and water eliminating (diuretic) properties. The herb is also known to be an effective galactagogue, or a substance that stimulates the production of breast milk. It has a long historical use of being used to stimulate milk production in cattle and, as the name suggests, in goats.

This herb contains guanidine which is the main synthesized active ingredient in the anti-diabetic drug glucophage (Metformin®). This medication is now one of the most commonly prescribed drugs in the treatment of type II diabetes and is also effective at decreasing the risk of development of the disease.[413, 414] Glucophage has also been shown to be effective in decreasing diabetes-related death such as heart attack and stroke.[415] Specifically, glucophage improves insulin sensitivity in muscle and liver and increases the number of insulin receptors.[416] This means that it helps to increase the ability of the hormone insulin to perform its job of getting blood sugar (glucose) from the blood into muscle and liver cells. When blood sugar cannot get into the liver or muscle remaining in the circulation too long, it ends up in fat tissue. Side effects of glucophage include weakness, fatigue, shortness of breath, nausea, dizziness, and in extreme long-term use possible kidney toxicity.

Galega officinalis has similar properties to glucophage and could be used to aid in promoting insulin sensitivity. Research has demonstrated that this herb initiates a reduction in blood sugar (glucose) levels without triggering the symptoms of hypoglycemia or low blood sugar.[417] Additionally, *Galega* has been found to aid the common diseases associated with diabetes such as small blood vessel disease that affects the eyes leading to cataracts, degeneration of the retina, and even kidney damage. Particularly for our focus here, some animal studies found that Goat's rue can cause a significant reduction in body weight.[418] If you are diabetic and on medication for diabetes, do not use *Galega officinalis* unless you consult with your healthcare provider. Be sure to have your blood sugar (glucose) levels monitored closely. Always look out for symptoms of low blood sugar.

A proper dose is between 50 and 100 mg of a leaf extract daily. For powdered herb, the dose is between 2 and 10 grams daily.

Green Tea and Green Tea Extract (EGCG)

The historical and scientific effectiveness of green tea to improve health has long been known and studied. Green tea has been associated with the following benefits:

> Making green tea your metabolic beverage of choice is a wise one.

- ❀ Modulates insulin sensitivity.[419]
- ❀ Increases fat burning.[420]
- ❀ Increases overall metabolism by 4 percent when coupled with caffeine.[421]

❧ Studies have shown that green tea extract and its active constituent epigallocatechins (EGCG) are effective for steady weight loss over time, particularly when coupled with exercise.[422] [423]

❧ Improves cholesterol.[424]

Making green tea your metabolic beverage of choice is a wise one. It can be taken hot or cold, sweetened or unsweetened. It is convenient, inexpensive, and healthy. There are a few cautions. Green tea is good for you, but only in moderation. While the polyphenols in green tea are credited with preventing heart disease and cancer, it seems they can cause liver and kidney damage if consumed in very large quantities.[425] Up to ten cups of green tea daily should not cause a problem, and supplements should be kept to effective but not excessive doses.

An excellent summary article by M. Nathaniel Mead reviewed several studies on the potential toxic effects of EGCG from green tea when taken in high amounts, particularly by those already suffering from liver damage. According to a Rutger's study, the concern is with doses higher than 500 mg daily.[426] However, other toxicological studies have concluded that "a no-observed adverse effect level of 500 mg EGCG preparation/kg/day was established."[427]

As for doses, use 150-300 mg daily of a standardized extract of green tea catechins (EGCG). I suggest adding in at least a cup or two of organic green tea daily for the added synergistic effects of the other compounds, including the caffeine. This will depend on your sensitivity to caffeine. It takes from 3 to 5 grams of tea to brew one cup. The best time to drink green tea is in the morning on an empty stomach, right before a high intensity, short duration interval workout.

Gudmar *(Gymnema sylvestre)*

This plant is native to central and western India, tropical Africa and Australia, and has been used in traditional Aryvedic medicine for centuries. When trying to control appetite and regulate blood sugar, this herb comes out on top.

Step 3: Supplements

For weight loss efforts, controlling appetite and sugar cravings can be a key to success. Craving and eating carbohydrates, particularly refined carbohydrates, is the true killer of any weight loss attempt. When the plant is placed directly on the tongue, the gymnemic acid content helps to decrease the taste of sugar,[428] thereby helping to reduce sugar cravings. This has to be done with the actual herb placed directly on the tongue; swallowing the pill form does not produce this effect. But swallowing a standardized extract directly has other blood sugar handling and weight loss benefits.

> **Craving and eating carbohydrates, particularly refined carbohydrates, is the true killer of any weight loss attempt.**

Studies have demonstrated the blood sugar lowering effects in both type I[429] (insulin dependent) and type II[430] (non-insulin dependent) diabetics, as well as the ability to lower hemoglobin A1C levels (the marker used to determine the severity of blood sugar regulation over time). Gymnemic acid molecules fill the receptor location in the intestine preventing sugar absorption, resulting in low blood sugar level[431] and decreased body fat.[432] When the blood sugar is regulated, it is easier to lose weight, improve mood and mental focus, and increase energy.

If you are taking insulin or hypoglycemic drugs such as Metformin®, monitor your blood sugar levels closely and consult with your healthcare provider before starting this herb.

The standard dose for gudmar is 400-600 mg daily of an extract standardized to contain 24 percent gymnemic acids. When trying to regulate blood sugar, splitting the overall amount into three doses can be helpful.

IV (Intravenous) and IM (Intramuscular) Nutrient Therapy

Oral nutrient therapy should always be considered the basic standard for nutritional support, whether for basic health or in an attempt to optimize your metabolic health. However, at times it is clinically relevant to consider IV (intravenous) nutrient therapy to deliver quality medicinal doses of nutrients. The advantages of IV Nutrient Therapy include being able to deliver high doses of nutrients in a consistent manner while avoiding liver metabolism completely.

IV therapy can be considered when the integrity of the gastrointestinal tract is compromised such as in conditions like Irritable Bowel Syndrome (IBS), Crohn's disease, and ulcers. IV therapy offers an excellent high dose nutrient therapy in acute conditions such as colds, flus, and in chronic conditions such as chronic fatigue syndrome, fibromyalgia, adrenal dysfunction, and cancer. Additionally, conditions such as high blood pressure, migraines, depression, allergies, and diabetes effectively respond to this therapy. IV nutrient therapy is also excellent at optimizing the metabolism, assisting detoxification and improving athletic performance.

One of the more typical IV nutrient combinations used is the Myers' cocktail. John Myers, a physician from Maryland, treated patients with intravenous nutrient therapy for over twenty-five years. After his death in 1984, Dr. Alan R. Gaby continued to treat his patients and is responsible for creating the term Myers' cocktail. The Myers' cocktail is composed of nutrients that are typically deficient in a variety of conditions. These nutrients include magnesium, calcium, the full array of B vitamins including B1, B2, B3, B5, B6, B12, and from 1,000 to 4,000 mg of vitamin C.

While vein injection spreads nutrients throughout the bloodstream, the direct injection of nutrients into muscles works well. IM nutrient therapy, such as B6/B12 shots, are also very effective at delivering two key B vitamins important for energy production, mood stabilization, and weight loss. Be sure to consider adding IV/IM Nutrient Therapy to your health regimen and seek out a qualified health practitioner who can safely and effectively administer this useful therapy.

Metabolic Spices

Here is a chance to add some very useful spice to your life. Did you know that adding these spices into your food could boost your metabolism, lower appetite, and balance blood sugar? Make sure they are fresh and have not been in your cupboard longer than six months. Do not underestimate the power of these simple and time-tested herbs:

- Cinnamon
- Cumin
- Ginger
- Turmeric
- Curry (Ginger, turmeric, cumin)
- Cayenne pepper
- Black pepper
- Chiles
- Chili powder
- Mustard seed powder

Milk Thistle (*Silybum marianum*)

Milk thistle is widely used in the U.S., Europe, and Egypt to support liver function and health and has been used for centuries across the globe. It has been studied extensively and continues to demonstrate its effectiveness and relative safety.

Milk thistle is thought to work by:[433, 434, 435]

- Preventing toxins such as alcohol or heavy metals from getting into liver cells.
- Improving liver cell regeneration.
- Acting as a free-radical scavenger and antioxidant.
- Modulating the immune response.

Since the liver plays a central role in overall body detoxification and has over 700 functions, keeping it clean and functioning normally is important for almost any health goal. Particularly, milk thistle can aid in gentle body detoxification that can aid in proper weight loss and improve energy.

Most clinical trials have used daily dosages of 420 to 480 mg of milk thistle's active ingredient *silymarin* divided into two or three doses daily. A monograph in *Alternative Medical Review*[436] suggests using a standardized extract (containing 70-80 percent *silymarin*) at 100-300 mg three times daily, which would range from 240 mg to 720 mg *silymarin* daily. Both animal and human studies have shown *silymarin* to be non-toxic. At high doses (> 1,500 mg per day) a laxative effect is possible due to increased bile secretion and flow.

Protein Supplements

Remember that nothing beats whole food choices of protein, especially clean and lean animal protein sources such as lean beef, poultry, and fish. But incorporating protein supplements is one of the best ways to optimize your health and ensure that you get adequate protein throughout the day. Use protein powders to:

- Increase your metabolism.
- Balance your blood sugar.
- Recover from exercise.
- Provide healthy convenient snacks.

Different protein powders have different digestive rates that influence your metabolism in different ways. Protein powders are ranked on their bioavailability to the body, meaning how well they are absorbed. Egg whites were given a ranking of 100 to create a standard. All other sources can be either more or less absorbable from that ranking.

Whey protein is very fast digesting and it quickly gets into your bloodstream. It has a bioavailability ranking of 104. This has benefits when you have just completed an exercise routine by helping you recover. However, because it absorbs more rapidly it is eliminated more rapidly, and may not provide long-term satiety. Whey protein powder has also been shown to have benefits to the cardiovascular and immune systems, and it helps increase lean body mass.

Casein powder is digested slowly and allows for a slower release of protein and amino acids that help to stabilize blood sugar. Its bioavailability is much lower than whey, at only 74, but this is an excellent type of protein powder to add in as a snack in between meals because it will stay with you longer. For those with milk sensitivities, this is not a good choice.

Egg white protein powder is a highly absorbed protein source containing all the amino acids. With a bioavailability of 100, it readily gets into the bloodstream.

Rice protein powder is created by isolating the protein from the brown rice grain. For a grain, the bioavailability is not as good as an animal source, but rice protein averages at a ranking of 83.

Pea protein bioavailability is only about 65. Larger amounts have to be consumed and it tends to be more expensive. However, if milk and egg sources need to be avoided for any medical or ethical reason, then this is a good option.

Be sure to find a protein supplement source that is of a high quality with the following characteristics:

- Where it comes from: If it is a dairy-based protein powder, be sure it originates from grass fed cows.
- How it's grown: Non-Genetically Modified Organism (GMO) for animal or plant-based protein powders.
- How it's processed: Triple cold press micro filtering is a superior method compared to the cheaper ion-exchange filtration processing which denatures the proteins by using acids and chemicals to separate whey from fats. Additionally, the product will contain no artificial flavors, colors, or preservatives.
- NEVER use soy protein powders, as they are goitrogenic (causing thyroid disease) and have estrogen-like compounds.

Yerba mate (*Ilex paraguayensis*)

Yerba mate is a popular South American beverage with mate bars as prevalent in South America as coffee bars in North America and Europe. It has been used historically as a tonic, diuretic, stimulant for fatigue, appetite suppressant, and a gastric aid. In Europe, and now popularly in the U.S., it is used for weight loss, physical and mental fatigue, nervous depression, and fatigue-related headaches. It also has been used to stimulate the immune system, for help with allergies, and to elicit a general cleansing effect for the body.

Regular use of yerba mate tea can be an integral part of any weight loss program and can stimulate your metabolism. This herb contains caffeine, theobromine, and theophyline. These constituents when combined have the interesting effect of relaxing smooth muscle while also stimulating the heart. People taking yerba mate often claim that they are alert but relaxed.

The caffeine content of an average 6 ounce yerba mate beverage is about 50-100 mg, where coffee in the same amount would be around 100-250 mg. Yerba mate has also proven to be very high in antioxidants[437,] [438] containing vitamins A, C, E, most B vitamins, biotin, and the minerals magnesium, calcium, iron, sodium, potassium, manganese, and sulphur.

The tea is very safe in moderate amounts. Extracts of the herb in capsules can be more potent and caution should be taken for those sensitive to stimulants and caffeine.

Depending on the quality of the tea, it can range from a very robust flavor to very bland. Try to find a supplier that harvests the mate leaves from trees growing in the wild. Effective amounts that help to lower appetite and increase energy are two to four cups of tea per day, depending on your tolerance to its stimulant potential.

Capsules of yerba mate extract can also be taken and are effective for appetite control. Take approximately 500 to 600 mg (of an 8:1 extract—look at the label) on an empty stomach before each meal. Each capsule of this type of extract is equivalent to one or two cups of tea.

Step 4: Balancing the Sex Hormones for an Optimized You

One of the most important steps to take for your metabolic health is to balance and/or replace your sex hormones, such as estrogen and testosterone. Menopause is a common condition for millions of women and the more recently understood andropause for men. When estrogen and testosterone continue to decline as we age, both men and women must take some time to first assess their deepest feelings about aging, then research the best way to approach their process of aging. We live at a time when it is possible to regain and retain control of the process of aging in order to achieve a maximum amount of happiness.

This section of the book outlines two concepts regarding sex hormones: balancing and replacement. There is quite a difference:

- Balancing implies working with your body to optimize how hormone is being produced and processed in your body naturally.
- Replacement refers to hormone replacement therapy from an outside medication source.

Sex Hormone Balance in Women

The first thing I want to address are nutritional considerations. When women come in to consult with me for hormone replacement therapy, they often ask about a specific diet that will help their hormonal imbalances. In fact, there are some specific choices that can be made to help benefit your hormonal balance and in turn optimize your hormone replacement therapy.

A Hormone Diet for Women: Cleaning up the Estrogen

Optimize your diet to balance your sex hormones by:

- Taking care to consume optimal animal protein sources. The flesh of animals raised in poor environments may contain synthetic hormones. If these hormones are present in food, they will either create or add to an imbalance.

- Chose free-range cultivated animals that are free from antibiotic and hormones. Only buy and cook wild caught fish. Use only raw or organic milk sources.
- Avoiding pesticides on fruits and vegetables. They act as synthetic estrogens which burden the body.
- Chose organic fruits and vegetables.
- Eating a diet high in clean protein sources, vegetables, and fruits to keep insulin and blood sugar regulated.
- Avoid soy products, particularly GMO soy.
- Engaging in regular diet cleansing to keep the liver functioning efficiently in order to metabolize excess hormone.
- Avoiding excess alcohol intake. It disrupts the normal ovarian production and rhythm of estrogen, progesterone, and testosterone.

Metabolizing Your Estrogen Properly

Your body produces a form of estrogen called estradiol (E2). This is the common form of estrogen used in hormone replacement therapy. When estradiol (E2) is metabolized, it converts into estrone (E1). Estrone (E1) has two versions that it can convert or metabolize into, either 2-hydroxyestrone, a less potent metabolite, or 16-hydroxyestrone, a more potent metabolite associated with increased risk of cancers of the uterus, breast, and prostate. If the ratio of 2:16 hydroxyestrone high, then the risk for breast cancer is lower.[439] The use of the 2:16 hydroxyestrone ratio has been shown to be a good predictor of future breast cancer risk in women.[440] In general, 16-hydroxyestrone is a cell-proliferative metabolite, which means it makes cells grow and multiply, increasing the risk for cancers. The 2-hydroxyestrone metabolite is an anti-proliferative metabolite. Even proliferative thyroid disease, such as goiter, has been associated with a low 2:16 hydroxyestrone ratio.[441] Obesity, tobacco use, chronic inflammation, pesticide exposure, and a diet low in antioxidants all lead to a lowered 2:16 hydroxyestrone ratio.[442]

Optimizing the 2:16 hydroxyestrone ratio can be done by:
- Exercising, which increases the levels of 2-hydroxyestrone.[443]

- Consuming cooked cruciferous vegetables such as broccoli, cauliflower, cabbage, bok choy, and arugula.[444]
  - Note: These cruciferous vegetables are also known goitrogens or foods that lower thyroid function. Cooking tends to eliminate the negative effects of these foods on the thyroid.
- Not smoking.
- Detoxifying through cleansing and lowering pesticide and toxin exposure.
- Lowering your body fat weight.
- Use Di-indol-methane (DIM), the active constituent in cruciferous vegetables that has been shown to improve the 2:16 hydroxyestrone ratio.[445]
  - Dose should be 150-300 mg daily through an encapsulated bioavailable form.

Strategies for Avoiding Environmental Synthetic Estrogens

In the U.S., you have the ability to choose many different ways of being a consumer. There are a multitude of choices for you and I suggest that you keep looking for ways to optimize your body and eliminate excess estrogens. Remember there is always hope.

The best ways to avoid being exposed to environmental estrogens are:
- Use glass or ceramics to store food and water; not plastic.
- Avoid perfumes, colognes or household air fresheners containing parabens. Know that natural perfumes are available.
- Do not microwave food in plastic containers or covered with plastic wrap.
- Do not leave plastic containers, especially drinking water, in the sun.
- Avoid synthetic fabric softeners.
- Use natural laundry soaps and dish detergents when possible.
- Avoid creams and cosmetics that contain parabens and stearalkonium chloride.

Step 4: Sex Hormones

- Avoid surfactants found in certain condoms and diaphragm gels.
- Avoid shampoo that contains estrogen or placental extracts.
- Sunscreen is one of the most common sources of environmental estrogen-like compounds including benzophenone-3, homosalate, 4-methyl-benzylidene camphor (4-MBC), octyl-methoxycinnamate, and octyl-dimethyl-PABA. There are multiple brands of natural sunscreens devoid of these harmful chemicals.
- Avoid herbicides. Use natural solutions for the garden such as vinegar and salt combined with water.
- Avoid birth control pills. Birth control pills contain synthetic estrogen that can become toxic with long-term use. If possible, use an alternative form of birth control.
- For a comprehensive list of environmental chemicals and where they are found, explore: http://www.ourstolenfuture.org/basics/chemuses.htm

Calcium and Magnesium

There are many nutritional supplements to consider for optimal health at any age. The chapter on supplements seeks to provide many answers in this direction. However, calcium and magnesium are particular supplements that are often discussed for menopausal women in regards to bone health.

The focus has always been on calcium to help with bone strength. Little attention has been given to magnesium and this could be leading to more health issues including increased cardiovascular disease and weaker bones.[446] But, as with most things in health, and in life, it is about a *balance* between the two.

Some important points about calcium:
- It acts as a blood clotter.
- It is a blood vessel constrictor.
- In excessive amounts it may contribute to increasing plaque in the arteries.

- It adds to the bone mineral portion of bone, but not the flexible protein portion of bone, thus making bones thicker, but more brittle if only calcium is taken.

  Some important points about magnesium:

- It is common to have a deficiency.
- It acts as a blood thinner.
- It is a blood vessel dilator.
- It works with estrogen to help the nervous system, helping with memory and protecting the brain.
- It adds to the flexible protein portion of bone, making bone more resilient to fracture.

In general, keep the ratio at least 2:1 of calcium to magnesium. A good starting place would be 1,000 mg of calcium and 500 mg of magnesium. Calcium needs vitamin D and the correct amount of magnesium to be utilized. An excess of alcohol, soda, and fluoride from tap water and toothpaste increases the need for magnesium. When supplementing with proper amounts of vitamin D and calcium, magnesium needs are increased.

Herbal Preparations for Sex Hormone Balancing and Restoration

Black Cohosh (*Cimicifuga racemosa*)

This is one of the most popular herbal supplements used for perimenopause and post menopause. This herb is native to Eastern North America and has been used in the U. S. for the treatment of gynecologic complaints and menopausal complaints for more than one hundred years. It can be particularly effective at helping with hot flashes, profuse sweating, insomnia, and anxiety. There is a substantial amount of evidence demonstrating the effectiveness of this herb on relieving the symptoms of menopause.[447, 448, 449] Black cohosh has even been found to have an equivalent benefit on improving both hot flashes and bone health as compared to hormone replacement therapy.[450]

Step 4: Sex Hormones

One of the most common misconceptions about black cohosh was that it was presumed to have estrogenic activity, making it possibly unsafe for menopausal women to use and also something to avoid during hormone replacement therapy. However, recent studies show no effect on blood hormone levels such as luteinizing hormone (LH), follicle stimulating hormone (FSH), prolactin, sex hormone binding globulin (SHBG), and particularly estradiol (E2).[451] Several animal studies using black cohosh extracts have found no estrogenic increases in the weight of the uterus or stimulation of vaginal and breast tissue.[452, 453, 454] The likely mechanism for black cohosh is its effects on serotonin receptors, not estrogen receptors.[455, 456]

What does all this mean for a menopausal woman? Black cohosh appears to be both safe and effective at helping with hot flashes, night sweats, sleeping difficulties, anxiety, and could be a good place to start with a supplement. Also, the addition of this herbal extract with natural hormone replacement therapy could be an excellent adjunct to improve symptoms and well-being. Very rarely do patients experience nausea, headaches, dizziness, breast pain, and weight gain. Never use black cohosh when pregnant or lactating as this can add in unwanted estrogen effects to the fetus or newborn.

Black cohosh comes in a standardized extract and your dose should be between 40-80 mg per day. As with many herbal supplements, be sure to give it time as it may take between four and twelve weeks before any benefits are seen.

Maca (*Lepidium meyenii*)

Lepidium meyenii (maca) is a root vegetable cultivated in the central Peruvian Andes that belongs to the *Brassica* (mustard) family. There has been a lot of attention given to this herb/food recently for its purported benefits with menopause, andropause, sexual desire, and potency. In fact, the herb has been used for centuries in the Andes to enhance fertility in humans and animals.[457, 458] Nutritionally, dried maca root is rich in amino acids, iodine, iron, and magnesium.[459] Maca has benefits for both men and women:

- Randomized control trial studies have demonstrated excellent results in sexual desire in men[460] independent of testosterone levels. In other words, maca stimulates sexual desire in men without increasing testosterone levels directly.

- In women, maca has also shown improvement in sexual desire and response[461] as well as improvement in sexual desire when using an SSRI anxiety medication such as Prozac®, Wellbutrin®, etc.[462] These types of medications are notorious for lowering sexual desire.

- Recent clinical trials have also suggested significant effects of maca for increasing sperm count and mobility, and improving sexual function in men.[463, 464]

- Maca has also been shown to reduce menopausal symptoms in women including hot flashes and night sweats.[465]

- Evidence exists that maca is also helpful with erectile dysfunction.[466]

This is an excellent herb to add into any supplement regimen when trying to improve a menopausal or andropausal situation. No adverse effects have been reported using maca. Because it is a food, generally there are no major concerns with its use.

Effective doses seem to be between 1,500-3,500 mg daily of dried maca powder, typically delivered in capsules. Results are usually achieved in twelve weeks or less. As with anything, start with a low dose and steadily increase daily until positive results are achieved.

Chronic Stress and Sex Hormones

Throughout this book the topic of stress is discussed in terms of affecting how we feel and how we react. This is especially true with sex hormone balance and production.

- Chronic stress leads to prolonged suppression of sex hormone production. This effect has been well demonstrated in ballet dancers, highly trained runners, and athletes of both sexes.[467, 468] These people have high levels of the stress hormone cortisol and adrenal glands

Step 4: Sex Hormones

that are in constant overdrive. In men, chronic stress leads to low testosterone levels and women usually develop menstrual disorders.

- ❧ Cortisol also inhibits the way that the pituitary gland communicates with the body to produce sex hormones and directly blocks the ability of the ovaries and testicles to produce estrogen and testosterone.[469]
- ❧ Stress hormones (such as cortisol) directly impact the body tissues that estrogen and testosterone target and render them resistant to stimulus.[470, 471] This means that stress blocks the testosterone and estrogen in your body from doing what it is supposed to do. When estrogen and testosterone are able to work their magic in your tissues, your symptoms of lack go away, allowing you to look, feel, and perform at your best.

Be sure to follow the advice described in the chapter on adrenal health where strategies on stress management and adrenal health help you to cope with chronic stress and optimize your sex hormones. Step 2 and Step 6 of the Metabolic Health Protocol also provide excellent stress reducing strategies.

Sex Hormone Balance in Men

First things first! If you are a man who has started reading this chapter and you skipped right over the above section on sex hormone balance for women, please stop to go back and read it. In fact, this is the first place that all men should start. You should understand the similarities with what women and men experience at this time in life. Understanding menopause and how to help it naturally will help you understand how to help andropause. Also, clean up the environmental estrogens and look into how your body is truly metabolizing estrogens, for the good or for the bad. One of the key reasons men have low testosterone and possibly even prostate issues is

> Understanding menopause and how to help it naturally will help you understand how to help andropause.

the constant insult of excessive environmental estrogens to our bodies. Do not underestimate the power of cleaning up your diet and personal environment because this can positively impact your testosterone levels and sexual performance. Environmental estrogens have been linked to erectile dysfunction,[472] reduced male fertility,[473] prostate cancer,[474] and testicular cancer.[475]

Optimizing Testosterone Levels Naturally

You should seek to increase your own body's ability to make testosterone as much as possible. The following strategies can be employed right away and also added later on, even if hormone replacement therapy has begun. But regardless, these strategies will always have benefit.

Implicit Power Motivation and Imagery of Winning

"Our deepest fear is not that we are inadequate. Our deepest fear is that we are powerful beyond measure. It is our light, not our darkness that most frightens us. We ask ourselves, Who am I to be brilliant, gorgeous, talented, fabulous? Actually, who are you not to be? There is nothing enlightened about shrinking so that other people won't feel insecure around you. And as we let our own light shine, we unconsciously give other people permission to do the same."

— Nelson Mandela, 1994 Inaugural Speech

I have always loved that speech from Nelson Mandela. He believed that people should seek out their personal power and success and always allow it to shine through, not at the detriment to those around you, but to their mutual advantage.

Hormones respond to our mental frame of reference and our imagination. Research has shown measurable increases in testosterone in response to simply *imagining* winning at a simple competitive task when the subjects were focused on assertiveness

> Hormones respond to our mental frame of reference and our imagination.

and individualized power.[476] This is a profound statement. It shows that our imagined will power can affect testosterone production, and assist in helping us to achieve success.

Spend time on imagining success in life and you can actually increase your testosterone levels!

REM Sleep

One of the best ways to optimize testosterone production is to simply get more sleep and particularly get more quality sleep. When we sleep, we enter into certain rhythms of Rapid Eye Movement (REM) that relate to deep sleep and dreaming. The nighttime testosterone production rhythm is related to deep sleep [477] and to REM/non-REM sleep cycles.[478] And as testosterone levels peak during sleep, it directly coincides with the onset of achieving REM sleep.[479] Be sure to see the section on sleep hygiene in Step 2 of The Metabolic Health Protocol and get to sleep!

Resistance Training

The chapter on metabolic exercise demonstrated that high intensity, short duration exercise positively effects hormone production, including testosterone. Research has shown that resistance exercise can increase testosterone production.[480, 481] The point here is to incorporate some form of weight bearing and resistance training into your exercise regimen in order to get your testosterone levels up. Remember, short bursts of intense physical activity is what keeps fitness levels optimal.

Factors That Interfere with Testosterone Production
Alcohol

One of the best ways to *lower* your testosterone production is to drink alcohol, particularly in excess. Alcohol affects testosterone in three ways:

- ❦ It increases the breakdown and removal of testosterone from the circulation.[482] This occurs because alcohol intake increases the enzyme testosterone reductase which is responsible for the normal breakdown of testosterone. Some of this enzyme is normal, but when it is in excess, testosterone is broken down too rapidly.

> One of the best ways to *lower* your testosterone production is to drink alcohol, particularly in excess.

❧ It decreases the production rate of testosterone. Interestingly, the testicles secrete enzymes to break down alcohol. These same enzymes are responsible for testosterone production. When alcohol is in the system in excess, the testosterone producing enzymes are occupied, thus decreasing testosterone production rates.[483] Making matters worse, alcohol increases the stress hormone cortisol,[484] which will also blunt testosterone production directly at the testicles.

❧ It increases Sex Hormone Binding Globulin (SHBG).[485] This is a protein produced by the liver that increases production with alcohol intake. SHBG is a transport protein that binds to testosterone. Some SHBG is normal, but too much lessens the ability of freed and unbound testosterone to get into the target cells of the body and produce changes that improve health.

Alcohol consumption is a personal choice and often very difficult for both men and women to avoid. If your goal is to optimize your testosterone production and improve your overall health, then keeping alcohol use to a minimum is advised. If you are able, avoid alcohol as much as possible to optimize testosterone levels. If you do choose to consume, keep the daily rate to no more than one to two six-ounce glasses of wine, one twelve-ounce beer, or one two-ounce shot of liquor.

Chronic Stress

I would hope that this comes as no shock to the reader that, yet again, chronic stress is related to something bad for your body. Stress kills. Stress makes you unhealthy. And yes, stress lowers testosterone production. The chronic stress hormone, cortisol, blocks testosterone production directly at the testicular level. Normally, a very important enzyme, 11ßHSD (11ß-hydroxysteroid dehydrogenase) converts active cortisol to inactive 11-dehydrocorticosterone. This inactive form of cortisol protects the important testosterone-producing Leydig cells in the

> The researchers of the Massachusetts Male Aging Study (MMAS) found that the loss of a spouse was associated with a ten-year aging-equivalent reduction in testosterone.

testicles, keeping testosterone levels up in the body. However, with chronic stress, high levels of cortisol will be produced and the 11ßHSD enzyme cannot keep up with the demand, and testosterone production suffers.

Other stressful life events that sometimes are uncontrollable can lower testosterone production. The researchers of the Massachusetts Male Aging Study (MMAS) found that the loss of a spouse was associated with a ten-year aging-equivalent reduction in testosterone.[486] So, keep your stress down to keep your testosterone optimized. Learn to cope. Follow the mental health suggestions found in this book.

Medications

Most men who come to see me are on medications for elevated blood pressure and elevated cholesterol. Alcohol is also a typical lifestyle choice of theirs that has contributed to the blood pressure and cholesterol issues. Ironically, it is these three substances that are associated with lowered testosterone levels in men. Other drugs/substances associated with lowered testosterone:

- Corticosteroids: anti-inflammatory medications.
- Finestaride (Propecia): hair loss and prostate cancer.
- Antidepressants (SSRI's, tricyclics, MAOI's).
- Chemotherapy: cancer treatment.
- Environmental toxins such as lead and particularly pesticides.

❦ Marijuana use.

Other factors that may have caused a low level of testosterone are:

❦ Past infections such as mumps, which affects the testicles.

❦ Removal of the testes due to cancer or trauma.

❦ Genetics. Some men just make less testosterone than others.

Diet and Nutritional Support for Sex Hormone Imbalances

One of the best diets to optimize testosterone levels while lowering estrogen is a high protein, low grain-based carbohydrate diet as explained in this book. Protein increases testosterone! This means clean, hormone and pesticide free sources of animal meats and fish that have been raised properly will yield the best results with optimizing testosterone and lowering estrogen levels.

Limit Phytoestrogens

Phytoestrogens are plant derived estrogen-like compounds. These compounds stimulate estrogen receptors on cells, acting similarly to the actual estrogen hormone. The highest phytoestrogen content would be from oily seeds (such as sunflower, safflower, canola, and soybean), soy products, cereals, breads, and legumes. Avoid and limit these foods as much as possible.

Plants contain these phytoestrogens as part of their natural defense against the overpopulation of herbivore animals by controlling male fertility.[487] And reports exist that phytoestrogen diets may cause reductions in human male fertility. [488, 489] However, another recent meta-analysis found that there is no connection with phytoestrogens and male fertility.[490] With conflicting scientific opinions, compounded with the problem of excessive estrogens in the environment, I believe it is important for men to limit their intake.

Step 4: Sex Hormones

Zinc

Zinc is one of the most important supplements for men's health with the highest concentrations in the prostate gland. This is one of the best minerals to add to your supplementation regimen. Some important points about zinc:

- It is a key mineral in male sexual function and a protective nutrient against prostate cancer.[491]

- Low testosterone and particularly low sperm counts may be signs of a zinc deficiency. Of the main biological trace elements, zinc, copper and selenium are important in reproduction in males and females. Zinc deficiency first impairs angiotensin converting enzyme (ACE) activity (an enzyme important for blood pressure control), and this in turn leads to depletion of testosterone levels and inhibition of spermatogenesis (sperm production).[492]

- Men with excessive estrogen levels despite normal testosterone levels may also lack this mineral.

- Zinc inhibits the activity of the 5-alpha reductase enzyme that irreversibly converts testosterone to dihydrotestosterone and may be helpful in the treatment of benign prostatic hyperplasia (enlarged prostate).[493]

- The phytic acid content of grains lowers zinc absorption, another reason to minimize grain-based carbohydrates in the diet.

- Oysters are the best sources of zinc of any food. Depending on the type of oyster, the average zinc content for one large oyster (about 16 grams) is about 15 mg with an appropriate ratio of copper at 1.0 mg.[494] Other forms of shellfish, beef, red meats, and nuts such as pumpkin seeds and sunflower seeds are also rich sources of zinc.

- We only absorb 20 to 40 percent of the zinc from our food.

- Excessive alcohol intake lowers zinc in the body.

If you use zinc as a supplement, always be sure to take it with copper. Zinc supplementation alone can lead to a copper deficiency.[495] The proper zinc-to-copper ratio is about 15:1. Doses of elemental zinc ranging from 100 to 150 mg per day for prolonged periods may lead to red blood cell (RBC) microcytosis (too small red blood cells), neutropenia (decreased white blood cells), and impaired immunity.[496]

Certain drugs and nutrients reduce zinc levels in the body by inhibiting its absorption or increasing its excretion. These include:

- Captopril (high blood pressure medication) and possibly other ACE inhibitors.[497]
- Oral contraceptives[498] (birth control pills).
- Thiazide diuretics.[499]
- H$_2$blockers[500] (such as Zantac®, Pepcid®, and Tagamet®) and proton pump inhibitors (such as Prilosec® and Prevacid®).
- Calcium.[501] [502]

Chose a form of zinc that is highly absorbable such as zinc picolinate, zinc citrate, zinc glycerate or zinc monomethionine. The doses listed here are elemental zinc amounts. Sometimes the milligram amount will be higher than the actual elemental zinc content.

To help increase lowered testosterone levels, consider 50 mg twice daily for a few months and have your blood levels of testosterone monitored. As a maintenance dose to keep the prostate healthy and estrogen lowered, consider 50 mg of elemental zinc daily.

Di-indoyl-methane (DIM)

At the beginning of this section, I mentioned how important it was for a man to keep estrogens in the body properly metabolized. The supplement DIM is one way to help with clearing unhealthy estrogen metabolites out of the body. It is the estrogens in a man's body that causes problems with the prostate. Take 150-300 mg daily of an encapsulated bioavailable form.

Herbal Medicine for Testosterone Enhancement and Lowering Estrogen

There are many herbal supplements that are touted as testosterone boosters and sexual libido enhancers. Some are better than others. I have placed emphasis on Long Jack *(Eurycoma longifolia)* or (Tongkat Ali)

(*Pasak Bumi*). Eurycoma longifolia, or otherwise known as Long Jack, is a Malaysian and Indonesian tree root possessing some peculiar benefits. Historically, the Indonesians and Malaysians have made a strong tea from the root to ward off disease and improve energy, libido, and sexual stamina. And currently, research is beginning to support the wonderful benefits of this herb. Tongkat ali has been found to be beneficial in fighting cancer[503] and possesses antibacterial[504] and antimalarial effects. [505, 506]

With respect to testosterone balancing, research has demonstrated that tongkat ali:

- Enhances sexual behavior and performance in rat models [507, 508] concluding the improvements are likely from increased testosterone levels.
- Improves testicular functioning and inhibits the effects of excessive estrogen.[509]
- Although the research is still limited, the likely mechanism of testosterone production is through Leydig cell stimulation in the testicles.[510]
- The *British Journal of Sports Medicine* published a research article that found tongkat ali increased muscle size and strength as compared to the placebo.[511]

Clinically, this herb has excellent potential. Many of my male patients have reported improving sexual libido and performance, as well as improved stamina in the gym. Another peculiar effect of tongkat ali is testicular appearance enhancement and increased volume. As men age and testosterone levels decline, the testicles have a tendency to shrink. Tongkat ali has the effect of stimulating the testicles, increasing blood supply and overall size.

Users of tongkat ali can experience a facial flush and a sensation of warmth from using the extract. This is a transient symptom that goes away from a few minutes to a few hours and often completely goes away when one gets used to taking the herb.

Throughout this book I have avoided naming particular brands or vendors concerning nutritional supplements and botanical (herbal) remedies. I want to be as objective as possible and focus on sound research and my honest clinical experience and opinion of the substance. I do not currently endorse any one brand or company. However, with respect to tongkat ali there are many counterfeit remedies available, particularly on the Internet, that are considerably ineffective at the least and potentially dangerous at the worst. With that, I highly recommend Sumatra Pasak Bumi, an Indonesian company who produces the herb correctly and safely. Their website is www.tongkatali.org.

The absolute minimum effective dose is 300 mg of a 1:50 extract. Any kind of extract that is smaller than this (such as a 1:10 or 1:20) or if it is the dried and ground root powder only, without being extracted, it will be ineffective. The dose can also range up to 2,000 mg of an extract of 1:200 potency, depending on your personal tolerance and need. Always start slowly and move up on the dose as needed. Typically, most men have success with between 300 and 1,200 mg of a 1:200 extract. Women can take it also and the dose can be left very low at 300 mg of either a 1:50 or 1:200 extract.

It is important to note that tongkat ali should be "cycled" when used. This means that the herb should be used daily for about three weeks on with one week off. This prevents the body from getting used to the herb and allows it to maintain its effectiveness. Another cycling option would be to take it five days on and two days off.

Hormone Replacement Therapy for Men and Women

Now that we have explored the basics on how to optimize sex hormones naturally, attention should be given to replacing these hormones when they remain low during menopause or andropause. The previous information is necessary to explore in order to lay a foundation to prepare you for hormone replacement therapy if needed or to enhance hormone replacement therapy once it has begun.

When sex hormones lower as we age, replacement may be the best choice for you. There are two types of hormone replacement therapy: conventional synthetic versions and natural Bioidentical Hormone

Replacement Therapy (BHRT). Synthetic versions such as Premarin® and others come with a higher associated risk of breast cancer and are not the type that I recommend. The focus here is on natural bioidentical hormone replacement therapy.

Delivery Methods for Sex Hormone Replacement for Women and Men

This section is organized based on the delivery method of hormone replacement. There are many different ways to get hormone into the body. Some are good, some excessive, some worthless, and some are superior. The best hormone delivery method is the one that works for you. Some of the delivery methods here will provide synthetic hormone, some provide both synthetic or bioidentical, and others tend to be for bioidentical hormone only. Since so much confusion exists between synthetic versus natural hormones, I include both for clarification.

Intramuscular Injections

This is an injection of sex hormone using a needle and syringe administered directly into the muscle. Both men and women can have testosterone or estrogen administered in this fashion.

For men, there are five injectable testosterone approved in the United States. These forms of injection are all synthetic:

- Aqueous Testosterone: very short acting (1-2 days).
- Testosterone Cyprionate: short acting (2-4 days).
- Testosterone Proprionate: short acting (2-4 days).
- Testosterone Enthanate: longer acting (7-10 days).
- Deca-Durabolin: longer acting, offering superior muscle pain relief (7-10 days).

Another form that is not yet approved in the United States is testosterone undeconate, a long-acting form of injectable testosterone produced and approved in Europe. I admit that the data on this form looks good in terms of its ability to maintain consistent testosterone levels for up to twelve weeks. This would be a marked improvement in the efficacy of testosterone injections, but it is still synthetic. Purportedly, testosterone undeconate has less negative side effects associated with it, and there is less liver involvement in the way it is processed.

> Injections cause an abrupt spike of testosterone and estrogen levels in men and women, and then an inevitable and marked rapid decline of the levels.

For women, there are both testosterone and estrogen injections which are both synthetic. A typical estrogen intramuscular injection is Depo-Estradiol, also known as estradiol cypionate. This is a 1 mg to 5 mg injection of synthetic estrogen that is administered once every three to four weeks. Testosterone injections for women are also administered in 50 mcg to 150 mcg monthly injections.

Here are the problems. Injections cause an abrupt spike of testosterone and estrogen levels in men and women, and then an inevitable and marked rapid decline of the levels. Of all of the types of delivery mechanisms, injections cause the largest fluctuation and the most inconsistent results. I have seen the lab results for both men and women showing extremely high levels of hormone well above the range or very low levels well below the range, depending on the time they had their blood drawn in relation to the time they had their injection. Additionally, the estrogen or testosterone injections are synthetic and can tax the liver over time. Rapidly flooding the body with hormone and then leaving it vacuous and depleted instantly causes additional physiological stress on the system.

Pills

Testosterone can come in a pill form in either a synthetic or bioidentical version. A typical synthetic pill used for testosterone replacement is methyltestosterone. This is one of the worst versions of testosterone replacement and even among conventional doctors it has fallen quickly out of fashion, although I have seen it occasionally prescribed. This particular type of oral preparation must travel through the liver to be activated causing liver toxicity over time. This is very well documented. Liver toxicity includes hepatitis (liver inflammation) and even liver cancer.[512, 513, 514] I would never suggest this type of testosterone for men or women.

A compounding pharmacist can put bioidentical estrogen, testosterone or progesterone in a pill form. Because it is bioidentical and natural to the system, it does not pose the same problems for the liver. However, it still has to go through the liver to be metabolized. The large problem with that is that the hormone gets broken down by stomach acid and the liver before it makes it to the general circulation. So, the delivery is not as easy and a larger overall dose is required.

I typically prescribe oral progesterone for women to protect the uterine lining. These doses range from 100 mg to 200 mg and are well tolerated by most women.

Trochies

Trochies, pronounced "tro-keys" is an industry term for an oral lozenge. It is created by a compounding pharmacist utilizing bioidentical hormones, including estrogen, testosterone, and progesterone. The trochee dissolves in the mouth and the hormone is delivered into the body sublingually or under the tongue and through the oral mucosa. The sublingual route is a very efficient way to deliver all types of substances into the body.

I always comment to my patients, "The great thing about trochies is they absorb really well. The bad thing about trochies is… they absorb really well." Trochies absorb very rapidly into the body creating a sudden spike

I always comment to my patients, "The great thing about trochies is they absorb really well. The bad thing about trochies is… they absorb really well."

of hormone that ultimately does not last. The large amount that has been delivered quickly metabolizes in the body leaving the hormone levels low again. I have seen countless estrogen and testosterone lab results that show almost no hormone in the system, even though the patient had taken the trochie within hours of the lab work. The levels of hormone will not stay in the body in a consistent, continuous fashion.

However, this does not mean that someone cannot benefit from this form of delivery. Some patients will respond very well to this form. Because it is specially compounded, the dose can be adjusted to attempt to optimize the situation for the patient's needs.

Creams and Gels

Hormones can be added to a cream or gel. Some of these substances are made by a compounding pharmacist while others are synthetic and are produced by pharmaceutical companies. Often, creams are associated with delivering natural bioidentical sex hormones such as progesterone or estrogen. Of all the different ways to give hormone to a patient, I would rank this at the bottom.

These are the problems with creams and gels:

- Many women find the creams oily, greasy, and messy. Clothing gets stained.
- Compliance is an issue, having to remember to not just put it on once or twice daily, but to actually rotate the area of skin where the cream or gel is applied.
- Rotation of the application site of a cream is needed because hormones from a cream tend to saturate the layer of fat under the skin, instead of getting into circulation.[515]
- Delivery of hormone into the blood is low.[516] I cannot begin to express the countless times I have seen poor response from patients to creams. Blood levels will be low and symptoms will be high. One double blind, placebo-controlled study utilizing various doses of progesterone cream (as high as 60 mg for six months) found no difference in symptomatic relief for women as compared to placebo.[517] Another study utilizing 32 mg of progesterone cream

in women concluded that it "does not seem to allow sufficient hormone to enter the body to achieve a biological effect on lipid levels (cholesterol), bone mineral metabolic markers, vasomotor symptoms (hot flashes and night sweats), or moods."[518]

🦠 Transference of the hormone from the person using it to another person, such as a spouse or child is high. Men can accidentally absorb some estrogen from their female partner if she had just applied the cream. This is even more concerning for women who may have excessive amounts of testosterone transferred from their male partner. A typical testosterone gel for men, Androgel®, can have a high rate of skin transference if the patient is not careful. In one example, I had a male patient applying a testosterone gel on his arms near the same time he would change his female infant's diaper. The child developed pubic hair leading to the initial assumption that she had a brain tumor, until it was determined it was simply from the testosterone gel transference. The child eventually improved. But be careful.

Creams and gels are not all bad, however. I have had some patients report good relief from the use of creams or gels. Some patients are very sensitive to adding in hormone into the body and topical creams are very gentle for this patient population. In the case of vaginal dryness, creams or gels can be a good solution. In the end, you need to find the best form of hormone delivery for you, and it may be a cream or gel.

Transdermal Patches

Hormone patches are delivered transdermally, or through the skin, in fairly steady doses throughout the duration of the patch life. Patches deliver hormone in very similar ways as a cream. However, the patch tends to deliver hormone more steadily over a longer period of time versus a cream or gel.

Hormone patches are usually replaced twice weekly for women to maintain hormone levels. In men, testosterone patches must be applied daily due to the larger amounts of hormone that men require.

Problems with the patch:

🌰 Compliance. Most patches, such as Vivelle®, need to be applied every third or fourth day, and often patients will forget to put it on, leaving hormone levels low for a stretch of time.

🌰 Adhesive allergies. For some sensitive patients, the adhesive used to keep the patch in place can cause irritation from mild to an actual burn on the skin.

The benefits of using a transdermal hormone replacement application such as a patch or cream includes:[519, 520, 521]

🌰 Hormones bypass the gastrointestinal tract and are absorbed directly from the skin into the blood circulation and get diffused to target organs before passing through the liver, so there is no "first-pass" liver metabolism issue.

🌰 Triglyceride levels in the lipid profile do not rise.

🌰 The positive effect on bone density may be quicker with transdermal patches and creams than oral pills.

Patches and creams are better suited for patients who have a medical history of:

🌰 Deep vein thrombosis.

🌰 Liver disease with abnormal liver function.

🌰 More serious osteoporosis with a higher risk of fractures.

🌰 High triglycerides.

🌰 Gastrointestinal and gall-bladder problems.

Subcutaneous Pellet Implants

After working in a busy practice largely devoted to subcutaneous pellet implants and subsequently treating thousands of men and women in this fashion, I am convinced it is one of the most superior delivery methods of hormone available. I have medically consulted with countless patients taking other forms of hormone delivery such as injections, creams, patches, and pills who did not consistently achieve good results from hormone replacement therapy until they received pellets.

In both men and women, this form of hormone replacement is potent, convenient, and consistent in delivering natural estrogen and testosterone to the body. Subcutaneous pellets are safe and natural to the system and are considered bioidentical, which means they possess the same biochemical shape as the hormones your body makes normally on its own.

Here are some common questions and answers about pellet therapy:

What makes pellets different from other forms of hormone delivery?

Subcutaneous pellets slowly dissolve over time providing a relatively consistent release of hormone. Other forms of hormone delivery simply cannot maintain a constant amount of hormone over time, leading to daily spikes and deficiencies of hormone.

What do the pellets look like?

Subcutaneous pellets are approximately the size of a grain of rice or smaller for women. Pellets for men are slightly larger, close to the size of an eraser head on a pencil.

Where do the pellets go in my body?

Pellets are placed subcutaneously (under the skin) on the side of the hip in an easy minor surgery procedure that takes less than five minutes. Other than some slight stinging that may occur with the anesthetic, it is a virtually painless procedure.

How long do the pellets last?

The pellets have an approximately three to six month life span before they dissolve completely and need to be replaced. How long they last depends on certain factors. People with a faster internal metabolic clearance rate, higher exercise rate, and high stress rate tend to utilize the pellets faster. However, this still depends as every person is different and even each insertion can have a slightly different lifespan.

Are pellets FDA approved?

When a compounding pharmacist makes pellets, they use FDA approved, USP (United States Pharmacopoeia) estradiol or testosterone materials. These materials are then placed in the form of a crystalline pellet in a particular dose fit for the patient that is *not* FDA approved. This is largely a technicality. However, there is an FDA approved testosterone pellet on the market called Testopel®.

Does scientific research support the efficacy and safety of pellet therapy?

Pellet therapy has been around since the 1930s, not long after both estradiol and testosterone were discovered and isolated in the laboratory. The research on this therapy is rich. One of the best places to find downloadable sources is www.hormonebalance.org.

Why doesn't my doctor know about hormone pellet therapy?

Despite the plethora of research and its long historical use, subcutaneous pellet therapy still remains outside of the typical standard of care for most doctors. Most mainstream medical journals will not have information about the therapy because it conflicts with the typical drug industry standards of synthetic medications.

Are there any side effects with the use of pellet therapy?

As with any medical procedure, side effects are potentially possible. Estrogen can lead to breast tenderness and uterine bleeding issues. Testosterone can potentially, but rarely, cause facial hair growth, acne, hair loss, and water retention, all to varying but reversible degrees. Progesterone can occasionally cause fatigue, nausea, dizziness, irritability, mood swings, and water retention. Most of these issues are handled by adjusting the dose of the hormone.

Step 4: Sex Hormones

Are there any complications with the pellet procedure?

If proper aftercare instructions are utilized by the healthcare provider and followed by the patient, then complications are very rare. When these instructions are not followed, then more potential exists for problems. The pellets can potentially extrude or pop out. Infection at the insertion site is also possible, but is easily handled with antibiotics. There can be pain in the area from a couple of days up to about a few weeks. Icing the area and taking anti-inflammatories can remedy this problem most of the time.

Is pellet therapy for me?

A large percentage of the patients that I consult with have already tried other forms of hormone replacement therapy and have not achieved good results. Patients are looking for complete relief of the menopausal or andropausal situation and are seeking a therapy that is not just effective, but convenient. Having a simple five-minute procedure done two to four times per year is often what most people are looking for. A consult with a qualified healthcare provider who understands hormone replacement therapy and particularly pellet therapy should help to determine the best personal choice for you.

In Conclusion: Is Hormone Replacement Therapy Safe For Me?

Every patient must make their own decision about how to proceed with incorporating hormone replacement into their lives. This should be done with proper medical counsel and diligent research and exploration. Reading this book is part of that research.

I do not have all the answers. But I can say that the proper use of natural bioidentical hormone replacement therapy can be an excellent adjunct to improve your health, state of mind, and overall well-being. And the use of natural bioidentical hormone replacement therapy has not at all been proven to be associated with serious disease. Ken Holtorff M.D. has written and published an excellent article[522] that explains and reveals the difference between synthetic and natural bioidentical hormone replacement therapy. Most of the controversy and fears associated with sex hormone replacement therapy, particularly for women, is predicated on the use of potent synthetic versions of sex hormones. Rebecca Glaser M.D. has written and researched the subject of bioidentical hormone replacement therapy, particularly on the subject of subcutaneous pellets, and her website is an excellent resource. Find it at www.hormonebalance.org.

The 2002 Women's Health Initiative studied synthetic estrogen and progestins and found a correlation with an increased risk of breast cancer. And even recently, in late 2010, yet again, another study on synthetic estrogen and progestins (i.e. Provera®), found that its use increases the risk for aggressive breast cancer.[523] These studies were not exploring natural hormone therapies, but potent synthetics.

For men, most of the controversy that still remains about using testosterone replacement comes from the extremely high amounts that body builders have been known to use. This type of abuse of testosterone and its derivatives has absolutely nothing to do with the normal physiologic use of testosterone in normal amounts. But, in some cases, with some doctors, the misunderstanding goes on.

Step 5:
Thyroid Hormone Treatment and Thyroid Gland Optimization:
A Revolutionary and Integrated Approach

Thyroid Gland Optimization

Take notice of the title of this step. The reason the word "revolutionary" is within the title is to show that this approach is in fact making a full circle back to an approach of thyroid gland and hormone treatment from years ago. Revolution implies sudden change, but also restoration to a point of origin. Historically, prior to the popular use of the TSH laboratory value and other political factors, physicians approached the thyroid patient with rationality that allowed the individual to experience optimal results and relief from the symptoms and conditions of thyroid disease. And "integrated" implies incorporating a multifaceted approach to human health and historical medical experience with the treatment of thyroid disease and a sub-optimal metabolism.

One of the first steps to improving your metabolic health is to improve the actual function of your thyroid gland as naturally as possible. This can and should be done whether you are on thyroid hormone medication or not.

If you believe your thyroid gland is sluggish based on a "borderline" diagnosis of hypothyroidism or "subclinical" hypothyroidism, then your first step should be to improve your thyroid gland function naturally and avoid the use of thyroid hormone medication all together. However, in some cases, attempting to optimize thyroid function conservatively will not be enough, and moving forward with thyroid hormone medication can be an effective, safe, and even instantaneous way

> One of the first steps to improving your metabolic health is to improve the actual function of your thyroid gland as naturally as possible.

of improving your overall metabolic health. Whether or not you are on a thyroid hormone medication, you will need to go through a process of optimizing your thyroid gland function naturally with nutritional and even herbal supplementation. This is just the best first step.

Thyroid Supportive Diet

Step 2 of The Metabolic Health Protocol and the chapter on metabolic diet clearly laid out an optimal lifestyle approach to eating that possesses the ability to improve thyroid health both directly and indirectly. This section gives advice on what to eat for a healthy thyroid gland.

The metabolic diet explained in this book is ideal for healthy thyroid function because:

- It reduces insulin resistance that in turn helps with the weight gain that is so common in hypothyroid (low thyroid function) patients.

- Hypothyroidism is related to insulin resistance, the precursor to type II diabetes[524] as well as altered insulin and carbohydrate metabolism.[525]

- It has a large focus on fruit and vegetable based fiber that helps to improve thyroid function, digestion, and elimination.

- The metabolic diet, which largely focuses on fresh and optimally-raised sources of animal proteins brings the unique asset of additional *natural* hormones. Red meat, due to its blood content, contains globulin-bound thyroid hormones and other naturally occurring hormones. Please do not confuse this with external synthetic hormones added to poorly raised animals for consumption. This is referring to the naturally occurring hormones that all mammals would have circulating in their system. Of course, we have evolved over millennia consuming these naturally circulating hormones and in fact may actually need this supplementation of hormones in our diets to naturally benefit and enhance our endocrine system. Also, the ancestral nature of the proposed metabolic diet contains a large amount and variety of plant vegetables including foods such as seaweed that actually contain natural hormone. In 2002, a Japanese publication reported the detection of physiologically significant amounts of thyroxine (T4) and triiodothyronine (T3), as well as DIT (T2) and MIT (T1) in the seaweeds Laminaria (Kombu) and Sargassum (Sargasso Weed).[526]

Specific Foods for Your Thyroid and Metabolic Health

The metabolic health plant of the sea is seaweed. This is one of the best foods to start if you have perceived thyroid imbalances or have many of the symptoms of hypothyroidism or low metabolism. Seaweed has been used as a botanical medicine for millennia by cultures from all over the world for hypothyroidism, goiter, weight loss, fatigue, feeling cold, nervousness and anxiety, and immune support. It is harvested on coastal shores worldwide, particularly Japan, Korea, and China.

One of the key reasons seaweed is so nutritious and beneficial is the large and complete array of minerals it contains. Seaweed contains large amounts of iodine, selenium, magnesium, sodium, potassium, and calcium. Specifically, seaweed has approximately 100 mcg of iodine per 5 grams. No land-based plant contains the abundance of minerals seaweed possesses. This is one of the reasons I recommend Celtic Sea Salt, as that salt also contains all eighty-two known minerals. However, even though Celtic Sea Salt is very complete in its mineral content, it is not as abundant as seaweed. Also, seaweed has a rich supply of vitamins A, B, B12, C, and even essential omega-3 fatty acids.

> The metabolic health plant of the sea is seaweed.

Thyroid Hormones in Seaweed

Seaweed has been shown to have physiologically significant amounts of the thyroid hormones T4 (thyroxine), T3 (triiodothyronine), T2 (diiodothyronine), and T1 (monothyronine).[527] It also has adequate amounts of T2, which when combined with one another, produce T4. T2 has been shown to have direct physiological metabolism enhancing effects on the body.[528, 529] The implications of the presence of thyroid hormone in seaweed are significant to understanding why seaweed is beneficial for so many hypothyroid patients. It also demonstrates that as a species, we are used to ingesting natural hormones from our diet, and may actually even require it for proper hormonal balance and health.

> Seaweed has been shown to have physiologically significant amounts of the thyroid hormones T4 (thyroxine), T3 (triiodothyronine), T2 (diiodothyronine), and T1 (monothyronine).

When seaweed is added to a supplement regimen of a patient taking thyroid hormone, the thyroid hormone medication dose may be able to be lowered or, in some cases, completely eliminated. This occurs with the use of iodine supplementation also, as explained in this book. Be sure to let your healthcare provider know if you start to use seaweed as this may lead to being over-stimulated on your thyroid hormone medication and the dose would need adjusting.

Adding Seaweed to Your Diet

Seaweed is a profoundly easy and extremely beneficial food source for your thyroid and metabolic health. In general, seaweed can be eaten in a variety of ways as a garnish to all types of foods. The best sources are raw, untreated seaweed, in pieces or powder, and not reconstructed flakes or sheets which are found in many Asian food stores. However, many Asian food stores will have raw, untreated dried seaweed available and this can easily be made into a powder in a food processor. There are many sources of this type of seaweed available to order on the Internet. The herbalist Ryan Drum suggests a mixture of seaweeds for optimal benefits, in a 2:1 ratio of brown seaweed to red seaweed. Varying the types of species in combination brings an eclectic array of benefits.

Always start slowly with seaweed when adding it into your diet or taking it as a dietary supplement. Some people may have some gastric irritation when first trying it, but this is uncommon.

Medicinal Use of Seaweed

Bladderwrack (*Fucus gardneri*) is a type of seaweed that has an extensive historical record of being beneficial for thyroid health and metabolism. This can be taken as loose powder and it acts as an excellent garnish for salads, soups, vegetables and even popcorn. It can also be added to smoothies and other juices. Putting it into a beverage makes it easier to get to a larger effective dose. Follow this guide for dosages:

- For medicinal purposes with the guidance of your healthcare provider, start with about 1 gram and increase by 1 gram per week until symptoms relieve or a maximum of 10 grams has been reached.
- For nutritional support and weight management, 1 to 5 grams daily.
- One teaspoon of powdered seaweed is approximately 3 grams.

The Metabolic Health Oil: Coconut Oil

This is by far one of the best oils you can consume, not just for your thyroid health, but for your entire body and metabolism. Coconut oil is a medium chained triglyceride (MCT) versus the long chain triglycerides (LCT) such as found in butter, lard, and other vegetable oils. Milk fat and palm oil are also considered medium chain triglycerides and real butter also contains some MCTs. MCTs easily pass into the gut without an energy requirement for digestion, and bypass the need for the liver and gall bladder to be involved with bile. Coconut oil contains many medium chain triglycerides, one of which is caprylic acid which has been shown to be very helpful in the treatment of candida (yeast) infections.

Coconut oil received very bad media attention in the late 1980s and inaccurately became associated with increasing heart disease. The campaign against coconut and even palm oil was launched and supported largely by the American Soy Association and other farmers that utilized vegetable-based oils. The falsehoods are not based on facts, science, or even health, but money.

Coconut oil is one of the most versatile and healthiest oils on the planet, demonstrating various benefits including:

❧ Antibacterial effects on diseases such as pneumonia,[530] candida (yeast),[531, 532] and MRSA (methicillin resistant *Staphilococcus aureus*).[533] It is also known to have antiviral properties.[534]

❧ Cardiovascular benefits that include decreased risk of coronary artery disease[535] and improved blood lipids (cholesterol).[536, 537]

❧ Improved digestion and absorption.[538, 539]

❧ Anticancer properties including breast cancer.[540, 541]

❧ Weight management and metabolism enhancement.[542, 543, 544, 545]

Coconut for Weight Management and Metabolism Enhancement

In 2002, the *Journal of Nutrition* published a review article[546] that examined all the published studies to date on MCT (Medium Chain Triglycerides) and weight management. They discovered that diets containing MCT result in:

❧ An increase in energy.

❧ Enhanced metabolism and caloric consumption.

❧ Satiety leading to a decrease in food consumption.

❧ Lowered body fat mass.

❧ An overall reduction in body mass.

Insulin will respond differently to MCT's such as coconut oil because it is digested so rapidly in the body. Other types of fats, such as the slower digested long chain triglycerides, circulate longer in the blood which stimulates a higher insulin response. The lowered insulin response from coconut oil contributes to an increased ability to lose body fat.

You should consume at least one or two tablespoons of coconut oil three times a day at meals. It mixes very well in smoothies and has a very mild coconut flavor. It is also an excellent oil to cook with because it has a higher heat tolerance than other oils. (Olive oil is considered to have a medium heat tolerance.) Be sure that your coconut oil is virgin and cold pressed to ensure the best quality and effectiveness.

Due to the lauric and caprylic acid content of the oil, this makes it very antimicrobial. For some people when they first take coconut oil, there could be a "die off" effect of certain microbes, particularly candida, which could lead to side effects such as headache and diarrhea. Be sure to start slowly with the oil, particularly if you are unhealthy. Increase the dose of the oil slowly over a few weeks and back off if you have any undesired effects. The diarrhea in and of itself is not necessarily a problem, but be sure to seek the advice of your healthcare provider.

Bruce Fife, N.D. has written extensively on the topic of coconut oil and I highly recommend his books. He has found that patients with hypothyroidism can actually increase their body temperature by one or two degrees due to the metabolism-boosting effects of the oil.[547]

Foods to Avoid: Goitrogens

Goitrogens are foods known to decrease thyroid function by inhibiting the synthesis of thyroid hormones within the thyroid gland. The most commonly consumed goitrogens are:

- Unfermented soybeans and soybean products such as tofu, soy milk, soybean oil, soy flour, soy lecithin. These are extremely common in many foods and touted as health food. When unfermented and highly processed, they are anything but health foods.
  - Unfermented soy products that contain isoflavones, such as genistein, inhibit the thyroid enzyme thyroid peroxidase which is necessary for producing the thyroid hormones T4 and T3.
  - It is important to note that fermented soy products, such as natto, miso, tempeh and tamari do not have the same thyroid-lowering affect that the more commonly used unfermented soy products have.
- Peanuts and peanut oil. (Remember: peanuts are not nuts, they are legumes.)

Soy products and peanuts are found in a multitude of packaged and prepared food products and people consume them all the time without even realizing it. Soy products and peanuts should be avoided in general as poor food choices for a multitude of reasons, but I will limit the discussion here to them simply being foods that are goitrogenic.

Other goitrogenic foods include the following and should be rotated and not eaten every day:

- Strawberries
- Cassava
- Pine nuts
- Millet
- Pears
- Peaches
- Spinach
- Bamboo shoots
- Sweet Potatoes

Vegetables from the *Brassica* family when eaten RAW are considered goitrogenic. Cooked or fermented versions do not have the same thyroid-lowering effects:

- Bok choy
- Broccoli
- Broccolini
- Brussels sprouts
- Cabbage
- Canola oil
- Cauliflower
- Chinese cabbage
- Choy sum
- Collard greens
- Horseradish
- *Kai-lan* (Chinese broccoli)
- Kale
- Kohlrabi
- Mizuna
- Mustard greens
- Radishes
- Rapeseed (*yu choy*)
- Rapini
- Rutabagas
- Tatsoi
- Turnips

Medications that Interfere with Thyroid Function

- Aspirin and other "salicylates" and anticoagulants such as Warfarin increase iodine excretion and can lead to hypothyroidism.
- The high blood pressure medication amiodarone, the anti-arrhythmia medication propropranol, and the bipolar disorder medication lithium all interfere with thyroid hormone production, its release, and conversion of T4 to active T3.
- The anti-seizure medications phenobarbitone (Barbita®), phenytoin (Dilantin®), and carbamazepine, (Tegretol®) as well as the antibiotic rifampin (Rifidin®) all destroy the thyroid hormones T4 and T3.

❧ Clomiphene (Clomid®) (fertility drug), cemetidine (Tagamet®) (ulcers), spironolactone (Aldactone®), and amphetamines (Adderall® for attention deficit disorder and narcolepsy) all increase TSH which could give a false positive for the diagnosis of thyroid disease.

❧ 5-hydroxytryptophan (5-HTP), growth hormone and bromocriptine all decrease TSH, which could give a false negative on the diagnosis of hypothyroidism and/or decrease the circulation of thyroid hormones.

❧ For a comprehensive list of medications and compounds that interfere with thyroid function, see http://www.thyroidmanager. org/Chapter5/5a-frame.htm.

Chemicals that Interfere with Thyroid Function

For a detailed look into the various chemicals that interfere with thyroid function, see the chapter on iodine in this book and refer to http:// www.thyroidmanager.org/Chapter5/5a-frame.htm as mentioned above.

❧ I would like to stress here again to avoid soft drinks completely as they contain polybrominated diphenyl ethers, a form of bromide that leads to decreased thyroid function and hypothyroidism. If consuming some form of carbonated beverage is imperative, choose carbonated water and add a small amount of natural fruit juice. Or, there are natural sodas available. But remember, for optimal function of your metabolic health, choose water as your beverage of choice.

Step 5: Thyroid

Other Environmental Hazards to Thyroid Function: X-rays and the Thyroid Gland

X-rays have been historically used for scalp ringworm (*Tinea capitis*), chronic acne, chronic tonsillitis, and asthma. Many of the patients who were treated with radiation for these maladies later developed goiters, nodules, hypothyroidism or thyroid cancers with most of problems occurring twenty to thirty years after exposure. I have patients who have received these treatments years ago and all of them have low thyroid function. One of them had thyroid cancer.

All x-rays or any type of radiation should be avoided when possible. However, routine x-rays at the typical low doses have shown little correlation with thyroid cancer.[548] On routine x-ray examinations, such as dental screenings, a lead neck collar should be considered to protect the thyroid.

Nutritional Supplementation

This is one of the most important facets of improving your thyroid gland function. As you've read, iodine is the most important nutrient for your thyroid.

The foods outlined in this chapter, particularly fresh sources of animal proteins and seaweed, provide an array of minerals that are excellent for your thyroid health including iodine, selenium, copper, zinc and others. These should be your frontline sources of these minerals and nutritional components. However, when access to these types of foods are limited, or if you want to ensure that you are getting adequate intake, supplementation is always an excellent way to provide these components. The key nutrients that have been shown to be effective in assisting thyroid gland function and optimizing thyroid hormone metabolism include:

- Zinc with copper
  - Zinc is important for increasing the production of the enzyme 5'-deiodinase which then converts inactive T4 thyroid hormone into active T3 thyroid hormone.
  - Dose: 30 mg zinc and 2 mg copper daily.
  - Zinc should always be given with copper to prevent copper deficiency.
  - The ratio is 15:1 zinc to copper.
  - Food sources of zinc are pumpkin seeds, oysters, mushrooms, liver, and meat.
- Selenium (optimal form: selenomethionine)

- Selenium assists in the production of 5'-deiodinase, the enzyme that converts inactive T4 thyroid hormone into the active T3 form.

- In a randomized control trial in seventy female patients with autoimmune thyroiditis having either anti-TPO and/or anti-TG antibodies measured in the blood were given 200 mcg of selenium daily. This produced a 40 percent reduction of anti-TPO in the selenium group versus a 10 percent increase in anti-TPO in the placebo group.[549]

- Dose: 400-600 mcg daily or 500 mcg twice daily for the first week, then 500 mcg once daily for the next week, then 200 mcg daily thereafter.

- Selenium and iodine should always be taken together. If iodine intake is high or adequate and selenium is low, then over-production of thyroid hormone may occur due to Graves' hyperthyroidism, or there *may be* an increased amount of oxidation of the thyroid producing antibodies and Hashimoto's thyroiditis may occur, but this is unlikely.

- A good food source for selenium is Brazil nuts. They contain around 50 mcg per nut. Mushrooms, fish, lobster, meat, eggs, and liver are all good sources.

- Tyrosine
  - Tyrosine is the key protein component of the thyroid hormone molecule.
  - Dose: At least 300 mg daily but optimally about 1 to 1.5 grams per day for adults.
  - Eggs, cheese, milk, meat, and poultry are all good sources of tyrosine.

- Iron
  - Iron deficiency impairs thyroid hormone synthesis by reducing activity of heme-dependent (iron dependent) thyroid peroxidase, the enzyme responsible for producing thyroid hormone. Iron-

deficiency anemia also interferes with the effectiveness of iodine supplementation.[550]

- Caution: Do not supplement with iron unless you have had a basic blood test to check for anemia. You should have blood iron and ferritin levels checked. Ferritin is the storage form of iron and is often overlooked by physicians when trying to determine iron deficiency. Checking iron levels alone is not as adequate as considering the ferritin levels.
  - Ferritin should be at least above 70 ng/mL.
- Dose and optimal form of iron: Iron should be consumed in an amino acid chelate form such as ferrous gluconate, which has better absorption and less tendency towards constipation. Ferrous sulfate is often prescribed but has the worst absorbability and it often causes constipation and should be avoided. Often, iron is dosed too low because of the difference between the total amount of iron with its attached protein or other molecule and the actual elemental iron or true iron content of a supplement. For example, ferrous gluconate contains 36 mg of elemental iron for every 325 mg tablet.
  - A good dose for iron deficiency anemia is about 100-150 mg elemental iron daily.
  - Taking iron with food can lower the absorbability of the iron,[551] so if you do not have any issues with stomach upset, then take the iron on an empty stomach. Using ferrous fumarate or gluconate usually does not bring the problems with stomach upset. However, take your iron with food to avoid stomach upset if this occurs.
  - Take your iron in divided doses to improve absorbability.[552] Larger doses of iron are more difficult to absorb.
  - Many medications interfere with iron, so avoid taking it with any medications, particularly thyroid hormone medication. Since iron interferes with thyroid hormone medication so severely, and that thyroid hormone should be taken in the

morning on an empty stomach, your iron supplements should be taken in divided doses at about noon and in the evening. Once you have achieved an adequate blood level of ferritin, then lower the iron to a maintenance dose of approximately 20 mg elemental iron; however, supplementation may not be needed if the diet is adequate in iron. Be sure to have your levels monitored and follow the advice of your healthcare provider. It can take several months for anemia to improve.

- Food sources: Beef, organ meats such as liver and kidney, nuts and seeds such as almonds, pumpkin seeds, cashews, and the herbs cinnamon, thyme, rosemary, and curry, dried figs and currants; shellfish such as clams, oysters, and mussels, and finally, blackstrap molasses.

Elemental iron content of various iron supplements:

- Ferrous sulfate (between 22 to 33 percent elemental iron): 65 mg elemental iron for a 325 mg tablet. Avoid this form.
- Ferrous gluconate (12 percent elemental iron): 36 mg elemental iron for a 325 mg tablet.
- Ferrous fumarate (33 percent elemental iron): 106 mg elemental iron for a 325 mg tablet.

Be cautious when you are taking iron. The oral lethal dose of elemental iron is approximately 200-250 mg/kg of body weight, which is over 13,000 mg of elemental iron for a 150 pound person. However, symptoms of acute toxicity may occur with iron doses of 20-60 mg/kg of body weight, or from 1,363 mg to 4,080 mg elemental iron for the same 150 pound person. Also, keep iron away from children.

Step 5: Thyroid

Herbal (Botanical) Medicines for Thyroid Health and Low Thyroid Function

Fucus vesiculosis (Bladderwrack)

This seaweed was reviewed above and is one of the most popular and effective seaweed botanical medicines for the treatment of low thyroid function. It was mentioned before in this chapter and warrants reminding of its potent benefits for thyroid health. Dose: 5 to 10 grams daily.

Commiphora mukul (Guggul)

This small tree has been used for thousands of years in traditional eastern Indian Ayurvedic medicine for its invigorating and weight loss properties. The resin from the commiphora mukul tree contains the active ingredient guggulsterone Z and guggulsterone E which have been found to increase iodine uptake and thyroid hormone production [553] and to increase conversion in the liver of the inactive thyroid hormone T4 into the active form, T3.[554] Enhanced thyroid hormone synthesis from guggulsterone use is also associated with enhanced activity of thyroid peroxidase and increased tissue oxygen uptake in the liver and muscle.[555]

Guggulsterones have also been shown to inhibit farnesoid X receptor.[556, 557] This inhibition enhances bile elimination, which in turn clears LDL (bad) cholesterol, triglycerides (fatty acids), and liver toxins. Guggulsterones are also associated with weight loss particularly when additional phosphates are incorporated.[558] Dose: With 2.5 percent guggulsterones at 750 mg daily (4 mg per pound of body weight).

> The resin from the commiphora mukul tree contains the active ingredient guggulsterone Z and guggulsterone E which have been found to increase iodine uptake and thyroid hormone production and to increase conversion in the liver of the inactive thyroid hormone T4 into the active form, T3.

Iris versicolor (Blue Flag)

Iris acts as a potent detoxifier of the thyroid gland and the liver and is known as a lymphagogue which means it helps to move lymphatic fluid in the body and organs. This herb is specifically indicated in thyroid enlargement (goiter) and in inflammatory conditions such as thyroiditis. This herb is potentially toxic at elevated amounts so keep the dose at recommended amounts and consult your healthcare provider regarding its use.

Dose: 750 mg daily.

Dietary Desiccated Thyroid Powder

So far in this chapter, I have described natural ways to enhance the function of the thyroid gland before even mentioning prescription thyroid medications. This is to emphasize that, whenever possible, the medical path of least invasiveness should be taken. It also emphasizes that even when thyroid medication is given, natural support for the thyroid gland, or any endocrine gland, is always a good idea and, in fact, may be necessary for optimal results. Dietary desiccated thyroid powder, you will see, walks the line between being a substance that both supports thyroid function as well as enhances the metabolism directly in a similar way as thyroid hormone medications.

When taken in high enough doses, dietary desiccated thyroid powder has the ability to enhance the metabolism directly through its medicinal effects. John C. Lowe D.C. has already published preliminary research confirming its metabolic enhancing effects and ability to relieve signs and symptoms of hypothyroidism.[559, 560] My clinical experience with this also confirms these findings.

It is important to note that dietary desiccated thyroid powder is a supplement and companies that manufacture and distribute these products make no claims to its medicinal effects or it being equivalent to natural desiccated thyroid hormone medications. However, the dietary thyroid "glandular" content provide potent and effective results for patients with hypothyroidism and/or conditions of lowered metabolism.

When Should I Use Dietary Desiccated Thyroid Powder?

- ❦ If you suspect and/or have confirmation of a lowered metabolism and/or signs and symptoms of hypothyroidism and are not yet on thyroid hormone medication.
- ❦ If you are on the borderline of a diagnosis of hypothyroidism and your situation is not yet severe.
- ❦ You are diagnosed with hypothyroidism and/or a condition of lowered metabolism such as fibromyalgia, and you have difficulty in obtaining a cooperating prescribing physician who either:
  - ❦ Keeps you on a form of thyroid hormone that is not working such as plain synthetic T4 or
  - ❦ You are kept on a dose of thyroid hormone that is too low to relieve you of your clinical signs and symptoms of hypothyroidism and/or lowered metabolism.

Dosing with Dietary Desiccated Thyroid Powder

The individual dose would be the least adequate dose to be effective at relieving the clinical signs and symptoms of the hypothyroidism (low thyroid function) and/or the lowered metabolism. On average, the dose can vary from 300 mg to a 1,000 mg or more, depending on the individual. The dose should be determined by you and your relief of symptoms based on the protocol outlined in the Metabolic Health Protocol in this book and with the guidance of your healthcare provider.

Thyroid Hormone Treatment: Hypothyroidism

If basic nutritional or herbal supplementation, or dietary desiccated thyroid powder are inadequate to maximize your thyroid gland health and/or your symptoms, you may need to move forward with thyroid hormone medication. If you are significantly hypothyroid (low thyroid function), have had part or all of your thyroid removed, or your thyroid was ablated (destroyed) due to radioactive iodine treatment for Graves' hyperthyroidism, and you have either been newly diagnosed and/or been on thyroid hormone medication for some time, you will need to start or continue with your thyroid hormone medication. But now it is time to figure out which type of thyroid hormone is the best choice for you and then maximize the actual dose so as to relieve you of your hypothyroid and low metabolism signs and symptoms.

> If basic nutritional or herbal supplementation, or dietary desiccated thyroid powder are inadequate to maximize your thyroid gland health and/or your symptoms, you may need to move forward with thyroid hormone medication.

What Type of Thyroid Hormone Medication Should I Use?

The short and concise answer is "the type that works for you." Too often, patients are forced into using one type of thyroid hormone medication, typically levothyroxine, or T4. The most popular brand of T4 is Synthroid®. The October 2008 issue of *AARP Bulletin* listed the fifty most prescribed drugs in the U.S. in that year. The fourth most prescribed drug was levothyroxine with 58.6 million prescriptions for a retail cost of $546 million. Synthroid®, the most popular brand of levothyroxine, ranked 26th and produced 23.3 million prescriptions at a retail cost of $515 million. This statistic demonstrates the absolute prevalence of hypothyroidism as an epidemic. It also shows how levothyroxine and particularly Synthroid® has the hypothyroidism market cornered. What I wish it demonstrated was that the prevalence of the prescribing of Synthroid® was due to its effectiveness. But, this is far from the reality.

Based on my experience, I have found that there is a basic tendency of thyroid hormone medication effectiveness. I rank them from most effective to least effective as follows:

- Natural Desiccated Thyroid Hormone
- Compounded T4/T3 preparations
- Plain T3
- Plain T4
- Plain T2

Step 5: Thyroid

Natural Desiccated Thyroid Hormone

I have found that the best type of thyroid hormone for most patients is natural desiccated thyroid hormone, such as Armour®, Nature Throid®, or Westthroid®. This type of thyroid hormone medication comes from a porcine (pig) source and is considered natural. It contains a complete array of thyroid hormones including the main thyroid hormones T4 and T3, and even T2 and T1, T0 (or tyrosine). T2 has limited activity and has been studied, and T1 and T0 have no known function but still make the product holistically complete and more bioavailable and absorbable. Most products that are closer to nature have a more complete effect on the human system. This is true of botanical (herbal) medicines that contain known active ingredients (that are often put into prescription medications) but also other naturally occurring substances that synergistically work in concert with the entire botanical medicine, making it more effective and ultimately producing less side effects.

Another key reason for the effectiveness of natural desiccated thyroid medications is due to the presence of a key thyroid hormone, T3, or triiodothyronine. As explained before in a previous chapter, T3 is the most potent, active form of thyroid hormone and delivers the best results for most patients.

> Another key reason for the effectiveness of natural desiccated thyroid medications is due to the presence of a key thyroid hormone, T3, or triiodothyronine.

Stability of Desiccated Thyroid

It has been touted by many endocrinologists and pharmaceutical companies that natural desiccated thyroid hormone such as Armour® and Nature Throid® are unstable and deliver inaccurate amounts of thyroid hormone leading to recalls of batches. As recent as 2005, Armour® thyroid had some batches recalled, but it had not been recalled before or since.[561]

However, in 2009, Armour® had some difficulties in formulation that temporarily halted production, but this had nothing to do with batch recall. Nature Throid® or Westthroid® have never been recalled and they have been producing natural desiccated thyroid since the 1930s. The leading choice of thyroid hormone by the endocrinology specialty is levothyroxine or T4, and there have been multiple recalls of this medication due to lack of potency. Between 1990 and 1997 alone there have been ten recalls of 150 lots worth of 100 million tablets due to content uniformity, sub-potency, and stability failures.[562]

The Physiologic Compatibility of Natural Desiccated Thyroid Hormone

The common argument against the use of desiccated thyroid hormone such as Nature Throid® is that the ratio of T4 to T3 of 4:1 within the medication is not physiologic for a human being. The opposition explains that humans have serum blood concentration ratios of T4 to T3 of 85.8 mcg of T4 to about 1.3 mcg of T3 or 65:1 which illustrates in their minds why T3 and desiccated thyroid hormone should not be used for hypothyroidism. But here are two facts regarding thyroid hormone physiology that they continue to ignore, even in the journals:

- One, production rates of T4 from the thyroid gland are 130 nmol/day/70kg body weight which equates exactly to 101.4 mcg (conversion rate for T4 is 1 nmol = 0.78 mcg) and T3 is 48 nmol/day/70kg which equates to 31.2 mcg (conversion rate for T3 is 1 nmol = 0.65 mcg), which is a ratio of T4:T3 of 3.25 to 1, far closer to the 4:1 ratio found in desiccated thyroid hormone.

- Two, the clearance rate of T3 from the blood is approximately twenty times more rapid than T4, which means that T3, the active form of thyroid hormone, will often be lower in the blood than T4 because it is busy doing its job at the cellular level.[563]

Dosing with Natural Desiccated Thyroid Hormone

It is important to note here also that the average dose for most patients on thyroid hormone, based on historical use,[564, 565, 566] and something that I have seen consistently in my clinical practice is two to four grains of natural desiccated thyroid hormone.

Each grain of natural desiccated thyroid contains 38 mcg of T4 and 9 mcg T3. So, two grains would have 76 mcg T4 and 18 mcg T3 and four grains would equate to 152 mcg of T4 and 36 mcg of T3. This compares to the above-mentioned normal thyroid hormone production rates of 101.4 mcg T4 and 31.2 mcg T3.

> It is important to note here also that the average dose for most patients on thyroid hormone, based on historical use,[564, 565, 566] and something that I have seen consistently in my clinical practice is two to four grains of natural desiccated thyroid hormone.

- ❧ A good starting dose is one grain of desiccated thyroid hormone. This dose can be increased by about a ½ grain every two to four weeks.

- ❧ I usually increase the dose by ½ grain increments on a three to four week basis. I believe this allows patients to truly get used to the thyroid hormone and the additional components of the metabolic health protocol.

Be aware that many of the elements of the metabolic health protocol, including the diet and exercise recommendations, the dietary supplements, and the additional hormone replacement therapies are all working on supporting both the metabolism and overall thyroid function. Therefore, a more steady and prudent approach to increasing the thyroid hormone dose has been more effective for the majority of my patients. Each patient is of course an individual, which necessitates occasionally increasing the dose either slower or faster.

Synthetic T4/T3 Combinations

The option exists to have a prescription of synthetic T4 and T3 combinations. One option is the manufactured prescription medication Thyrolar® which is a synthetic product combining levothyroxine (T4) and triiodothyronine (T3) in a ratio of T4 to T3 of 4:1.

These types of prescriptions are best formulated by a compounding pharmacist and are reasonably priced. Compounding allows for titration of the dose to very exact specifications for each individual patient. Many patients will need a ratio of T4:T3 of 4:1, but others may need a 3:1 ratio to improve. Compounding allows for this, where a manufactured T4/T3 product such as Thyrolar® does not.

- ❷ A good starting dose is 40 mcg of T4 and 10 mcg of T3 in a single compounded instant release pill.
- ❷ The dose can be increased every two to four weeks by 20 mcg T4 and 5 mcg T3 at a time.

The term "synthetic" does not necessarily mean it is inferior or unsafe. In fact, these types of synthetic thyroid hormones are actually bioidentical, being the exact biochemical structure of the hormone that your thyroid produces. But, they are still isolated hormones that are synthetically derived versus natural desiccated thyroid hormones that are derived from a natural source containing the complete array of all the thyroid hormones.

> Compounding allows for titration of the dose to very exact specifications for each individual patient.

Plain Synthetic T3

In some circumstances, patients will have better results with plain synthetic T3. Particularly, patients being treated for fibromyalgia, hypometabolism or thyroid hormone resistance, will react better to plain synthetic T3. For these conditions, I believe that it is important to start with natural desiccated thyroid hormone initially, and if after a few months of little to no improvement, then a switch to T3 would be prudent. It still may be the decision of the physician to start these types of patients initially on T3 and this is still a good clinical decision.

> In some circumstances, patients will have better results with plain synthetic T3.

- ❧ A good starting dose is 25 to 40 mcg.
- ❧ The dose can be increased every two to four weeks by 20 to 30 mcg.

Plain Synthetic T4

Rarely, patients will not tolerate T3 therapy in any amount or type (compounded T4/T3 combinations or natural desiccated thyroid) and prefer to stay with synthetic T4. This occurs less than 5 percent of the time in my practice. The intolerance to T3 can be due to severe adrenal fatigue, hypoglycemia (low blood sugar) or simply an intolerance and sensitivity to the T3. T4 can be used and I prefer to have it compounded by a professional at a compounding pharmacy. A compounding pharmacist allows the dose to be titrated to an exact dose, providing more flexibility and individual tailoring for the patient.

The average dose of levothyroxine is about 200 to 400 mcg, which equates to two to four grains of desiccated thyroid hormone. In general, the dose can be increased by 50 mcg in monthly increments.

Plain Synthetic T2 Added Into a T4/T3 Combination Product

Typically, the thyroid hormone T2 is thought to have little to no cellular activity. However, there has been more research showing that T2 possesses some real metabolic activity and this was mentioned in the section on seaweed.

T2 appears to work directly on mitochondrial respiration,[567] which increases energy rapidly. T3 and T4 thyroid hormones work on increasing oxidative phosphorylation and its related enzymes, which results in increased energy, but somewhat slower. T2 will increase energy within one hour, where it takes about twenty-four hours for T3 to cause an increase in energy.[568] In respect to the actual potency of T2 in comparison to other thyroid hormones, depending on the study, it is anywhere from five to twenty-five times less potent in comparison to the potent active thyroid hormone T3.[569, 570]

> Typically, the thyroid hormone T2 is thought to have little to no cellular activity. However, there has been more research showing that T2 possesses some real metabolic activity

Of course, when taking seaweed and/or natural desiccated thyroid hormone medication, you are taking T2 as it naturally occurs in these substances. However, T2 could be added to a compounded T4/T3 product to make it more complete and better mimic natural desiccated thyroid hormone, such as Armour® or Nature Throid®.

More on Dosing Thyroid Hormone

This is one of the most controversial and confusing subjects for physicians and patients alike. The summary answer to the question of "How do I determine the best thyroid hormone dose?" is: Follow the clinical signs and symptoms that a patient presents with and not solely thyroid hormone laboratory analysis.

Therefore, a patient needs to be monitored closely with a healthcare provider who is willing to take the necessary time to apply integrative clinical rational reasoning to an individual case. Monitoring is done by determining if the patient still presents with many of the signs and symptoms of hypothyroidism or, simply, if they are improving or not. This is not necessarily a difficult thing to do, nor is it easy. It just takes a keen eye and a willingness to understand that higher doses of thyroid hormone can be extremely effective and very safe.

Step 5: Thyroid

Here is a summary of the basic thyroid hormone dose ranges for various types of thyroid hormone medications:

Thyroid Medication	Average Effective Dose
Natural Desiccated Thyroid (Nature Throid®, Armour®)	2-4 Grains (120-240 mg)
Compounded T4/T3	80 mcg T4 & 20 mcg T3 to 160 mcg T4 & 40 mcg T3
Plain T3 (liothyronine, Cytomel®)	50-100 mcg
Plain T4 (levothyroxine, Synthroid®)	200-400 mcg

Monthly Monitoring

A patient can have their thyroid hormone dose increased on a monthly basis that normally allows for their body to adapt to a dose. Along the way, symptoms are monitored using questionnaires, basic clinical questioning, and measurable signs such as basal body temperature, pulse rate, blood pressure, and Achille's tendon reflex time. The healthcare provider will monitor these symptoms, but the patient also must pay attention to help determine if improvement is taking place.

- For natural desiccated thyroid hormone, the dose is typically started at ½ to one full grain and then increased on a monthly basis by ½ grain increments. Since the average dose is two to four grains, the appropriate dose can be achieved in 2 to 6 months in many cases. When going through a comprehensive protocol of enhancing your metabolism and overall health, improvements are steady and complete on many levels.

- Another approach to determining your dose is to work with a healthcare provider who is willing to have your dose increased more rapidly, depending on your unique situation. For natural desiccated thyroid, the dose can be started at ½ grain and then increased by ½ grain increments every three to four days until symptomatic relief is achieved. It is important to not go over four grains until the hormone is in your system at that dose for at least a month. This approach allows for a more rapid improvement of symptoms, but runs more of the risk of becoming over stimulated from a thyroid hormone excess. Use this method very carefully.

- When using T4/T3 compounded formulations, the dose can be started at around 40 mcg T4 and 10 mcg T3 and then increased by 20 mcg T4 and 5 mcg T3 every month.

- When using plain T3 compounded formulations, the dose can be started at around 25 mcg and then can be increased by 10-20 mcg monthly.

- With plain T4, 75 to 100 mcg is an appropriate starting dose and then can be increased by 50 mcg monthly.

- When using T4/T3 compounded formulations, the dose can be started at 40 mcg T4 and 10 mcg T3. It will be important to work with a healthcare provider who will prescribe the T4 and T3 separately and then prescribe 10 mcg T4 and 5 mcg T3 in a large bottle to allow for flexibility in increasing the dose. The dose should be increased by 20 mcg T4 and 5 mcg T3 every three to four days until a maximum dose is achieved of 160 mcg T4 and 40 mcg T3.

- When using plain T3 compounded formulations, the dose can be started at around 25 mcg and then increased by 5 mcg amounts every three to four days until symptomatic relief is achieved or a 50 mcg maximum is reached before clinical assessment takes place. Once 50 mcg of T3 is reached, the same strategy could be employed again to reach a necessary higher dose.

- With plain T4, the same strategy as above is applied, starting at around 100 mcg and then increasing by 50 mcg increments every three to four days.

Step 5: Thyroid

Hashimoto's Thyroiditis

This condition is a chronic autoimmune inflammatory process of the thyroid gland that leads to hypothyroidism (low thyroid function). If a patient has this condition, it can be more challenging to help with just natural thyroid hormone medication. Because of the erratic inflammatory nature of this condition, patients will have chronic flare-ups of inflammation within their thyroid glands leading to such things as sudden fatigue, a choking sensation, and enlargement of the thyroid gland.

In essence, the chronic inflammation needs to be treated and this can be done with certain natural substances. There is a certain gene called Nuclear Factor Kappa B or NF Kappa B that is responsible for generating an inflammatory cytokine called COX-2. Influencing the NK Kappa B gene to slow down how much COX-2 it produces may be able to help with overall inflammation in the body including the thyroid gland.[571, 572]

There are some natural ways to down-regulate Nuclear Factor Kappa B and lower the inflammation in Hashimoto's:

- Resveratrol
  - Resveratrol is found in grapes, fruits, and root extracts of Japanese Knotweed (Polygonum cuspidatum) and has been found to have anti-inflammatory, cell growth-modulatory, and anti-cancer effects.[573] The clinical implications of the use of resveratrol are beginning to be studied en masse.[574]
  - Suggested dose: 300 mg daily up to 1,500 mg daily in certain situations.
- Quercitin
  - This is a plant-derived flavanoid found abundantly in many vegetables and fruits particularly green tea, capers, and berries. It is also associated with lowering Nuclear Factor Kappa B.[575]
  - Suggested dose: 100-200 mg three times daily.
- *Boswellia* (frankincense):
  - *Boswellia* has been used effectively in multiple types of inflammatory-type conditions such as arthritis, inflammatory bowel disease, as well as thyroiditis. [576]
  - Suggested dose is 250 mg daily.
- Vitamin D:
  - This book explores vitamin D in detail. Vitamin D has been found to decrease Nuclear Factor Kappa B.[577]
  - Suggested dose is 5,000 to 10,000 IU daily and monitor levels of 25-OH vitamin D.

❧ *Iris versicolor.*
  ❧ As mentioned earlier, this is an excellent herb to decrease the inflammation within the thyroid gland.
  ❧ Suggested dose: 750 mg daily.

Hot and Cold Alternating Compresses for Thyroiditis (Swollen Thyroid)

Hydrotherapy is a time-tested, efficient, and effective way to improve circulation and health. When applied to the thyroid in this fashion, the temperature contrast creates a pumping action from the contracting cold and dilating heat. This moves blood and lymphatic fluid, lowering inflammation and stimulating function of the gland. Here's how to do it:

❧ First get two large bowls ready, one filled with ice water and the other with very hot water.
❧ Place a small towel in each bowl.
❧ Start by applying the wet but wrung-out hot towel over the thyroid/neck area for three minutes and then contrast with thirty seconds of cold.
❧ Perform five cycles of this two times daily.
❧ Always end with cold.
❧ Be sure to keep the contrast of temperatures high to truly influence the movement of lymphatic fluid.

Step 5: Thyroid

Hyperthyroidism Treatment

If you have hyperthyroidism (high thyroid function) and you present with the typical symptoms of cardiac abnormalities including elevated heart and/or palpitations, shaking, tremors, profuse sweating, and bowel distress including diarrhea, consult your doctor immediately. The acute cardiac problems of hyperthyroidism can be life threatening.

Conventional Treatment Options

Radioactive iodine ablation is the most common treatment for hyperthyroidism. The use of radioactive iodine is the most direct and immediate treatment for lowering the symptoms associated with hyperthyroidism so it is the first choice by most conventional doctors. The radioactive iodine is given in a pill and immediately goes to work in lowering the excessive thyroid hormone synthesis, but also starts to permanently destroy the thyroid gland. Patients having this type of treatment will need to be on lifelong thyroid hormone medication.

Surgical Removal of the Thyroid

If a large goiter and/or a suspicious and large thyroid nodule is present, then a thyroidectomy, or removal of the thyroid, may be indicated to help with the hyperthyroidism. Sometimes a part or the entire thyroid is removed. Because the entire gland is removed and is no longer contributing any amount of thyroid hormone, these types of patients tend to need larger amounts of thyroid hormone replacement to feel normal.

Antithyroid Drugs

The medication known as Propothiouracil (PTU) inhibits the processing of iodine by the thyroid gland thus inhibiting thyroid hormone synthesis. It also inhibits inactive T4 to active T3 conversion. The typical course of treatment for this medication is up to two years or more to be effective. The incidence of developing future hypothyroidism in patients using PTU is high.

PTU has the potential to be liver toxic and this should be monitored very closely if a patient undergoes this type of treatment. The risk for liver toxicity for this drug should not be underestimated. In 2009, new black box warnings were made mandatory for this drug. A black box warning is given to prescription drugs that may cause serious adverse effects. This drug should be limited to adults over the age of forty and avoided during pregnancy if

> The incidence of developing future hypothyroidism in patients using PTU is high.

possible. PTU is the third most likely drug associated with the need for liver transplant.

Methimazole (Tapazole)

This medication inhibits thyroid hormone synthesis but does not interfere with the conversion of inactive T4 to active T3. Considerable debate surrounds optimal dosage and duration. If medications are going to be used in the case of a child's treatment, then this drug would be the lesser of two evils. However, it still has associated side effects such as rash, itching, hives, abnormal hair loss, and skin pigmentation. This medication is also associated with liver toxicity, but not to the same extent as PTU. Women who are pregnant, trying to get pregnant or who are breast feeding should avoid this medication.

Most of my patients who have had a history of hyperthyroidism come to me after

they have already undergone a more aggressive and immediate conventional treatment such as radioactive ablation or removal of the thyroid gland. They are then in a hypothyroid (low thyroid function) state and dependent on lifelong thyroid hormone treatment.

I see less hyperthyroidism (high thyroid function) for a couple of reasons. One, hyperthyroidism is not as common as hypothyroidism and therefore does not present as often in general. Two, the symptoms of hyperthyroidism often present in a very acute and severe manner leading patients immediately to their conventional doctor where the treatment options are focused on killing or removing the thyroid gland. However, alternative options exist in the treatment of hyperthyroidism.

Alternative Treatment Options for Hyperthyroidism

There are several dietary considerations for hyperthyroidism. Essentially, all of the foods that are listed as goitrogenic and were suggested to be avoided for hypothyroidism (low thyroid function) should be consumed. Additionally, many of the recommendations for hypothyroidism above, such as coconut oil, can also be effective. The basic principle of a wholesome diet and focusing on the basic pillars of health thoroughly described in "The Metabolic Health Foundation" are perfect foundational starts for helping with hyperthyroidism.

Iodine is helpful with hyperthyroidism. I have had excellent results with using iodine in medicinal doses for hyperthyroidism. Be sure to review the chapter on iodine for the specific historical premise behind the use of iodine. But as a review, iodine has the wonderful affect of balancing thyroid function in either a low or high functioning situation.

Dosing of iodine for hyperthyroidism should be gradually increased from approximately 12.5 mg daily to doses as high as 100 mg or more daily to reduce the symptoms of hyperthyroidism and begin to normalize lab values. I have had many subclinical hyperthyroidism patients who could keep their TSH values normalized as long as they stayed on their iodine at the appropriate effective dose.

Bugleweed (*Lycopus virginicus*)

This herb from the mint family has consistently been a traditional herbal treatment for hyperthyroidism and is known to decrease pulse rate and blood pressure in hyperthyroid patients. Studies on *Lycopus* has shown it to reduce excessive thyroid hormone levels[578] as well as being effective at inhibiting the receptor-binding and biological activity of Graves' immunoglobulins or TSI (thyroid stimulating immunoglobulins), and thereby reducing excessive production of thyroid hormone.[579]

The dose for *Lycopus* should be gradually increased over time, to see what is most effective

> Studies on *Lycopus* has shown it to reduce excessive thyroid hormone levels as well as being effective at inhibiting the receptor-binding and biological activity of Graves' immunoglobulins or TSI (thyroid stimulating immunoglobulins), and thereby reducing excessive production of thyroid hormone.

for the individual. For a liquid tincture extract, start with twenty drops or 1 mL of a 1:3 extract. An average dose is about 150 drops or 7.5 mL of a 1:3 extract. The whole plant can be used also at about 1 to 2 grams per day.

Lemon Balm (*Mellissa officinalis*)

Another plant from the mint family, this herb is often combined with *Lycopus* for hyperthyroidism. Traditionally, it has been used for nervous conditions such as anxiety and insomnia, and elevated blood pressure and palpitations which commonly accompany hyperthyroidism. *Mellisa* has also been shown to decrease the binding of TSI (thyroid stimulating immunoglobulins) that further stimulates the thyroid gland to produce excessive thyroid hormone.[580]

The dose should be gradually increased over time, depending on symptomatic relief. For a liquid extract, start with ten drops or 0.5 mL and gradually increase over time. An average effective dose is forty to fifty drops or 2-2.5 mL of a 1:3 extract.

Additional Considerations for Hyperthyroidism

If cardiac symptoms persist while seeking any type of treatment for hyperthyroidism, such as elevated heart rate, erratic heartbeat, skipping beats or arrhythmias, elevated blood pressure or chest or arm pain, consult your healthcare provider immediately. Proper monitoring and possible medications or treatments may be necessary and this should not be underestimated.

Step 5: Thyroid

Step 6:
Strengthening the Adrenals to Fight Fatigue and the Results of Chronic Stress

Once again, Dr. Cristina Romero-Bosch:

More than 80 percent of the American public suffer from some level of adrenal dysfunction[581] as a result of our industrialized life style; rush to work, rush to eat, rush to rush. And, with a medical system that separates people into a state of disease or health, there is little consideration for people who are feeling *unwell*. When you find that you are running on empty, do not seem to fit into any conventional concept of disease and suspect adrenal dysfunction, there are steps to take to accurately diagnose and treat your adrenal glands.

Making an Assessment

Be an advocate for your own health and successfully take the discussion to your physician's office for further assistance on adrenal dysfunction treatment by clearly describing the parameters you are using to support your working diagnosis. Adrenal function testing can be divided into two categories: simple physical examination and laboratory testing.

Physical examination should include findings such as pupillary constriction, low blood pressure, orthostatic hypotension and physical signs and symptoms such as dry hair and skin and hypoglycemia. Begin by completing the Adrenal Fatigue questionnaire found in Appendix 7 to determine if further investigation is merited. If you conclude that your symptoms support your suspicion of adrenal dysfunction then request your physician perform these adrenal specific exams:

Pupillary Constriction: The constriction (closing) of the pupil (black center of the eye) is measured by detecting the contraction of the pupil in response to light. Your physician will note that your pupil is slow to close or oscillates in attempt to constrict with bright light.[582] The pupil is unable to hold a constriction despite light being directed into the eye.

Low Blood Pressure (hypotension): In adrenal dysfunction low blood pressure accompanied by slight dizziness or even headache with change in position is common. However, if you have treated or un-treated high blood pressure (hypertension) this does not exclude a diagnosis of adrenal dysfunction but does indicate an additional disease process affecting your cardiovascular system.

Orthostatic hypotension: Orthostatic (standing up) hypotension (low blood pressure) is measured

> **The most specific test for confirming adrenal dysfunction is a salivary Adrenal Stress Index as it provides a picture of circadian production of cortisol.**

at two intervals with a change in position. You will be asked to have your blood pressure measured while you are lying down and then again immediately after rising. A sudden drop in blood pressure when you stand up from a sitting, squatting, or supine (lying) position is termed orthostatic hypotension.

The most specific test for confirming adrenal dysfunction is a salivary Adrenal Stress Index as it provides a picture of circadian production of cortisol. Serum (blood) and urine measures of cortisol test for disease states like Addison's and Cushing's, but do not evaluate patient levels that are neither diseased nor optimal. And, it is within this low-normal high-normal cortisol production that adrenal dysfunction can be found. Remember that adrenal dysfunctions (including adrenal fatigue) are not recognized by conventional medicine as a "true" disease. Free cortisol has been found to be more accurately representative of cortisol production than serum (blood test) as it is a measure of hormone levels inside the cell versus urinary or serum levels which indicate cortisol levels outside the cell.[583, 584] A morning serum cortisol may be acquired as an initial screening. However, this value has been found over-estimated in research studies suggesting that in the presence of symptoms a salivary adrenal assessment is necessary despite normal serum cortisol readings. Salivary testing usually includes four daily cortisol readings (typically around 6:00 a.m., noon, 4:00 p.m., 11:00 p.m.) as well as other adrenal hormones such as DHEA-s, progesterone and even pre and post-prandial (before and after eating) insulin.

Understanding the Role of Lifestyle Changes

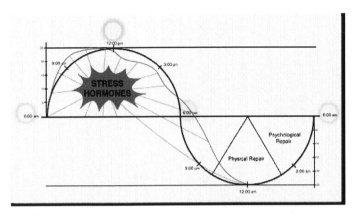

Figure showing normal cortisol circadian rhythm.

The wonderful thing about treating the adrenal glands is that they are truly responsive to a little TLC (yes, I do mean Tender Loving Care) and heal with ease. As a physician, treating adrenal dysfunction is a chance to really look like a hero. But in reality, most of the "secrets" to healing the adrenals are based on guiding patients to changing some of the most basic daily activities that are causing and aggravating adrenal dysfunction. Simply said, lifestyle factors are the true key to restoring adrenal function and preventing relapse. How often do you do the following: multi-task, leave the TV on while you sleep, skip meals, avoid drinking water, reach for sugary snacks, smoke, go to sleep too late? Identifying and correcting taxing lifestyle components will launch your adrenal repair program and help ensure maintained success.

To begin treating adrenal dysfunction I recommend becoming better aware of the causes of adrenal strain; determine which lifestyle factors can be immediately addressed and take steps to do so. To achieve this, I always recommend making a list. Lists are such an easy way to organize any intention from an overwhelming feat into manageable steps. Take this as an opportunity for you to strengthen your "pre-diagnosis" and facilitate your discussion with your physician. By going to your doctor's visit having already recognized and initiated lifestyle changes you may find your time with your physician to be more efficiently used and focused on additional testing.

Consider going to visit your doctor with a series of adrenal concerns ranging from "wired but tired," dizziness when rising from seated position, difficulty losing weight, and fatigue not alleviated by sleep. You explain to your physician

> Most of the "secrets" to healing the adrenals are based on guiding patients to changing some of the most basic daily activities that are causing and aggravating adrenal dysfunction.

you recognized your sleep hygiene was not optimal, your relationship with your work supervisor was stressful, and you had been skipping breakfast. And upon correcting these factors you are still concerned about your cortisol production as your symptoms have not been alleviated. Your physician may be more inclined to thoroughly evaluate your adrenal function despite their suspicion that everything is "normal." If nothing else, your physician will respect that you are being proactive about your health and you are not simply making the diagnosis for them.

So, how do you determine what lifestyle changes you should be making to get the repair program started? Make a list of all the aspects of your life that are taxing you in some way—remember that we discussed in a previous chapter that not all stressors are negative so feel no guilt if you include a new born child, an aging parent, or a promotion that requires extra hours at the office. The purpose of this list is to guide you towards your optimal hormone zone, so be honest with yourself. This list will help you realistically distinguish the things that you can and want to change from the things that you cannot or do not want to change. From here another list can be made to determine the "end-date" for the things that cannot be currently changed but are draining your adrenals. In establishing an end-in-sight perspective you may find them more tolerable and that alone will help decrease their adrenal burden.

Once you have listed the aspects of your life that need eliminating or better controlling, take time to make a list of the lifestyle habits you already have that help rejuvenate your adrenals (mid-day power naps, lunch time walks, Saturday morning yoga, a wonderful confidant, watching your child play sports, etc.). Remember to take the time to congratulate yourself for a job well done and to learn what about these activities works for you and can be reproduced with more frequency throughout the week.

Taking control over perceived stressors is paramount to feeling less stressed; therefore, recognizing the importance of changing the things you can, and eliminating the things you can't will result in an immediate sense of empowerment and that in itself is healing. Changing your lifestyle is not an act of punishment but an opportunity to better know yourself so that you can make daily changes that better meet your life needs, goals, and dreams by preserving your health to make these ideals reality.

In Summary:
- ❧ List of Energy Drainers (physical and emotional)
  - ❧ Change the things you CAN immediately change.
- ❧ List of End-Dates for Energy Drainers that can't be changed immediately
  - ❧ Understand that anything can be "tolerated" for a bit longer.
- ❧ List of Energy Givers (physical and emotional)
  - ❧ What can be learned from these positive elements?

Blood Sugar Control

The primary lifestyle change that must be adopted to repair and sustain healthy adrenal function is appropriate regulation of blood sugar. This is the simplest and most cost effective way of reducing daily

> The primary lifestyle change that must be adopted to repair and sustain healthy adrenal function is appropriate regulation of blood sugar.

adrenal assaults *and* is entirely within your control. The cortisol produced by the adrenal glands has a significant effect on blood sugar levels, so eating habits play a major role in moderating the condition. Remember that cortisol helps regulate blood sugar and as a result constant dips in blood sugar levels from infrequent eating demands intervention from the adrenals.

These simple diet recommendations will make a significant difference for your adrenal health and begin to immediately alleviate symptoms.

- Eat breakfast within an hour of waking up.
  - Choosing to consume grains only at breakfast is a poor way of balancing blood sugar and lessening the burden on the adrenals.
  - Breakfast does not have to be a large meal if you find that you are not experiencing clear hunger signals upon rising. Focus on protein and good fats to regulate blood sugar after overnight fasting.
- Eat meals high in protein to better balance sugar metabolism.
  - Having an early lunch and then a mid-afternoon snack will keep blood sugar stable and decrease cortisol demand.
- Snack on high protein snacks every two to three hours.
  - A protein snack such as eggs, yogurt, protein shakes in between meals further supports blood sugar control.
- Limit grains to no more than one daily serving or less.
  - Refined sugars should be eliminated as much as possible with complex carbohydrates taking their place in no more than one serving daily.
- Enjoy a small protein/healthy fat snack about one or two hours before bedtime.
  - Having a light snack of protein and good fats before bedtime will help with irregular cortisol during the evening and help prevent interrupted sleep.
- Elimination of caffeine during your adrenal repair program.

> • In adrenal fatigue caffeine can have a taxing affect by increasing cortisol production in a system that cannot tolerate the additional demand affect by demanding an increase in cortisol release that the tired gland cannot tolerate further depleting the individual when the caffeine wears off.[585]
>
> ❷ Make time to make prepare meals and then eat them.
>
> > • Homemade meals are more likely to respect your dietary restrictions. Meals eaten at home around the dinner table encourage slower eating and aid digestion through proper chewing and elimination of stimulants like TV, work or standing up.

Eliminating Food Sensitivities

Diet is defined as food you eat on a regular basis and is a concept independent of the notion of deprivation.[586] A healthy diet is very individualized as it depends on your food sensitivities and allergies as well your specific nutritional demands. Food sensitivities are mediated by Immunoglobulins G[587] (IgG) which are delayed reactions that can take up to seventy-two hours to express themselves making it challenging to find a pattern in the foods you are eating that are leading to symptoms. Therefore, a blood test of IgG food sensitivities is required to properly determine your specific food eliminations. The role that any allergy or sensitivity has on adrenal health is related to the inflammatory response caused by the histamine releasing allergic response. Cortisol, being a primary anti-inflammatory hormone, is released with excess frequency in a body that is over-exposed to inflammatory foods. Remember that these foods may actually be "good" for you and typically will

The role that any allergy or sensitivity has on adrenal health is related to the inflammatory response caused by the histamine releasing allergic response.

be able to be reintroduced after approximately three months of digestive repair and food elimination. Eliminating these taxing foods will efficiently decrease the burden on your over-worked adrenals.

Sleep Patterns

During sleep hours the body repairs itself and resets metabolic equilibrium. Remember the circadian rhythm of healthy adrenal hormone secretion is based on the twenty-four-hour circadian rhythm of the sun. Sleep hygiene must be respected while rehabilitating the adrenals. Therefore, setting a bedtime no later than 10:30 p.m. and a wake time no later (or earlier) than 5:30-6:00 a.m. is necessary for rehabilitation and maintenance of healthy adrenal function. Many patients will tell me that they feel most productive during the late evening and it is important to remind them not to let this second wind kick in as it will aggravate your morning exhaustion. And, if you are having difficulty waking periodically, especially with a sense of anxiety, it may be that your blood sugar is dropping and is stirring you to rise. This is where the pre-bed snack helps by regulating blood sugar so that you are not awoken with hypoglycemia.

Consider redefining your bedtime routine. Focus on activities that reduce stress, body temperature, and exposure to light and sound. Typically, in the evening we watch stimulating or depressing TV like the news or a dramatic series on the couch with full bellies or perhaps still snacking on cortisol raising high-carbohydrate foods. Then, we go to bed with all the lights on for reading or even fall asleep with the television on expecting a deep sleep. We fail to recognize these habits as micro-stressors increasing our evening cortisol. Instead, consider using the evening as a pampering time, like the old Calgon® commercials suggested to let yourself be

> Setting a bedtime no later than 10:30 p.m. and a wake time no later (or earlier) than 5:30-6:00 a.m. is necessary for rehabilitation and maintenance of healthy adrenal function.

taken away.[588] The use of herbal teas, a relaxing magazine, a stroll around the block and an evening shower that ends on cold water are excellent "spa like" therapies that you can incorporate into your evening routine. These tools should not be considered luxuries but must be recognized as medical recommendations that can be instantly added to your daily living as part of your adrenal repair program. In Summary:

- ❧ Wake no earlier than 5:30 a.m. but no later than 6:30 a.m.
  - ❧ Feel free to take an early morning nap after being awake for a couple of hours and after having breakfast.
- ❧ Sleep no later than 10:30 p.m.
  - ❧ Avoid staying awake too long so that your second wind never hits.
- ❧ Pre-bed snack: high protein and good fats to prevent nocturnal hypoglycemia.

Physical Activity

Exercise has been shown to improve stress management, prevent tissue damage and inflammation by reducing obesity and weight related disease, and by stimulating a healthy metabolism through muscle mass stimulation. However, strenuous physical activity and certain endurance exercises can further impair adrenal function.[589] There is increasing evidence that excessive exercise is related to acute and chronic diseases. This correlation is more profound in females and is evidenced by an increase in incidences of "exercise-related female reproductive dysfunction." These events in both genders include infertility, eating disorders, osteoporosis, coronary heart disease, and euthyroid "sick" syndrome. Since

> Strenuous physical activity and certain endurance exercises can further impair adrenal function. There is increasing evidence that excessive exercise is related to acute and chronic diseases.

we have thoroughly established the relationship between the adrenal, sex and thyroid hormone it is safe to correlate that if strenuous exercise can negatively impact sex hormone and thyroid hormone then it indirectly, if not directly, is affecting the adrenal hormones as well.

When being treated for adrenal dysfunction, consider shifting away from long distance running and biking or competitive training such as for a marathon. Interval training, stretch exercise, and meditative grounding practices like yoga are better indicated during the adrenal repair stage. Most importantly, find exercises that you enjoy. The thirty to sixty minutes you spend on yourself should be used in pleasure.

Relaxation

Whether it is a "staycation," daily meditation or an hour of soap operas you must establish routine methods of relaxation to succeed in adrenal repair. In Chinese medicine, adrenal fatigue is considered a kidney deficiency and is often treated by pressing acupressure points between the medial malleolus (inner bone on the ankle) and the Achilles tendon.[590] This is a wonderful easy massage that you can give yourself to support your adrenal health by massaging the area daily. Whatever your choice, remember that relaxation is a vital part of your health and has been clearly associated with longevity and increased quality of life.[591]

Nutritional Remedies
Magnesium Citrate

Next to potassium, magnesium is the second most abundant nutrient inside cells and is involved in enzyme activity, energy production, and nerve conduction. Energy, or Adenosine-5'-triphosphate – the cell's energy transporter (ATP), is created through magnesium's involvement in cellular respiration and is directly involved in muscle contraction to create ATP. Magnesium initiates the chain reaction of adrenal hormone production. Magnesium supplementation for four weeks in overweight individuals led to distinct changes in gene expression and proteomic profiling consistent with favorable effects on several metabolic pathways.[592] Magnesium also acts as a muscle relaxer that assists in the sensation of relaxation, decrease in pain, and better control of tissue damaging inflammation. It is best taken at night for optimal absorption and increased benefit from the muscle and mood relaxation. As is the case with most nutrients, when taken grouped together or with food, the co-factor nutrients and digestive enzymes increase their absorption. Effervescent magnesium that has been completely dissolved in water seems to be best absorbed, but regardless dosing around 400 mg daily will positively affect magnesium levels.[593]

During times of stress, emotional or physical, your body's demand for antioxidants increases making an increased supply of these nutrients beneficial for coping and healing.[594] Remember these nutrients work synergistically together; therefore, increased magnesium supplementation taken along higher levels of vitamins C and B5 pantothenic acid will assist in your rehabilitation of your adrenal dysfunction. The concept of supply and demand always applies to your nutritional levels. As your metabolic needs increase due to achieving improved metabolic health or to increased demand from stressful illness so must your nutritional supplementation. You may find that taking magnesium periodically throughout the day when your adrenal dysfunction is particularly evident will bring you relief through muscle and emotional relaxation.

Vitamin C

Vitamin C is the most important nutrient regarding adrenal function because of the direct correlation between adrenal hormone release and vitamin C levels.[595] Vitamin C levels are not stored in the body due to their being water-soluble and each person has different levels of need and bowel tolerance. It is commonly said that

> Vitamin C is the most important nutrient regarding adrenal function because of the direct correlation between adrenal hormone release and vitamin C levels.

vitamin C should be taken to bowel tolerance to determine your tolerated dose; meaning dose Vitamin C in 500 mg increments every one or two hours until you have loose watery stools. This amount indicates what dose of vitamin C you should consider taking during times of increased stress. Vitamin C can be a useful supplement to take when you are treating adrenal dysfunction and especially adrenal fatigue as it helps increase the baseline level at which oxidative damage begins as a result of prolonged stress. For many, this level reaches up to 5,000 mg dosed in 500 mg increments throughout the day during peak stress time.

Pantothenic Acid (Vitamin B5)

The family of B vitamins works synergistically and taking them in a complex enhances their effect. B5 is the nutrient most related to adrenal function for its involvement in the production of adrenal hormones when it converts into co-enzyme acetyl A (a part of the Krebs's cycle which produces cellular energy).[596,597] It is also required for almost every energy production biochemical pathway in the body. You should use a daily B complex formula as the B vitamins are water-soluble and therefore, like vitamin C, not stored in the body. Recommendations of an additional dose of B5 in adrenal supportive preparations should generally provide a B5 dose of approximately 500 mg a day with one or two doses per day during times of increased stress.

Melatonin

Melatonin is secreted by the pineal gland and functions to regulate circadian rhythm and induce sleep. Melatonin circadian secretion in patients with adrenal dysfunction has been shown to be significantly lower compared to healthy individuals. Studies also have

> Melatonin circadian secretion in patients with adrenal dysfunction has been shown to be significantly lower compared to healthy individuals.

shown that nightly administration of 2 mg of melatonin increased the DHEA-s: cortisol ratio after six months of treatment.[598] Melatonin is a natural antioxidant, has been shown to effectively aide in inducing sleep, and can be safely taken for acute relief up to 6 mg nightly to assist with the wired but tired symptoms of adrenal dysfunction.[599] (See Step 2 of The Metabolic Health Protocol for more information on melatonin and sleep hygiene.)

Selenium and Zinc

Zinc is a mineral that is absolutely vital to living, and even a small deficiency can cause health problems. It is found in every cell in the body and it stimulates the activity of about one hundred enzymes—substances that promote biochemical reactions in the body. Zinc helps to maintain a healthy immune system, is necessary for wound healing, helps to maintain your sense of taste and smell, and is needed for DNA synthesis. It aids in regulating hormones, can help to maintain prostate health, and can even increase fertility. Zinc helps prevent and heal cold sores, and also aids in the body's absorption of minerals. It can improve the health of your skin and hair, and can even reduce the appearance of acne. Zinc has also been shown to help heal ulcers and can help you maintain a healthy digestive tract. It is also an antioxidant mineral, and reduces the damage caused by free radicals. It can revitalize the functioning of the thymus gland that is crucial for a strong immune system. It can help you to recover faster from colds and flu.

Trace minerals are vital for adrenal function by directly supporting hormone production, decreasing inflammatory cascades, and acting as co-factors for other nutrients.[600, 601] Selenium is a major component in antioxidant activity and

> Trace minerals are vital for adrenal function by directly supporting hormone production, decreasing inflammatory cascades, and acting as co-factors for other nutrients.

adrenal hormone production.[602] Studies show that low levels of selenium result in decreases levels of adrenal hormone production like DHEA-s.[603] To ensure proper adrenal activity and to decrease need for cortisol production through a decrease in inflammation selenium supplementation is suggested. Zinc is an immune stimulating trace mineral that is vital for adrenal function, it is essential for immune function and management of mental stressors. For dosing information on zinc and selenium, see Step 5 of The Metabolic Health Protocol.

Phosphatidylserine

Phosphatidylserine is an amino acid (protein) found in foods such as organ meats, fish, animal meat, white beans, and soybeans.[604] Phosphatidylserine aides in stunting ACTH secretion that stimulates cortisol release. It is useful in the early stages of adrenal dysfunction/fatigue by helping reduce hormonal request for excessive cortisol production. It may also aide in stress reduction.[605] I recommend phosphatidylserine in my patients that are in the early stages of adrenal dysfunction and are over-producing cortisol at inappropriate times with nightly bedtime doses starting at 50-100 mg.

There are many wonderful food sources of these nutrients and the perfect thing about consuming nutrients in whole food form is that they naturally come with the co-nutrients that tend to aide in their absorption and activity.[606] Magnesium is found highest in whole grains, nuts, and spinach. Vitamin C is found highest in fruits and veggies like papaya, broccoli,

> It is useful in the early stages of adrenal dysfunction/ fatigue by helping reduce hormonal request for excessive cortisol production.

bell peppers, and oranges. Selenium is high in shellfish, Brazil nuts, and sunflower seeds. Oysters and almonds are two wonderful sources of zinc. Deciding what whole foods can be part of your medicinal replacement for any nutrient is going to again be dependent on our particular food sensitivities/allergies, personal belief systems leading to dietary restriction, or other health concerns.

Hormonal Medications
Dietary Desiccated Adrenal Glandulars

Dietary desiccated adrenal glandulars refer to raw animal organs and glands that have been extracted, freeze-dried and formulated into nutritional supplements for the treatment of dysfunction in that particular human gland or organ. These are commonly formulated for the treatment of thyroid, adrenal or pituitary dysfunction. Glandulars are believed to contain many nutritive substances aside from hormones, but since there are limited studies using glandulars it is difficult to say specifically what in the tissue extract is healing to the body. Anecdotal evidence and glandular formulations with additional adrenal supportive herbs and nutrients enhance the therapeutic effect of dietary desiccated glandulars. Dietary desiccated adrenal glandulars contain some cortisol but the dose will vary between manufacturers. This is not a prescription medication. With glandulars, dosing would need to follow the recommendations from the manufacturer and the guidance of your healthcare provider. Since they are believed to contain cortisol however a general recommendation would be that you are not receiving more than 10 mg of hydrocortisone equivalence without a physician's supervision.

Hydrocortisone

Cortisone is a very useful tool for treating adrenal dysfunction that is in late stages of adrenal fatigue. Upon receiving an Adrenal Stress Index indicating low cortisol production I will recommend hydrocortisone in doses ranging from 2.5 mg to 20 mg usually in divided doses to represent healthy circadian production of cortisol. This is a prescription medication. It is important to distinguish the difference between short term physiologic dosing of cortisone to pharmaceutical, and often chronic use, of hydrocortisone or other steroid derivatives. When using low dose hydrocortisone to repair adrenal fatigue salivary samples of cortisol production are taken every three to six months, patient symptoms are monitored and the adrenal gland is being supported through concomitant therapies in the form of nutrients and herbs. Prednisone is a synthetic corticocosteroid drug that is commonly used for immune suppression.[607] Remember that prednisone is physiologically four times more potent than hydrocortisone and hydrocortisone is chemically equivalent to the cortisol your body is producing.[608] The dangerous side effects of glucocorticoid therapy is not seen with physiologic dosing meaning that the dose is gentle enough to encourage normal hormone function rather than suppress gland/organ activity.[609]

A note from Dr. Robinson: It is important to make the correlation of adrenal fatigue and chronic fatigue syndrome, particularly in the context of using hydrocortisone as an adjunct therapy. Essentially, adrenal fatigue and chronic fatigue syndrome clinically present as the same condition, with slight differences in categorization. Low physiologic doses of hydrocortisone, as discussed and suggested here, has been shown to be safe and effective in the treatment of chronic fatigue syndrome.[610] [611] [612] [613] [614] [615] [616] I would encourage patients and clinicians to follow the medical literature references to dispel some of the myths that surround the use of hydrocortisone.

Herbal Medicine

Dosing depends on adrenal state and size of patient. This will be true with most herbs as they are incredibly helpful but only when dosed at medicinal levels. This "medicinal level" unfortunately varies with patients. If you are not using a single herb remedy then follow the recommended manufacturer's dose or consult your physician.

Licorice (*Glycyrrhiza glabra*)

Licorice is a fabulous herb that has an affinity for working with the adrenals by directly inhibiting the liver's processing of hydrocortisone resulting in blocked breakdown and therefore increased circulating levels in the blood. Since the adrenals work on the negative feedback signals discussed in another chapter, elevated cortisol levels in the blood helps to slow down the pituitary's release of ACTH which in turn helps the adrenal gland get a break from constant ACTH stimulation.[617] A decrease in ACTH stimulation results in less cortisol being requested from the adrenal gland. This relief from cortisol production makes licorice a key player in herbal treatment protocols for adrenal dysfunction.

Glycyrrhiza is an herb in its own category due to its multitude of uses and its desirable taste. It is a nourishing, anti-inflammatory, anti-microbial, adrenal supporting plant. Licorice also inhibits 5-beta-reductase, an enzyme that regulates cortisol and aldosterone metabolism. This allows licorice to slow the release of corticosteroids as well as slow down the biological half-life of cortisol and aldosterone making them available longer.[618]

I recommend licorice liquid tincture to be dosed thirty drops (1/2 teaspoon) two to six times daily depending on the level of repair needed. It is important to monitor blood pressure changes, fluid retention, or sudden increases in cortisol with licorice supplementation so physician supervision is recommended. Few adverse effects have been reported with this ancient herb when used in moderate doses. It is however contraindicated in patients with high blood pressure, heart, liver, or kidney disease due to its excreting of potassium in the urine.[619]

Very high doses of 50 grams per day can result in hypertension (high blood pressure).[620] The doses discussed here are not anywhere near this excessive amount. To avoid concern, as this really is a wonderful plant, I simply recommend regular blood pressure monitoring, complete metabolic panel blood testing and regular discussion with your physician.

Ashwaganda (*Withania somnifora*)

Withania somnifora, commonly called by its Ayurvedic name ashwaganda, has been used as an adaptogen, diuretic, anti-inflammatory, and sedative.[621,622] An adaptogen is a substance that helps a living organism adapt to stressors (environmental, physical, or psychological).[623] Ashwaganda's active chemical constituent is known as withaferin A and has been found to increase sex hormones testosterone and progesterone.[624] In addition to helping relieve adrenal gland responsibility by promoting sex hormone production, ashwaganda has been used for the treatment of anxiety because of its reported benefits in lowering coritsol.[625] Unfortunately, like with many botanicals, there are very limited clinical trials but there are many in vitro experiments suggesting that ashwaganda's health benefits extend to supporting the immune system, the central nervous system, and inflammatory conditions like cancer. There are contraindications with pregnant women as abortifacient properties have been reported.[626] Also, because it does not have an offensive bitter taste it is an easy additive to any herbal preparation. *Withania somnifera* (ashwaganda) is by far my favorite plant; it is a lovely and gentle but assertive and incredibly effective.

Step 7:
Freedom from Prescription Medications

Prescription medications are sometimes necessary to maintain balance. Many times, they are not. The unwavering need and dependency on prescription medications to maintain a sense of health is pervasive in the conventional medical community and the American culture. As I have stated before, our social culture dictates our medical culture. Our social norm of instant gratification and limited time, concern or knowledge of how to take care of ourselves on all integrated levels leaves us inevitably unhealthy. And our medical culture, emboldened and empowered by the submission we provide, further exacerbates the problem by offering us the one limited solution that our social construct will allow: prescription medications.

> Prescription medications often hinder your way towards personal responsibility and freedom. The medications can actually limit choices in terms of realizing optimal health.

Prescription medications often hinder your way towards personal responsibility and freedom. The medications can actually limit choices in terms of realizing optimal health. The side effects and chemical load to the system can be very dangerous and life threatening at times.

Here are some interesting and mind-opening statistics about prescription medications:[627]

- Total Number of Retail Prescription Drugs Filled at Pharmacies in 2008
    - 3,649,468,866
- Total Retail Sales for Prescription Drugs Filled at Pharmacies in 2008
    - $215,115,456,488
- Retail Prescription Drugs Filled at Pharmacies (Annual per Person) in 2008

● 12.0 prescriptions per person with an average cost of $58.44 each or $701.28 per person

Fortunately, this social norm is changing on many fronts. The fact that you are reading this book proves that. There are five steps to the process of eliminating prescription medications from your life. There is hope and I believe fervently that the pendulum is swinging in the direction toward personal responsibility and awareness of health in a holistic and integrated fashion. The more we understand and practice this, the easier it will become to limit our need for most prescription medications. The first step in becoming free from unneeded prescription medications is awareness. You are achieving that now by making yourself informed.

> **You are in control of your health and your healthcare decisions with the guidance of your healthcare provider.**

The second step is to start a dialogue with the healthcare provider you see who prescribes medications for you. In some cases, you will not be able to get off of certain prescribed medications. You may only be able to limit the dose. But explore the possibility that you may be able to eliminate certain drugs altogether. Always be honest with your healthcare provider about your symptoms and reactions to the drugs and supplements you are taking. I could give countless examples of patients not telling their other physicians that they are also seeing a naturopathic physician because of wanting to avoid ridicule, consternation or even fear of being released from the other physician's practice because the doctor does not agree with an alternative approach. I fully understand and sympathize with these patients who want to avoid that type of negative reaction from their trusted healthcare provider, but honesty is always the better position to take. I believe this keeps the patient safe, as more options remain open for all involved. Also, if a patient is keeping information from another healthcare provider it causes me to wonder if they are keeping information away from me. So, be honest and open with all healthcare providers who are working to treat you.

With all of that said, you are in control of your health and your healthcare decisions with the guidance of your healthcare provider. You should also feel free to seek out additional professional advice and alternative opinions about your health and any and all prescription medications you take so you remain fully informed and replete with choices.

The third step is to make a choice and a decision. When you have sought out all the options and have established a rapport with a trusted healthcare professional, you must decide and be willing to go forward with the work that may be involved to wean off the dependency of some medications. Your physiology will likely go through some changes. Other times, the transition can be very easy. Every individual case is different. Either way, you must be committed and ready to choose a lifestyle that will support you being off of the medication, if this is possible.

The fourth step is to support and prepare your body for the transition off of prescription medications. This step, the preparation, is the most important. My mission in writing this book was to bring you the concept of improving your overall health status by incorporating new lifestyle choices, improving diet, and balancing hormone deficiencies. There are key nutrient supplements and herbal medicines that can act to replace the need for certain medications in certain situations.

The fifth step is to wean yourself off your medications with the guidance of your healthcare provider. Once your system is prepared and certain alterations in lifestyle have been made, you will be ready to remove the prescription medication over time. Be sure to transition slowly, with the advice of your healthcare provider, and never throw away your medication until you are certain the transition has been made smoothly with no adverse effects, and your healthcare provider gives permission.

Step 7: Rx Freedom

Knowing When You're Ready to Stop Filling Your Prescriptions

With the guidance of your prescribing physician and any additional healthcare provider you have on your team, you should be able to come to a conclusion about the timing. Also, I believe that many patients seem to intuitively know when it is time based on how they feel or how they are reacting to other complimentary treatments. For example, let's say that you begin to address your health issues when you are thirty pounds overweight, do not exercise, and are on high cholesterol medication. Through the good diet choices you've made you lose fifteen to twenty pounds and have been engaging in consistent exercise for a month or more. Your lab results have shown a significant decrease in your cholesterol level and your increased energy and happiness indicate that you will continue on the path. At that point, going off your cholesterol medication could be warranted.

Cases of Hypothyroid and/or Hormone Imbalances

It is important to note that all too often these patients have been prescribed medications due to poor management of hormone imbalances and under-treated hypothyroidism. I have many examples of helping patients relieve themselves of the burden of multiple prescription medications simply because they were on synthetic thyroid hormone at inadequate doses or their estrogen or testosterone were low. For example, if the body is not functioning optimally due to low thyroid hormone, then many conditions will arise that result in physicians prescribing additional medications for the new symptoms that would not be needed if

> I have many examples of helping patients relieve themselves of the burden of multiple prescription medications simply because they were on synthetic thyroid hormone at inadequate doses or their estrogen or testosterone were low.

the dose were adequate. Once natural thyroid hormone is prescribed at effective doses for proper stimulation of the metabolism the need for medications to treat these thyroid deficiency related conditions becomes unnecessary.

When patients have the guidance of a healthcare provider trained in looking at the body in a holistic manner who also understands pharmacology, then a comprehensive plan can be created to eliminate the need for many prescription medications. Here are some examples of medications that are often given by medical doctors (or those who practice conventional medicine) for conditions related to poor lifestyle choices, inadequate diet/nutrition, hormone imbalances, hypothyroidism, and lowered metabolism.

- Pain medications
- Cholesterol medications
- Hypertension (high blood pressure) medications
- Depression and anxiety medications: SSRIs such as Prozac®
- Migraine medications
- Mixed amphetamines: such as Adderall®
- Attention Deficit Disorder: such as Ritalin®
- Insulin resistance and type II diabetes medications such as Metformin®
- Allergy medications

Conclusion

Writing this book was my wish to clarify one of the most confusing concepts in medicine: hormones. Let *The Hormone Zone* be a guide, or perhaps a beacon, for you, the weary traveler. And in reading this book you have traveled on a long journey, through the body, the mind, the emotions, and the spirit. It could be said that this book is about hormones and how to balance them as naturally as possible, but it is much more than that. The conclusion of this book is merely the beginning, as every step on your health journey really is only the beginning of another process, another day, another opportunity. Before reading this book you met the very large obstacles of the unknown and now find yourself in the quintessential center of *The Hormone Zone*, more informed and more prepared to make sense of it and yourself.

Appendix 1: Internet Resources

Sex Hormone and Thyroid Hormone Balance:

John Alexander Robinson, N.M.D. www.yourhormonezone.com

This website offers insights into a full array of health topics covering the physical, mental, emotional, and spiritual aspects of our beings. The website and blog offer patients updated information on hormone therapy, thyroid solutions, nutritional advice, weight loss strategies and much more.

SottoPelle® www.sottopelletherapy.com

Gino Tutera, M.D., FACOG, has revolutionized the use of subcutaneous hormone pellet implants and the way male and female sex hormones are replaced and properly balanced.

Rebecca Glaser, M.D. www.hormonebalance.org

Dr. Glaser is an ardent researcher and promotes the proper use of bioidentical hormone replacement therapy. Her website is full of references and information for the savvy consumer looking for the details.

Metabolic Rehabilitation and Fibromyalgia Specialists:

John C. Lowe, D.C. www.drlowe.com

From his website: "Dr. John C. Lowe is a fibromyalgia, thyroid, and metabolism researcher and a board certified pain management specialist. As Director of Research for the Fibromyalgia Research Foundation, he has spearheaded the scientific study of two related topics: the metabolic causes of fibromyalgia, and the relief of fibromyalgia symptoms through the treatment approach he developed and named 'metabolic rehabilitation.' He is author of the internationally acclaimed book *The Metabolic Treatment of Fibromyalgia*, considered by many the most important document ever published on fibromyalgia."

His website contains a wealth of information regarding the rational and effective treatment of thyroid hormone deficiency. This is both a patient and physician resource filled with multiple commentaries by Dr. Lowe regarding his experience with treating hypometabolic states such as hypothyroidism and fibromyalgia.

Cristina Romero-Bosch, N.M.D.   www.iluminartherapy.com

From her website: "Cristina Romero-Bosch, NMD is a graduate of Southwest College of Naturopathic Medicine in Tempe, Arizona. After receiving her doctorate degree in naturopathic medicine, Dr. Bosch was selected among a nationwide pool of physicians to become the sole resident in Integrative Medicine at Yale University's Prevention Research Center Griffin Hospital and University of Bridgeport College of Naturopathic Medicine. She lectured extensively on the relationship between Metabolic Health and chronic endocrine conditions like Fibromyalgia and Hypothyroidism."

Dr. Bosch has now brought her unique specialized training to Scottsdale, Arizona where she focuses on restoring proper metabolic health for patients with thyroid conditions, chronic and adrenal fatigue, fibromyalgia and those hoping to optimize their health. Her North Scottsdale office, Iluminar, offers an integrated medical approach that prioritizes establishing a relationship with the patient to determine their unique metabolic needs. She is one of the few physicians utilizing the ReeVue® machine that accurately measures resting metabolic rate (RMR) which, if low, supports a diagnosis of hypothyroidism (low thyroid function) despite normal thyroid labs offering options to patients that have otherwise found little assistance. At Iluminar, Dr. Bosch aims to guide all patients towards happy, healthy living through education, inspiration and cutting edge Metabolic Rehabilitation.

Thyroid Patient Advocates:

Mary Shoman http://thyroid.about.com

From her website: "Patient advocate and writer Mary Shomon transformed her own 1995 thyroid diagnosis into a mission to educate and empower other patients who struggle with thyroid, autoimmune, and weight loss challenges… Unfortunately, doctors tend to think of thyroid disease as a mundane, easy to diagnose, easy to treat, one-size-fits-all problem. Patients, however, recognize that the truth is far more complex, and that effective treatment requires innovation, and often includes not only conventional approaches, but nutritional and lifestyle changes. My motto and battle cry is clear: 'We're patients. . . *not* lab values!' We deserve to feel well!"

Mary Shoman is a beacon of reason and hope for all hypothyroid patients. She brings her journalistic approach to the forefront of her tireless campaign for helping hypothyroid patients. This site provides patients with hope and a deeper understanding of hypothyroidism and what to do about it. I endorse it fully.

To Find a Thyroid Doctor Near You:

http://www.thyroid-info.com/topdrs/

This is an excellent source to find a thyroid doctor well-versed in many of the alternative perspectives offered in this book.

Stop the Thyroid Madness: www.stopthethyroidmadness.com

From their website: "Thyroid Madness Definition:

1. Treating hypothyroid patients solely with T4-only meds

2. Dosing solely by the TSH and the total T4, or using the outdated 'Thyroid Panel'

3. Prescribing anti-depressants in lieu of evaluating and treating the free T3

4. Telling thyroid patients that desiccated natural thyroid like Armour is 'unreliable,' 'inconsistent,' 'dangerous' or 'outdated.'

5. Making lab work more important than the hypo symptoms which

scream their presence.

6. Failing to see the OBVIOUS symptoms of poorly treated thyroid, and instead, recommending a slew of other tests and diagnoses [and I add: 'Prescribing more unnecessary medications unrelated to the true cause.']"

This website is an excellent patient advocate resource promoted and maintained by patients who have really done their homework. They are forcing the conventional medical establishment to reexamine the effectiveness of thyroid hormone treatment. It promotes the necessary concept that patients are ultimately in charge of their health. Healthcare providers are coaches providing guidance for patients while on their personal health journey.

Alternative Medical Support Thyroid Newsgroup Website
www.altsupportthyroid.org

Yet another complete thyroid support Internet source that outlines a rational approach to thyroid hormone treatment including the promotion of natural desiccated thyroid hormone and T3. The links are also very useful.

Professional Organizations and Resources:

The American Association of Naturopathic Physicians (AANP) www.naturopathic.org

From their website: "Founded in 1985, the American Association of Naturopathic Physicians (AANP) is the national professional society representing licensed or licensable naturopathic physicians who are graduates of four-year, residential graduate programs. Each of the six schools in North America is either accredited, or is a candidate for accreditation by an agency of the United States Department of Education. Located in Washington, DC, the AANP has 38 official State Affiliates across the country. Our membership consists of more than 2000 student, physicians, supporting and corporate members who collectively strive to expand access to naturopathic medicine nationwide.

"A licensed naturopathic physician (N.D.) attends a four-year graduate-level naturopathic medical school and is educated in all of the same basic sciences as an M.D., but also studies holistic and nontoxic approaches to therapy with a strong emphasis on disease prevention and optimizing wellness. In addition to a standard medical curriculum, the naturopathic physician is required to complete four years of training in clinical nutrition, acupuncture, homeopathic medicine, botanical medicine, psychology, and counseling (to encourage people to make lifestyle changes in support of their personal health). A naturopathic physician takes rigorous professional board exams so that he or she may be licensed by a state or jurisdiction as a primary care general practice physician."

A Naturopathic Doctor will provide you with a rational and holistic approach to treating you as an individual and not simply a disease. If you seek a healthcare professional that will understand an alternative approach to treating thyroid disease (or any disease for that matter), then a Naturopathic Doctor will fill this need.

Broda Barnes Foundation: www.brodabarnes.org

From their website: "The Broda O. Barnes, M.D. Research Foundation, Inc. is a not-for-profit organization dedicated to education, research and training in the field of thyroid and metabolic balance. Broda O. Barnes, M.D., Ph.D. dedicated more than 50 years of his life to researching, teaching and treating thyroid and related endocrine dysfunctions in this country and abroad. During his many years of research and practice, two of his many significant discoveries were: The development and use of thyroid function blood tests left many patients with clinical symptoms of hypothyroidism undiagnosed and untreated. Patients taking thyroid replacement therapy have much better improvement of symptoms with natural desiccated thyroid hormone rather than synthetic thyroid hormones."

Broda Barnes was a giant among men, revealing a true rational approach to diagnosing and treating hypothyroidism. Much of the information we have today regarding thyroid physiology comes from his pioneering work. The site has some information on hypothyroidism, but much of its benefit comes from the additional book resources they provide access to.

The Endocrine Society www.endo-society.org

From their website: "Founded in 1916, The Endocrine Society is the world's oldest, largest, and most active organization devoted to research on hormones and the clinical practice of endocrinology. The Society works to foster a greater understanding of endocrinology amongst the general public and practitioners of complementary medical disciplines and to promote the interests of all endocrinologists at the national scientific research and health policy levels of government."

I am an active member of this organization. They offer evidence-based scientific approaches to endocrinology including thyroid disease. This is the main organization of the Endocrinology specialty. The views within the organization follow mostly traditional and conventional guidelines, but they offer scientific discourse on all subjects.

Thyroid Disease Manager www.thyroidmanager.com

From their website: "Thyroid Disease Manager@ offers an up-to-date analysis of thyrotoxicosis, hypothyroidism, thyroid nodules and cancer, thyroiditis, and all aspects of human thyroid disease and thyroid physiology. It provides physicians, researchers, and trainees (as well as patients) around the world with an authoritative, current, complete, objective, free, and down-loadable source on the thyroid. This website is directed to helping physicians care for their patients with thyroid problems."

A very in depth and technical website that provides physiological and scientific information regarding thyroid function and disease.

Diet Recommendations:

Paleolithic Diet www.thepaleodiet.com

This is the main website for information on Paleolithic nutrition promoting the research and book that started it all by Dr. Loren Cordain.

More Paleolithic Diet information www.paleodiet.com

Specific Paleolithic Diet Recipes:

A simple web search can provide you with more specific Paleo diet recipe ideas than you could eat in a lifetime, so have fun. But here a couple of good places to start:

www.thepaleodiet.com

http://paleofood.com/

Coconut Oil Resources:

Coconut Research Center:

Bruce Fife, N.D., has written many books on the subject of the wonderful benefits of coconut oil. Explore his excellent website at: http://www.coconutresearchcenter.org/index.htm

Organic Food Choices:

In general, Whole Foods, Trader Joe's, and Sprouts have excellent choices for organic produce and organic meats. This is a good place to start and convenient for many people. Be sure to shop between each of them to see who has the better prices at the time.

When possible, support your local organically grown produce or meats. For locally grown produce in Phoenix, Arizona go to:

http://az.naturesgardendelivered.com/index.php

For a comprehensive list of organic meat, fish, and produce sellers go to: http://www.greenpeople.org/OrganicMeat.html

Real Raw Milk:

A Project of the Weston A. Price Foundation:

http://www.realmilk.com/.

This provides a wealth of information about the health benefits and safety of consuming nonpasteurized, raw milk products. My family consumes raw milk obtained from reputable sources in Arizona and we've enjoyed optimal results and great taste.

For an excellent report regarding the science behind the benefits, safety and political history of Raw Real Milk read: "Supplemental Report in Favor of Grade A Raw Milk: Expert Report and Recommendation." By Dr. William Cambell Douglas Jr., M.D. and Aajonus Vonderplanitz, Scientific Nutritional Researcher. Available at: http://www.karlloren. com/aajonus/p15.htm

Another excellent website about Raw Real Milk and health in general: http://www.drrons.com/raw-milk-health-benefits.htm

Nutritional Organizations:

The Price-Pottenger Nutrition Foundation: http://www.ppnf. org/catalog/ppnf/index.htm

From their website: "The Price-Pottenger Nutrition Foundation (PPNF) is a non-profit educational resource providing access to modern scientific validation of ancestral wisdom on nutrition, agriculture, and health for 57 years. Originally known as the Weston A. Price Memorial Foundation, we serve as the guardian for the precious archival material from the research of Weston A. Price, DDS and Francis M. Pottenger, Jr., MD, and most of the great nutrition pioneers of our time, as well as maintaining a library of over 10,000 historical and contemporary references."

The Weston A. Price Foundation: http://www.westonaprice.org/splash_2. htm

The Weston A. Price Foundation is a nonprofit, tax-exempt charity founded in 1999 to disseminate the research of nutrition pioneer Dr. Weston Price, whose studies of isolated nonindustrialized peoples established the parameters of human health and determined the optimum characteristics of human diets. Dr. Price's research demonstrated that humans achieve perfect physical form and perfect health generation after generation only when they consume nutrient-dense whole foods and the vital fat-soluble activators found exclusively in animal fats.

Iodine Information:

Guy Abraham, M.D. www.iodine4health.com

This website is an excellent resource for not only breast cancer therapy but the concept that the toxic halide bromide is related to iodine deficiency and thyroid disease.

http://www.breastcancerchoices.org/bromidedominancetheory.html

Appendix 2: Naturopathic Medicine Defined

The principles of naturopathic medicine and natural healing modalities have roots from thousands of years ago. However, as a distinct profession, Benedict Lust, a prominent physician from New York who was originally from Germany, founded it in 1902. The profession went into near extinction by the 1950s when the atomic age ushered in a more reductionistic view of science in general and in medicine specifically. The use of miracle drugs such as penicillin dominated the medical culture. By the 1970s, a lack of solution to rising chronic disease led to the public demanding more results from the failing medical model. Naturopathic medicine and other natural based systems of healing offered a solution to this crisis, and the profession started to reemerge. Today, due to the efforts of thousands of physicians and patients, naturopathic medicine has emerged as an integral part of the healthcare system.

The current scope of practice and training for naturopathic medicine is broad and includes traditional conventional medical diagnostics, botanical or herbal medicine, homeopathic medicine, nutrition, physical medicine including basic orthopedics and advanced manipulation, traditional Chinese medicine and acupuncture, environmental medicine and detoxification practices, counseling and stress management, minor surgery, and when applicable, the ability to prescribe drugs.

Naturopathic medicine is a distinct system of primary care medicine. Its distinction lies in two key areas; one, in its principles of practice and two, its underlying philosophy of practice.

The six principles listed below give rise to a medical practice that emphasizes the individual and engenders empowerment towards greater responsibility in personal healthcare.

1. First Do No Harm—*Primum Non Nocere*

The first and most important principle in all medical practices, particularly within the philosophical tenets of naturopathic medicine. Naturopathic medicine utilizes therapies that are both effective and safe.

2. The Healing Power of Nature—*Vis Medicatrix Naturae*

This is a key tenet of naturopathic medicine and refers to the innate and inherent ability of the body to heal itself. The *Vis Medicatrix Naturae* is a concept elaborated in the writings of Hippocrates and is not unlike the concept of chi or qi, or prana, or any other concept of a life-generating and sustaining force.

3. Discover and Treat the Cause—*Tolle Causam*

Naturopathic physicians seek to treat the underlying cause of disease. Symptoms are viewed as natural expressions of healing which guide the physician towards a holistic view of the patient that reveals the true cause.

4. Treat the Whole Person—*Tolle Totum*

We are whole beings, with mental, emotional, spiritual and physical dimensions that must be viewed while trying to help any condition.

5. The Physician is a Teacher—*Docere*

The physician must help and guide the patient towards newer understandings about themselves and their health. The physician must teach, and with that commitment he or she must also be a perpetual student for the benefit of the patient.

6. Prevention as the best cure—*Preventire*

Through education and lifestyle changes, the naturopathic physician can lead the patient towards preventing disease processes before they occur or reoccur. Physicians can assess risk factors early on and intervene appropriately to prevent illness.

Upon these six unifying principles, adopted in 1989 by the American Association of Naturopathic Physicians (AANP), prominent thinkers in naturopathic philosophy and policy, naturopathic doctors Jerad Zeff and Pamela Snyder articulated a Therapeutic Order that expounds upon basic naturopathic philosophy.

Naturopathic Therapeutic order:

1. Establish the conditions for health.
   a. Identify and remove disturbing factors.
   b. Institute a more healthful regimen.
2. Stimulate the healing power of nature (vis medicatrix naturae): the self-healing processes.
3. Address weakened or damaged systems or organs.
   a. Strengthen the immune system.
   b. Decrease toxicity.
   c. Normalize inflammatory function.
   d. Optimize metabolic function.
   e. Balance regulatory systems.
   f. Enhance regeneration.
   g. Harmonize with your life force.
4. Correct structural integrity.
5. Address pathology: Use specific natural substances, modalities, or interventions.
6. Address pathology: Use specific pharmacologic or synthetic substances.
7. Suppress or surgically remove pathology.

From Zeff J, Snyder P. Course syllabus: NM51 71, Naturopathic clinical theory. Seattle: Bastyr University, 1997-2005. ("The actual therapeutic order may change, depending on the individual patient's needs for safe and effective care. The needs of the patient are primary in determining the appropriate approach to therapy.")

This Therapeutic Order allows the physician to approach the clinical situation in a patient-centered fashion utilizing the least invasive measure when possible but providing the avenue for more heroic measures if needed. In the end, the patient receives the best possible care that provides true healing of the entire system.

Currently, fifteen states and five provinces in Canada license and regulate the practice of naturopathic medicine including Alaska, Arizona, British Columbia, California, Connecticut, Hawaii, Idaho, Kansas, Maine, Manitoba, Montana, New Hampshire, New York, Nova Scotia, Ontario, Oregon, Saskatchewan, Utah, Vermont, and Washington. Washington, D.C., Puerto Rico, and the U.S. Virgin Islands also have licensing laws for naturopathic doctors. In the great state of Arizona, naturopathic doctors enjoy a broad scope of practice and are fully licensed primary care physicians and many health insurance plans offer coverage of naturopathic medical services.

Appendix 3: Thyroid Hormone Conversion Charts

The following chart is a basic guide for converting from one form of thyroid hormone to another. This chart is a guide only and your individual dose adjustment will be necessary. It is important to understand that desiccated thyroid products such as Armour® or Nature Throid® are highly bioavailable and absorbable. Natural desiccated thyroid contains additional weak thyroid hormones that make the product more whole and effective. The major active thyroid hormones such as T4 and T3 are present in measurable amounts, but the weaker, inactive hormones T2, T1, and calcitonin found in smaller amounts theoretically contain some activity. With that said, many patients who are on a particular dose of Levothyroixine (T4) may need a slightly smaller equivalent dose of Armour® or Nature Throid® in the beginning stages of treatment.

Drug	Thyroid Tablets, USP (Armour® Thyroid, Nature Throid®)	Liotrix Tablets, USP (Thyrolar®)	Liothronine Tablets, USP (Plain T3, Cytomel®)	Levothyroxine Tablets, USP (Plain T4, Unithroid®, Levoxyl®, Levothroid®, Synthroid®)
Approx. Dose Equivalent	1/4 grain (15 mg)	¼		25 mcg (.025 mg)
Approx. Dose Equivalent	1/2 grain (30 mg)	½	12.5 mcg	50 mcg (.05 mg)
Approx. Dose Equivalent	1 grain (60 mg)	1	25 mcg	100 mcg (0.1 mg)
Approx. Dose Equivalent	1 1/2 grains (90 mg)	1 1/2	37.5 mcg	150 mcg (0.15 mg)
Approx. Dose Equivalent	2 grains (120 mg)	2	50 mcg	200 mcg (0.2 mg)
Approx. Dose Equivalent	3 grains (180 mg)	3	75 mcg	300 mcg (0.3 mg)

Nature Throid® is a registered trademark of Western Research Laboratories, Inc.

Armour®, Thyrolar® and Levothroid® are registered trademarks of Forest Pharmaceuticals, Inc.

Appendix 4: Thyroid Neck Examination

The American Association of Clinical Endocrinologists provides a method to check your thyroid gland. This is an excellent screening process and should be a habit for everyone, particularly women, due to the high prevalence of thyroid disease in females. Checking your thyroid should be as routine as the monthly self-examination of breast tissue. Here's how:

- Get a glass of water and a hand-held mirror.
- With the mirror in your hand, study the area of your neck just below the Adam's apple and immediately above the collarbone. That is the location of your thyroid gland.
- While focusing on this area, tip your head back.
- Take a drink of water and swallow.
- As you do, look at your neck. Be on the lookout for bulges or protrusions in this area when you swallow. Be careful not to confuse the Adam's apple with the thyroid gland. The gland is closer to the collarbone.
- Repeat this process a few times if you suspect anything.
- If you do see any bulges or protrusions, you should see your physician. Your thyroid gland may be enlarged, or you may have a nodule. In any case, it should be checked for cancer or thyroid disease.

    Source:
http://www.aace.com/public/awareness/tam/2006/pdfs/NeckCheckCard.pdf

Of course, this examination is designed as a home screening tool for patients. This examination does not replace the routine need for patients to have a doctor perform an annual thyroid exam and any other necessary imaging and blood work analysis.

Appendix 5: The Safety, Efficacy, and Historical Use of Bioidentical Hormone Replacement Therapy

Patients ask me every day, "If this is so effective of a therapy, why don't more doctors know about it and want to prescribe it for their patients?" The short answer to this complex question is "money." It must be understood that the pharmaceutical industry is driven by the manufacture, marketing, and medical distribution of synthetic pharmaceutical drugs. Only unique synthetic biochemical structures can be patented. Products such as estrogen or testosterone, which occurs naturally in the body cannot be patented. Naturally occurring substances such as the extract of a plant also cannot be patented. Therefore, it is not in the interest of the pharmaceutical companies to endorse natural medications or substances that cannot be patented simply because they do not lead to the generation of significant revenue. If bioidentical hormones (made of naturally occurring substances) were patentable, a financial push to use them and fund extensive marketing strategies for them would have emerged years ago. Presently, pharmaceutical companies do not want to involve themselves in naturally occurring substances that contradict the synthetic pharmacopeia mindset that generates money now and with future synthetic drugs.

Although pharmaceutical companies focus their promotion on manufactured synthetic products, they actually manufacture bioidentical hormones without using the term "bioidentical." For example, Prometrium® contains bioidentical progesterone in dosage strengths of either 100 mg or 200 mg. The technical description provided by the European manufacturer Solvay Pharmaceuticals, Inc. explains "Progesterone is synthesized from a starting material from a plant source and is *chemically identical* to progesterone of human ovarian origin." (Emphasis added.) [628]

Confusion About HRT Safety

A tremendous storm of confusion was produced when a study from the University of Texas M.D. Anderson Cancer Center announced in December of 2006 that breast cancer incidence in the United States had dropped more than 7 percent and that this drop related to the fact of millions of women deciding to avoid hormone replacement therapy following the results of the Women's Health Initiative (WHI) in 2002.[629] There are two key problems with the interpretation of this set of data and its correlation to the cessation of hormone replacement therapy.

- ❧ We cannot directly infer that the decrease of breast cancer diagnosis had anything to do with adding or eliminating hormone replacement therapy. Breast cancer is a disease that takes time to develop and measurement of a single year's incidence does not allow for direct correlation to a disease process that takes many years to develop.

- ❧ If we attempt to correlate a relationship with the lowered breast cancer risk to a rapid cessation of hormone therapy, then we must understand that it was synthetic hormones that were discontinued and therefore synthetic hormones would be correlated to the breast cancer risk and not bioidentical hormones. This is true because most women were using synthetic hormones prior to the revealing WHI results of 2002 and not compounded or manufactured bioidentical hormones. In fact, since 2002 compounded bioidentical hormones had the largest amount of public awareness and were seen as a safer alternative to synthetic hormones due to the WHI results. Therefore, the decrease could be interpreted as being due to women stopping synthetic hormones and starting *en masse* compounded and manufactured bioidentical hormone therapy.

A Long History of Use

There is nothing new about bioidentical hormones. Their history is rich, beginning when bioidentical hormones were first isolated as far back as the 1920s. Ruzicka achieved the synthesis of bioidentical testosterone from cholesterol in 1936.[630] Estrogen and progesterone were both isolated and synthesized as early as 1929.[631] Bioidentical subcutaneous pellets have been used continuously since 1939 at the University of Georgia Medical School, reporting no adverse effects or increased risk of harm.[632] When used in proper physiologic doses, bioidentical hormones are effective and safe. Vast empirical clinical evidence disproves harm and demonstrates effectiveness. Conversely, synthetic hormones are foreign to the body and may lead to the harmful health risks we associate with synthetic hormone replacement therapy such as an increased incidence of breast cancer, myocardial infarction (heart attack) and blood clotting that leads to stroke.[633]

Gino Tutera, M.D., FACOG, an Arizona gynecologist and expert in the use of bioidentical hormone replacement therapy with subcutaneous pellets, performed an excellent clinical observational study of 973 women using estradiol (estrogen) pellets. The average length of treatment was ten years but some women in the study had been using estradiol pellets for up to twenty-five years. The study revealed that estradiol pellet treatment created no increased risk for breast or ovarian cancer. In fact, the study showed that bioidentical estradiol may have decreased the risk for those diseases.[634] Having worked personally in the same setting since 2006, witnessing thousands of "patient years" on this therapy, I have not seen an *increase* in breast or uterine cancer outside of the actual nationwide averages.

Not All Estrogens Are Made the Same

Synthetic hormones, such as the now known potentially disease-causing estrogen diethylstilbestrol (DES), are so different that it never gets converted to the original bioidentically shaped hormone, but induces powerful and deleterious "estrogenic effects" on the body.[635, 636] The risk of breast cancer for DES-exposed women over age forty was 1.9 times the risk of breast cancer for unexposed women of the same ages. Also, oral synthetic estrogens are known to increase clotting factors due to the processing that must take place in the liver. This increased clotting raises a woman's chances for stroke and death.[637]

Bioidentical Hormones: Regulated, Safe, and Effective

Bioidentical hormones are created by state regulated compounding pharmacies but have not gone through the FDA approval process for each individual compounded prescription. However, compounding pharmacies use FDA approved materials certified by the United States Pharmacopeia (USP) in all of their compounded medications. Compounding pharmacies were in existence long before larger pharmaceutical companies began to dominate the prescription landscape through manufacturing synthetic medications. In fact, compounding has been approved and regulated by state boards of pharmacy since the Food, Drug, and Cosmetic Act was passed in 1938. All ingredients of compounds come from manufacturers or re-packagers who must be FDA registered and meet FDA specifications for safety and purity. The materials used are FDA approved and certified and cataloged by the United States Pharmacopeia (USP), but each specific prescription they fill based on a physician's request is *not* approved. The pharmacists have the training and ability to compound known FDA approved pharmaceuticals or FDA approved manufactured medications and provide the flexibility of specific dosage and unique delivery of the medication that may vary from typical manufacture in delivery (gel, cream, tablet, etc.) and in dosage.[638] In fact, when any FDA approved medication is altered into another delivery system (gel, cream, tablet, etc.) it must be compounded into an alternate dose not available through the manufacturer. Therefore, the newly compounded dose, that differs from the manufacture is not FDA approved.

For example, a physician would like to use a specific FDA approved medication for a child. That medication went through the FDA approval process only as a 20 mg tablet minimum dose. But, due to the unique need of the child, the physician wants to lower the dose to 5 mg and put it into a liquid form. This amount and form of the medication would not be FDA approved because it differs from the form and dose that gained original FDA approval. But the medication used was still FDA approved as safe to be used by children.

Compounded bioidentical hormones have not undergone the FDA approval process, but the materials used are USP materials that are FDA approved. It is just that the combination of materials and perhaps the form of delivery and dose amount has not been approved for that unique compound. It would be impossible for the FDA to approve a uniquely compounded prescription for each individual patient. The role of the healthcare professional in knowing what to prescribe and in what form and amount is where the responsibility lies. And when the patient is honest with the healthcare provider, safe medications can be beautifully and expertly designed for each individual.

Compounding Creates Flexibility and Choice

A medication prepared by a pharmaceutical company produces a limited number of dosages including hormones, implying a one-size-fits-all approach to dosing. A compounding pharmacy has the ability to prepare a bioidentical hormone prescription, or any medication, to a specific dosage indicated by a prescribing physician, resulting in a clinical approach wholly unique to that individual. Bioidentical hormones of any type, including subcutaneous hormone pellets, are produced by an FDA-approved compounding pharmacy using strict compounding guidelines and independent lab analysis to determine potency and dosage variance.

Semantics and Definitions

Many FDA approved bioidentical hormones are available by prescription. Some examples include 17-beta-estradiol (Estrace®, Climara®), estrone (Ortho-Est®, Ogen®), and micronized progesterone (Prometrium®, Prochieve® 4%). These prescription medications can be further researched at www.rxlist.com. Each of these bioidentical formulations come in specific doses that went through the FDA approval process for the specific dose tested. The doses for FDA approved bioidentical hormones are supposedly safe and effective. For example, bioidentical Estrace® comes in three specific FDA approved doses of 0.5 mg, 1 mg and 2 mg. But an alternative dose of a compounded bioidentical prescription of estradiol, which is present in Estrace®, would not be FDA approved. The real contention then is whether any particular dose of a bioidentical hormone differs from what is typically manufactured, not whether there is safety or efficacy of that bioidentical hormone. We are then left with a debate about compounding bioidentical hormones and not really the safety or efficacy of the bioidentical hormone per se.

Compounding versus Manufacturing

Since the 1990s, the FDA has claimed that compounding has been illegal since the Federal Food, Drug, and Cosmetic Act was passed in 1938 establishing compounding as a legal and sanctioned professional practice. The FDA claims that all compounded medications need to be considered new drugs and go through the same extensive approval process a manufactured drug endures.

A landmark ruling in August of 2006 in favor of upholding compounding practices quelled the FDA fervor. The U.S. District Court Judge in Midland, Texas, Robert Junell explained: "If compounded drugs were required to undergo the new drug approval process, the result would be that patients needing individually tailored prescriptions would not be able to receive the necessary medication due to the cost and time associated with obtaining approval… It is not feasible, either economically or time-wise, for the needed medications to be subjected to the FDA approval process. It is in the best interest of public health to recognize an exemption for compounded drugs that are created based on a prescription written for an individual patient by a licensed practitioner." [639, 640]

It is important to note that not all medications widely used by physicians and prescribed to patients have undergone the FDA approval process. The popular thyroid hormone medication Synthroid® avoided

FDA approval for 46 years until 2002, yet was prescribed almost exclusively by endocrinologists and physicians for the treatment of hypothyroidism during that time. Interestingly, there are multiple compounds that are commonly used today that are either prescribed or given over the counter that did not go through the FDA approval process. The following footnote reference provides a link with a list of common medications that were grandfathered in after the 1938 revision of the 1906 Food and Drug Act.[641] These medications did not technically go through the FDA approval process and are commonly used today.

The pharmaceutical companies produce medications that are responsible for saving lives and improving the quality of lives. They are also responsible for a multitude of deaths due to medications that were FDA approved and supposedly safe. A 1998 meta-analysis in the Journal of the American Medical Association (JAMA) showed that 106,000 deaths occur annually due to adverse drug effects, with a ten year estimated total of 1.06 million deaths.[642] The cost to the American public was $12 billion.[643] This point illustrates that the use of FDA approved medications do not automatically disprove harm and dictate efficacy, nor does it indicate that it was these products that directly caused these deaths. It does demonstrate that just because medicines undergo a rigorous process of approval and research, it does not mean that no harm exists for the public. This of course applies to the use of compounded or manufactured bioidentical hormones. Yet, there is no evidence to show that bioidentical hormones cause long-term negative effects to those using them when prescribed by a healthcare provider. The obvious biological evidence that bioidentical hormones are safe and effective at preventing disease is the lowered incidence of disease in younger populations when endogenous hormones are at their peak.

When the facts have illuminated the definitions and when historical and scientific rigor have united with common sense and practical utility regarding these bioidentical hormones, we will be left with the true root of this contention. When the truth is revealed we see that the contention is not about safety, efficacy, science, medicine or even health. It is about the manufacturing of hormones and medications versus the compounding of hormones and medications and the resulting financial implications. As a society, do we deem the manufacturer of medications as the purveyor of medical truths and advice shrouded in FDA approval? Or do we see the doctor, ensconced within the Hippocratic oath and a lifetime of medical education, as the protector of a patient's health? With this debate, we are faced with an attack on one of the most intimate of social relationships, the doctor-patient relationship.

Summarized Points

- Bioidentical hormones have an extensive history of use spanning more than eighty years.
- Bioidentical hormones are synthesized and are therefore not a naturally derived substance but specifically are synthetically produced exact copies of hormones found in the body.
- Compounded bioidentical hormones are not independently FDA approved, but use FDA approved materials certified by the USP.
- Manufacturers produce FDA approved bioidentical hormones and are available in various limited doses and multiple delivery systems.
- Not all medications prescribed regularly by physicians are FDA approved, but those medications are derived from FDA approved materials certified by the USP.
- All medical devices, practices, and medications cannot be proven to be safe. We can only disprove their harm. Compounded bioidentical hormones have a historical record of lack of harm.
- An extensive amount of documented research exists using bioidentical hormones for more than eighty years disproving harm.
- Compounding pharmacies are regulated by each state.
- There are distinct differences between synthetic and bioidentical hormones.

Appendix 6: Top 50 Prescribed Medications in 2008

Here is the complete list of the top 50 prescribed medications for 2008 from the October 2009 *AARP (American Association of Retired Peoples) Bulletin.* Take note that many of these medications were given for conditions related to a lowered metabolism and/or poor diet and lifestyle:

1.	Hydrocodone	(pain)
2.	Lisinopril	(hypertension)
3.	Simvastatin	(high cholesterol)
4.	Levothyroxine	(hypothyroidism)
5.	Amoxicillin	(bacterial infection)
6.	Azithromycin	(bacterial infection)
7.	Lipitor®	(high cholesterol)
8.	Hydrochlorothiazide	(edema/hypertension)
9.	Alprazolam	(anxiety/depression)
10.	Atenolol	(hypertension)
11.	Metformin®	(type II diabetes)
12.	Metoprolol Succinate	(hypertension)
13.	Furosemide oral	(edema/hypertension)
14.	Metoprolol tartrate	(hypertension)
15.	Sertraline	(depression)
16.	Omeprazole	(ulcers/reflux)
17.	Zolpidem tartrate	(insomnia)
18.	Nexium®	(ulcers/reflux)
19.	Lexapro®	(depression)
20.	Oxycodone	(pain)
21.	Singulair	(asthma)

22.	Ibuprofen	(pain/inflammation)
23.	Plavix®	(blood clotting)
24.	Prednisone oral	(allergies/inflammation)
25.	Fluoxetine	(depression)
26.	Synthroid®	(hypothyroidism)
27.	Warfarin	(blood clotting)
28.	Cephalexin	(bacterial infection)
29.	Lorazepam	(anxiety)
30.	Clonazepam	(epilepsy/anxiety)
31.	Citalopram HBR	(depression)
32.	Tramadol	(pain)
33.	Gabapentin	(epilepsy/pain)
34.	Ciprofloxacin HCl	(bacterial infection)
35.	Propoxyphene-N	(pain)
36.	Lisinopril	(hypertension)
37.	Triamterene	(edema/hypertension)
38.	Amoxicillin	(bacterial infection)
39.	Cyclobenzaprine	(muscle injury/spasm)
40.	Prevacid®	(ulcers/reflux)
41.	Advair®	(asthma)
42.	Effexor XR®	(depression)
43.	Trazodone HCl	(depression)
44.	Fexofenadine	(allergy)
45.	Fluticasone nasal	(allergy)
46.	Diovan®	(hypertension)
47.	Paroxetine	(depression/anxiety)
48.	Lovastatin	(high cholesterol)
49.	Crestor®	(high cholesterol)
50.	Trimethoprim	(bacterial infection)

Appendix 7: Questionnaires

Andropause: Aging Male Survey (AMS)

Which of the following symptoms apply to you at this time? Please rank each symptom on the space to the left using numbers from 0 to 5.

0 = none, 1 = very mild, 2 = mild, 3 = moderates, 4 = severe, 5 = very severe

_____ 1. Decline in your feeling of general well-being (general state of health, subjective feeling)

_____ 2. Joint pain and muscular ache (lower back pain, joint pain, pain in a limb, general back ache)

_____ 3. Excessive sweating (unexpected/sudden episodes of sweating, hot flushes independent of strain)

_____ 4. Sleep problems (difficulty in falling asleep, difficulty in sleeping through, waking up early and feeling tired, poor sleep, sleeplessness)

_____ 5. Increased need for sleep, often feeling tired

_____ 6. Irritability (feeling aggressive, easily upset about little things, moody)

_____ 7. Nervousness (inner tension, restlessness, feeling fidgety

_____ 8. Anxiety (feeling panicky)

_____ 9. Physical exhaustion/lacking vitality (general decrease in performance, reduced activity, lacking interest in leisure activities, feeling of getting less done, of achieving less, of having to force oneself to undertake activities)

_____ 10. Decrease in muscular strength (feeling of weakness)

_____ 11. Depressive mood (feeling down, sad, on the verge of tears, lack of drive, mood swings, feeling nothing is of any use)

_____ 12. Feeling that you have passed your peak

_____ 13. Feeling burned out, having hit rock-bottom

_____ 14. Decrease in beard growth

_____ 15. Decrease in ability/frequency to perform sexually

_____ 16. Decrease in the number of morning erections

_____ 17. Decrease in sexual desire/libido (lacking pleasure in sex, lacking desire for sexual intercourse)

Scoring:

17-26 or less: None. Andropause or low testosterone is highly unlikely.

27-36: Slight. Andropause is possible as a mild condition.

37-49: Moderate. Andropause is moderate in possibility and condition.

50+: Severe. Andropause is highly likely and severe in condition.

Sources:

http://www.aging-males-symptoms-scale.info/

http://www.issam.ch/

Hypoglycemia Questionnaire

This form is designed to determine if you suffer from hypoglycemia or low blood sugar. Check all that apply. If you are experiencing many of these symptoms, then hypoglycemia may be a problem for you.

Symptoms of Hypoglycemia

- Sudden fatigue
- Anxiety
- Depression
- Headaches
- Difficulty concentrating
- Sweating, including palms
- Tremors and shakiness
- Excessive hunger
- Abdominal discomfort and bloating

Conditions Associated with Hypoglycemia

- Adrenal dysfunction
- Alcoholism
- Anxiety
- Pituitary issues
- Insulin resistance
- Hypothyroidism

Reasons for Hypoglycemia

Skipping meals: This is one of the main reasons for hypoglycemia. Avoiding meals and not eating in a regular fashion places an unnecessary burden on your system and takes you further away from your goals.

Increased metabolism: When you are undergoing any kind of treatment that enhances your metabolic rate, such as the things that are described in this book, then hypoglycemia can become more of an issue. *As the metabolic rate increases, the demand for a steady stream of nutrients and sugar becomes more imperative.* When your metabolic rate is slower, people can get away with skipping meals and taking nutritional supplements. But as you place demand on your physiology with increased thyroid, adrenal and sex hormones, then old patterns of eating will not work and hypoglycemia can ensue.

Note: The symptoms of hypoglycemia listed above are very similar to the symptoms of excessive thyroid hormone stimulation. Often, when a patient believes they may be overstimulated by their thyroid hormone medication it can in fact be issues of hypoglycemia. This is not always the case so be sure to contact your healthcare provider to help determine what is clinically occurring.

Determining Hypoglycemia

One method to determine hypoglycemia is to have a fasting glucose blood test that can determine where your blood sugar is while fasting for at least twelve hours. However, an even more accurate method is to purchase an inexpensive blood glucose monitor at a drug store and monitor your blood sugar throughout the day and specifically when you are having symptoms. If your blood sugar is below 80 mg/dL while having symptoms, and your symptoms relieve after you eat, then you likely are dealing with hypoglycemia. Be sure to contact your healthcare provider about this.

What to do for Hypoglycemia

- Reduce refined sugars and most grain-based carbohydrates, as described thoroughly in this book.
- Eat three meals plus two snacks daily, spreading out your food over the day.
- Limit alcohol.
- Limit caffeine intake, *if you are sensitive.*
- Add in nutritional and herbal supplements. In general, the basic supplements described throughout this book provide the proper nutritional foundation to balance blood sugar. Here are a few specific nutritional considerations for hypoglycemia and blood sugar regulation:
  - Chromium picolinate (400-600 mcg/day)
  - Biotin (7,000 to 15,000 mcg daily/day)
  - Gymnema (*Gymnema sylvestre*) Leaf 75% gymnemic acid (150 mg/day)
  - Bitter Melon (*Momordica charantia*) Fruit Extract 40:1 (50 mg/day)
  - Vanadium (as vanadyl sulfate) (950 mcg/day)

Hypothyroid Symptom Questionnaire

Which of the following symptoms apply to you at this time? Please rank each symptom on the space to the left using numbers from 0 to 5.
0 = none, 1 = very mild, 2 = mild, 3 = moderate, 4 = severe, 5 = very severe.

Dermatological

Dry skin	__/5
Course skin	__/5
Itchy skin	__/5
Dry, coarse hair	__/5
Thinning/loss of hair	__/5
Thinning eyebrows	__/5
Brittle or ridges on nails	__/5
Excess wax in ears	__/5
Decreased sweat	__/5
Paleness of skin or lips	__/5
TOTAL	**__/50**

Metabolic

Lethargy (low energy)	__/5
Sensation of cold	__/5
Heat intolerance (not hot flashes)	__/5
Slow speech(not memory)	__/5
Weight gain with little food intake	__/5
Lack of appetite	__/5
Lack of libido	__/5
TOTAL	**__/35**

Dryness (sicca)

Dry eyes	__/5

Dry skin	__/5
Dry mouth	__/5
Dry nose	__/5
Dry sinuses	__/5
Dry vagina	__/5
TOTAL	**__/30**

Gastrointestinal

Constipation	__/5
Diarrhea	__/5
Irritable bowel syndrome	__/5
GERD (reflux disease)	__/5
TOTAL	**__/20**

Reproductive

Delayed menstrual Flow	__/5
Excessive menstrual Flow	__/5
Painful menses	__/5
Impotence (men only)	__/5
TOTAL	**__/15/5**

Mental/Emotional well-being

Depression	__/5
Irritability/mood swings	__/5
Nervousness	__/5
Anxiety	__/5
Impaired memory	__/5
Impaired focus	__/5
TOTAL	**__/30**

Cardiovascular/ Respiratory

Chest pain	__/5
Palpitations	__/5
Atrial fibrillation	__/5
Chronic cough of _unknown_ reason	__/5
Airflow obstruction (non smokers)	__/5
Shortness of breath on physical exertion	__/5
Shortness of breath in general	__/5
TOTAL	**__/30**

Swelling

Swollen ankles	__/5
Swollen wrists	__/5
Swollen eyelids	__/5
Swollen, thick tongue	__/5
Swollen face	__/5
TOTAL	**__/25**

Musculoskeletal

Muscle weakness	__/5
Unexplained tingling or numbness	__/5
Body aches	__/5
Muscle pain	__/5
Joint pain	__/5
Carpal tunnel syndrome	__/5
Plantar fasciitis	__/5
TOTAL	**__/35**

Sleep

Difficulty getting to sleep	__/5
Difficulty staying asleep	__/5
Wake unrefreshed	__/5
Sleep apnea	__/5
Snoring	__/5
TOTAL	**__/25**

Past medical diagnosis of:

__Hypertension

__High cholesterol

__Infertility/Multiple Miscarriage

__Anemia

__Hypothyroidism

__Thyroid Nodules

__Goiter

__Hashimoto's thyroiditis

__Fibromyalgia

__Chronic Fatigue Syndrome

__Adrenal Fatigue

__Lupus

__Diabetes Type I

__Insulin Resistance

__Celiac's disease

__Multiple Sclerosis

__Rheumatoid arthritis

__Sjogren's disease

__Positive ANA

__Polycystic Ovarian Syndrome

__Fibrocystic Breasts/Dense Breasts

__Live, work, or grow up near a nuclear power plant

__Currently taking Lithium or amiodarone (Cordarone)

Menopause Symptom Questionnaire

Which of the following symptoms apply to you at this time? Please rank each symptom on the space to the left using numbers from 0 to 5. 0 = none, 1 = very mild, 2 = mild, 3 = moderate, 4 = severe, 5 = very severe.

Vasomotor Symptoms

Hot flashes/flushes	__/5
Night sweats	__/5
Hot/cold sensation	__/5
TOTAL	**__/15**

Mental

Poor memory	__/5
Difficulty focusing	__/5
Difficulty concentrating	__/5
Feeling disoriented	__/5
TOTAL	**__/20**

Emotional

Irritability	__/5
Mood swings	__/5
Cry easily	__/5
Anxiety	__/5
Depression	__/5
Feelings of dread/doom	__/5
TOTAL	**__/30**

Nervous System

Trouble getting to sleep	__/5
Trouble staying asleep	__/5
Itchy, crawly skin	__/5

Electric shock feeling in skin	__/5
Numbness/tingling of extremities	__/5
Restless leg syndrome	__/5
Headaches	__/5
Dizziness	__/5
Loss of balance	__/5
Ringing in the ears	__/5
Burning tongue	__/5
TOTAL	**__/55**

Musculoskeletal

Sore joints	__/5
Sore achy muscles	__/5
Increased tension in muscles	__/5
Poor response to exercise	__/5
TOTAL	**__/20**

Genitourinary

Irregular timing of periods	__/5
Long periods (>10 days)	__/5
Short periods (< 3 days)	__/5
Heavy flow	__/5
Scanty flow	__/5
Vaginal dryness	__/5
Incontinence	__/5
TOTAL	**__35**

Cardiac

Irregular heart beat	__/5
Palpitations	__/5
TOTAL	**__/10**

Metabolism

Fatigue	__/5

Lack of libido   __/5
Weight gain   __/5
TOTAL   **__/15**

Gastrointestinal

Indigestion   __/5
Flatulence   __/5
Nausea   __/5
Bloating   __/5
TOTAL   **__/20**

Other

Breast tenderness   __/5
Allergies   __/5
Thinning hair (head)   __/5
Loss of hair (pubic, body)   __/5
Increase in facial hair   __/5
TOTAL   **__/25**

Related Conditions

Hypothyroidism	Yes	No
Osteopenia (mild bone loss)	Yes	No
Osteoporosis (severe bone loss)	Yes	No
High blood pressure	Yes	No
High cholesterol	Yes	No
Fibromyalgia	Yes	No
Chronic fatigue syndrome	Yes	No

Metabolic Syndrome Questionnaire

Metabolic Syndrome is a condition related to insulin resistance which is the inability of insulin to do its job of shuttling in sugar from the blood into the cells. Weight gain and disease occurs over time. Particularly, this condition can make it very difficult to lose weight and optimize your health.

This form has two parts. One is a checklist of basic questions that lead to an increased risk for Metabolic Syndrome. Two is a checklist of technical questions that are based on body measurements and blood laboratory analysis.

Part One: Lifestyle Risk Factors and Past Medical History
- ❏ Current or past history of prolonged stress
- ❏ Lack of consistent exercise
- ❏ Over the age of 50
- ❏ Past or current diagnosis of liver disease
- ❏ Past or current diagnosis of heart disease
- ❏ Past or current diagnosis of diabetes mellitus
- ❏ Past or current diagnosis of PCOS (polycystic ovarian syndrome)
- ❏ Hirsutism: abnormal amounts of facial and body hair in women
- ❏ Acanthosis nigricans: This is a brown or black hyperpigmentation of the skin usually found in body folds, such as in the folds of the side or back of the neck, the armpits, groin, forehead, and around the abdomen.

Part Two: Body Measurements & Blood Laboratory Analysis
- ❏ Elevated waist circumference. Men: Equal to or greater than 40 inches (102 cm), Women: Equal to or greater than 35 inches (88 cm).
- ❏ Raised triglycerides: A level greater than 150 mg/dL (1.7 mmol/L), or being treated for this lipid abnormality.

- ❑ Reduced HDL (good) cholesterol: A reading less than 40 mg/dL (1.03 mmol/L) in males, or less than 50 mg/dL (1.29 mmol/L) in females, or being treated for this lipid abnormality.
- ❑ Raised blood pressure: systolic blood pressure greater than 130 or diastolic blood pressure greater than 85 mm mercury, or on medication for previously diagnosed hypertension.
- ❑ Raised fasting blood glucose (sugar): greater than 100 mg/dL (5.6 mmol/L), or previously diagnosed type II diabetes. If fasting blood glucose is greater than 5.6 mmol/L or 100 mg/dL, an OGTT Glucose Tolerance Test is strongly recommended but is not necessary to define presence of the syndrome.
- ❑ Urinary albumin excretion ratio greater than or equal to 20 µg/min or albumin: creatinine ratio greater than or equal to 30 mg/g.
- ❑ Body mass index (BMI) greater than 30 kg/m2.

Additional blood test factors:
- ❑ Elevated C-reactive protein (CRP)
- ❑ Elevated hemoglobin A1C (hA1C)

If you have many of these risk factors, particularly abdominal obesity with elevated blood pressure and cholesterol, then Metabolic Syndrome is likely and you should consult with your healthcare provider about this condition. You will need to treat this condition by enhancing your metabolic health and consider utilizing the information found in this book.

Overstimulation by Thyroid Hormone Evaluation Form

This form determines if your body is in a state of overstimulation by thyroid hormone. Which of the following symptoms apply to you at this time? Please rank each symptom on the space to the left using numbers from 0 to 5.

0 = none, 1 = very mild, 2 = mild, 3 = moderate[s], 4 = severe, 5 = very severe.

Cardiac/Pulmonary

Shortness of breath at rest	__/5
Shortness of breath (exercise)	__/5
Irregular heart beat	__/5
Elevated heart rate	__/5
TOTAL	**__/20**

Neurological

Tremors, shaking	__/5
Poor concentration	__/5
Brain fog	__/5
Insomnia	__/5
Moodiness	__/5
Nervousness/agitation	__/5
Racing thoughts	__/5
Rapid talking	__/5
TOTAL	**__/40**

Genitourinary

Absent or irregular menses	__/5

Metabolism/Musculoskeletal

Fatigue	__/5
Heat intolerance	__/5

Excessive sweating	__/5
Rapid weight loss	__/5
Increased appetite	__/5
Muscle weakness	__/5
TOTAL	**__/30**

Dermatological

Thinning hair	__/5
Warm moist skin	__/5
Red and itchy skin	__/5
TOTAL	**__/15**

Gastrological

Frequent bowel movements	__/5
Unexplained diarrhea	__/5
TOTAL	**__/10**

Important Points:

- Signs and symptoms of over-stimulation from thyroid hormone can actually be very similar to an inadequate thyroid hormone dose.
- Fill the form out before you start using thyroid hormone to provide a baseline.
- Fill the form out at each evaluation period to provide comparison.

Related Conditions:

- Hypoglycemia, or low blood sugar. In patients who are taking thyroid hormones, an imbalanced diet can make them believe that the symptoms come from the drug instead of the food—not getting enough protein or skipping a meal altogether. The signs and symptoms of hypoglycemia are very similar to the clinical presentation of thyroid hormone over-stimulation.

- ❷ Benign familial tremor. This benign neurological condition presents with bilateral hand tremors and possibly head shaking.
- ❷ Menopause or andropause. The signs and symptoms of inadequate or excessive estrogen and/or testosterone can mimic many of the signs and symptoms of over-stimulation. Hair loss is a typical sign of excessive testosterone.

Clinical Signs:
- ❷ Axillary (arm pit) basal body temperature over 98.2 F.
- ❷ Heart rate *consistently* above 90 beats per minute at rest.
- ❷ Hyperreflexia (fast reflexes), particularly the Achilles tendon reflex.
- ❷ Abnormal EKG, particularly an increased QRS voltage from pervious EKG's.
- ❷ Suppressed TSH value (too low), but this is suggestive, not definitive.
- ❷ Elevated Total and Free T4 and Total and Free T3, but these again are suggestive, not definitive.

Adrenal Fatigue Questionnaire

For the following sections, please rank your symptom, condition, or situation according to the categories below and enter a number from

0 = none/never

1 = very mild/rarely/monthly

2 = mild/sometimes/a few times monthly

3 = moderate/often/a few times weekly

4 = severe/almost daily

5 = very severe/always/daily

Metabolic System

____ I have difficulty getting up in the morning despite adequate sleep.

____ I have low energy before the noon meal (approximately 11:00 a.m.)

____ I have low energy in the late afternoon between 3:00-5:00 p.m.

____ I usually feel better after 6:00 p.m.

____ I get a "second wind" of energy late at night (after 11:00 pm)

____ I like to stay awake late to get my second wind.

____ I need to rest after any type of mental, physical, or emotional stress

____ I have a decreased tolerance for cold.

____ TOTAL

Musculoskeletal System

____ I have a weak back and/or weak knees.

____ TOTAL

Immune System

____ Frequent cold and flus (more than 2 annually)

____ It takes me a long time to recover from illness.

____ TOTAL

Cardiovascular System

____ I have consistent palpitations.

____ I suffer from mitral valve prolapse

___ I get swelling in the extremities, such as the ankles.

___ I get dizzy or have blurry vision when standing up rapidly from a sitting or lying   position.

___ TOTAL

Reproductive/Urological System

___ I have irregular menstrual periods caused by stress.

___ I suffer from PMS. (Premenstrual syndrome)

___ I urinate more frequently than before and get up at night.

___ I have lowered libido (sexual desire).

___ TOTAL

Neurological System

___ I have poor mental focus that is affected by stress.

___ I feel faint often.

___ I have frequent headaches.

___ I am sensitive to bright light.

___ I tend to shake or am nervous when under pressure.

___ I have constant hand or head tremors.

___ TOTAL

Psychological

___ I worry often.

___ I have vague feelings of being generally unwell for no apparent reason.

___ I have an impending sense of doom.

___ I feel depressed like nothing is "worth it."

___ I have a decreased tolerance towards others.

___ I become stressed easily.

___ I have poor recovery from physical or emotional stress.

___ TOTAL

Diet

___ I become mentally confused or shaky if I miss a meal.

____ I crave sugar, sweets, or desserts often.

____ I must use stimulants, such as coffee, to get started in the morning.

____ I need caffeine (chocolate, tea, coffee, soda) to get me through the entire day.

____ I crave food high in fat and feel better when eating high-fat foods.

____ I often crave salt and/or foods high in salt.

____ I feel worse if I eat sweets and no protein for breakfast.

____ I do not eat regular meals.

____ I eat fast food often.

____ I feel worse if I eat high potassium containing foods (like bananas, figs, raw

potatoes), especially if I eat them in the morning.

____ I restrict my salt intake.

____ I have meals at irregular times.

____ TOTAL

Lifestyle factors

____ I tend to be a perfectionist and "type A" personality.

____ My life contains insufficient enjoyable activities.

____ I do not take vacations. (At least two full weeks per year.)

____ I have an addictive personality.

____ TOTAL

Sleep patterns

____ I have trouble getting to sleep.

____ I tend to wake early (approximately 3:00 to 5:00 a.m.) and have trouble getting back to sleep.

____ My best, most refreshing sleep often comes between 7:00-9:00 AM.

____ TOTAL

Alleviating features

____ I have symptoms that improve after eating.

____ I feel better after spending time with my friends.

___ I feel better after a vacation, but quickly decline when normal life resumes.

___ I often feel better if I lie down.

___ Regular meals decrease the severity of my symptoms.

___ TOTAL

___ SUBTOTAL / 280 Possible points

For these sections, give yourself 1 (one) point for a "yes" answer and 0 points for a "no" answer. A yes answer would apply if you have the condition now or in the past.

Physical signs

___ I have dermatographism (a white line appears on my skin for at least a minute if I run my fingernail over it).

___ I have an area of pale skin around my lips.

___ The skin on the palms of my hands and soles of my feet tends to be red/orange in color.

___ I have dry skin.

___ Small irregular dark brown spots have appeared on my forehead, face, neck and shoulders.

___ The fat pads on palms of my hands and/or tips of my fingers are often red.

___ I bruise easily.

___ I have tenderness in my back near my spine at the bottom of my rib cage when pressed.

___ I have low blood pressure (around 90/60 or below)

___ TOTAL

Related conditions

___ Chronic fatigue syndrome

___ Restless leg syndrome

___ Chronic allergies

___ Chemical sensitivities

___ Raynaud's syndrome

___ Hypoglycemia (low blood sugar)

___ Long term, high dose steroid use

___ Chronic skin conditions (i.e., psoriasis)

___ Fibromyalgia

___ Irritable bowel syndrome (IBS)

___ Chrohn's disease

___ Post traumatic stress disorder (PTSD)

___ Bulimia or anorexia nervosa

___ Drug or alcohol abuse.

___ Type 2 diabetes (Insulin resistance)

___ Thyroid disease (hypo- or hyperthyroidism)

___ Rheumatoid arthritis.

___ Sensitive to pharmaceutical medications and/or nutritional supplements

___ Mononucleosis or Epstein Barr virus (EBV)

___ TOTAL

___ SUBTOTAL / 28 Possible points

___ *GRAND TOTAL / 308 Possible points*

Scoring:

A score of 45 or below: Adrenal fatigue is unlikely

A score of 46 – 95: Mild adrenal fatigue

A score of 96 – 154: Moderate adrenal fatigue

A score of 155 or above: Severe adrenal fatigue: Consider actual Addison's disease

Endnotes

1   Liu C, Aloia T, Adrian T, Newton T, Bilchik A, Zinner M, Ashley S, McFadden D (1996). "Peptide YY: a potential proabsorptive hormone for the treatment of malabsorptive disorders.". Am Surg 62 (3): 232–6.

2   Van der Lely AF, Tschop M, Heiman ML, Ghigo E. Biological, physiological, pathophysiological, and pharmacological aspects of ghrelin. Endocrine Reviews. 2004;25:426–457.

3   Williams KW, Scott MM, Elmquist JK (March 2009). "From observation to experimentation: leptin action in the mediobasal hypothalamus". Am. J. Clin. Nutr. 89 (3): 985S–990S.

4   Knutson KL, Spiegel K, Penev P, Van Cauter E (June 2007). "The metabolic consequences of sleep deprivation". Sleep Med Rev 11 (3): 163–178.

5   Dell, D. L. and D. E. Stewart. 2000. Menopause and mood: Is depression linked with hormone changes? Postgraduate Medicine vol. 108, no. 3.

6   Yaffe K, Sawaya G, Lieberburg I, Grady D. Estrogen therapy in postmenopausal women: effects on cognitive function and dementia. JAMA. 1998 Mar 4;279(9):688-95.

7   Epperson, C. N. et al. 1999. Gonadal steroids in the treatment of mood disorders. Psychosomatic Medicine 61:676-689.

8   The Writing Group for the PEPI Trial. Effects of estrogen or estrogen/progestin regiments on heart disease risk factors in postmenopausal women. The Postmenopausal Estrogen/Progestin Intervention (PEPI) Trial. JAMA. 1995; 273: 199–208.

9   Popiela T, Kulig J, Klek S, et al. Enzyme therapy in patients with advanced colorectal cancer. Przegl. Lek. 2000;57 Suppl 5:138-139.

10   Salvati F, Pallotta G, Antilli A, et al. [MACC plus thymostimulin (TP-1 Serono) therapy of small cell bronchogenic carcinoma. Clinico-immunologic evaluation of the results of a randomized trial]. G Ital Chemioter. 1984;31(1-2):185-189.

11   Taylor AL, Finster JL, Mintz DH. Metabolic clearance and production rates of human growth hormone. J Clin Invest. 1969 Dec;48(12):2349-58.

12   Koppelman MCS et al. Effect of Bromocriptine on affect and libido in hyperprolactinemia. Am J Psychiatry 1987; 144: 1037-1041.

13   Heini, A.F. and Weinsier, R.L. 1997. Divergent trends in obesity and fat in patterns: the American paradox. American Journal of Medicine 102(3):259-64.

14   Kipnis, David. Effect of Diet Composition on the Hyperinsulinemia of Obesity. NEJM, 1971.

15   Kyrou I.,Tsigos C. Stress hormones: physiological stress and regulation of metabolism. Curr Opin Pharmacol., 2009 Dec;9(6):787-93. Epub 2009 Sep 14.

16   Jönsson, et. al. Agrarian diet and diseases of affluence ☐ Do evolutionary novel dietary lectins cause leptin resistance? BMC Endocrine Disorders 2005, 5:10. Available: http://www.biomedcentral.com/1472-6823/5/10

17   Veniant MM, LeBel CP: Leptin: from animals to humans. Curr Pharm Des 2003, 9:811-818.

18   Considine RV, Sinha MK, Heiman ML, Kriauciunas A, Stephens TW, Nyce MR, Ohannesian JP, Marco CC, McKee LJ, Bauer TL: Serum immunoreactive-leptin concentrations in normal-weight and obese humans. N Engl J Med 1996, 334:292-295.

19   Meyers, et. al. Serum leptin concentrations and markers of immune function in overweight or obese postmenopausal women.J Endocrinol. 2008 Oct;199(1):51-60. Epub 2008 Jul 9.

20   Simeons A. The action of chorionic gonadotropin in the obese. Lancet 1954; 2: 946-947.

21   Chorionic gonadotropin in weight control. A double-blind random cross-over study of the effectiveness of human chorionic gonadotropin (HCG) vs. placebo in a weight reduction program [JAMA. 1976]

22   Bosch B, Venter I, Stewart RI, Bertram SR. Department of Medical Physiology and Biochemistry, University of Stellenbosch, Parowvallei, CP. Human chorionic gonadotrophin and weight loss. A double-blind, placebo-controlled trial. S Afr Med J. 1990.

23   Available: http://www.asbp.org/resources/uploads/files/HCG%20Position%20Statement.pdf

24   Lijesen GK, Theeuwen I, Assendelft WJ, Van Der Wal G. The effect of human chorionic gonadotropin (HCG) in the treatment of obesity by means of the Simeons therapy: a criteria based meta-analysis. British journal of clinical pharmacology 1995; 40: 237-243.

25   S. Boyd Eaton. The ancestral human diet: what was it and should it be a paradigm for contemporary nutrition? Proceedings of the Nutrition Society (2006), 65, 1–6. Available: http://www.mattmetzgar. com/matt_metzgar/files/ancestralhumandiet.pdf

26   Bogert LJ, Nutrition and Physical Fitness, Philadelphia: Saunders, 1939:437.

27   Lindeberg S, Cordain L, Eaton SB. Biological and clinical potential of a Paleolithic diet. J Nutr Environ Med. 2003;13;149-160.

28   Eaton SB, Konner M. The Paleolithic Prescription: a program of diet & exercise and a design for living. New York: Harper & Row Publishers; 1988.

29   Eaton SB, Eaton SB III. Paleolithic vs. modern diets – selected pathophysiological implications. Eur J Nutr. 2000;39;67-70.

30   Cordain PhD, Loren. "The Paleo Diet." John Wiley and Sons, Inc. Hoboken, New Jersey. 2002.

31   Lindeberg S, Cordain L, Eaton SB. Biological and clinical potential of a Paleolithic diet. J Nutr Environ Med. 2003;13;149-160.

32   S. Boyd Eaton. The ancestral human diet: what was it and should it be a paradigm for contemporary nutrition? Proceedings of the Nutrition Society (2006), 65, 1–6. Am J Clin Nutr 2005;81:341–54. Available: http://www.mattmetzgar.com/matt_metzgar/files/ancestralhumandiet.pdf

33

34   Available: http://www.ppnf.org/catalog/ppnf/TraditionalDietsSimilarities.htm

35   Batmanghelidj. Science or Attitude? Science in Medicine Simplified 2: 1-4, June 1991.

36   Boschmann, M. Journal of Clinical Endocrinology and Metabolism, December 2003; vol. 88: pp. 6015-6019.

37   Douglas Jr., M.D., William Cambell, and Aajonus Vonderplanitz. Supplemental Report in Favor of Grade A Raw Milk: Expert Report and Recommendation. Scientific Nutritional Researcher. Available: http://www.karlloren.com/aajonus/p15.htm

38   Grassi D, Necozione S, Lippi C, et al. Cocoa reduces blood pressure and insulin resistance and improves endothelium-dependent vasodilatation in hypertensives. Hypertension 2005;46:398-405.

39   Taubert D, Roesen R, Schomig E. Effect of cocoa and tea intake on blood pressure: a meta-analysis. Arch Intern Med 2007;167:626-34.

40   Taubert D, Roesen R, Lehmann C, et al. Effects of low habitual cocoa intake on blood pressure and bioactive nitric oxide: a randomized controlled trial. JAMA 2007;298:49-60.

41   Buijsse B, Feskens EJ, Kok FJ, Kromhout D. Cocoa intake, blood pressure, and cardiovascular mortality: the Zutphen Elderly Study. Arch Intern Med 2006;166:411-7.

42   Kris-Etherton PM, Derr J, Mitchell DC, et al. The role of fatty acid saturation on plasma lipids, lipoproteins, & apolipoproteins: I. Effects of whole food diets high in cocoa butter, olive oil, soybean oil, dairy butter, & milk chocolate on the plasma lipids of young men. Metabolism 1993;42:121-9.

43   Gaitan E. Goitrogens in food and water. Annu Rev Nutr 1990;10:21-39.

44   Doerge DR, Sheehan DM. Goitrogenic and estrogenic activity of soy isoflavones. Environ Health Perspect 2002;1 10(suppl):349-53.

45   Lakshmy R, Rao PS, Sesikeran B, Suryaprakash P. Iodine metabolism in response to goitrogen induced altered thyroid status under conditions of moderate and high intake of iodine. Horm Metab Res 1995;27:450-4.

46   Andersen S, et. al. Changes in iodine excretion in 50-69 year old denizens of an Artic society in transition and iodine excretion as a biomarker of the frequency of consumption of traditional Inuit foods. Am J Clin Nutr 205;81:656-63.

47   Eisenstein J, Roberts SB, Dallal G, Saltzman E: High protein weight loss diets: are they safe and do they work? A review of the experimental and epidemiologic data. Nutr Rev60 :189– 200,2002 .

48   Available: http://en.wikipedia.org/wiki/Metabolic_equivalent

49   Ottosson ET. AL. (2000). Effect of Cortisol and Growth Hormone on Lipolysis in Human Adipose Tissue. J Clin Endocrinol Metab. 85(2):799-803.

50   Crawford ET AL. (2003). Randomized Placebo-Controlled trial of androgen Effects in Muscle & Bone in Men Requiring Long-Term Glucocorticoid Treatment. J Clin Endocrinol Metab. 88(7):3167-3176.

51   Bjorntorp ET AL. (1997) Hormonal Control of Regional Fat Distribution. Hum Reprod. Suppl 1:21-25.

52   Gladden (2004). Lactate Metabolism: A new paradigm for the third millennium. Journal of Physiology. 558(1):5-30.

53   Chawalbinska-Moneta ET AL (1996). Threshold increases in plasma growth hormone in relation to plasma catecholamine and blood lactate concentrations during progressive exercise in endurance-trained athletes. European Journal of Applied Physiology. 73(1-2):117-120.

54   Godfrey et. al. The exercise-induced growth hormone response in athletes. Sports Medicine. 33(8):599-613. 2003.

55   Turner et. al. Effect of graded epinephrine infusion on blood lactate response to exercise. J Appl Physiol,79(4):1206-11. 1995.

56   Takahashi et. al. Relationship among blood lactate and plasma catecholamine levels during exercise in acute hypoxia. Applied Human Sci,14(1):49-53.1995.

57   Kaiser et. al. Effects of acute beta-adrenergic blockade on blood and muscle lactate concentration during submaximal exercise. International Journal Sports Med, 4(4):275-7. 1983.

58   Osterberg et. al. Effect of acute resistance exercise on postexercise oxygen consumption and resting metabolic rate in young women. International Journal of Sport Nutrition and Exercise Metabolism.10(1):71-81. 2000.

59   Schuenke et. al. Effect of an acute period of resistance exercise on excess post-exercise oxygen consumption: Implications for body mass management. European Journal of Applied Physiology. 86:411-417. 2002.

60   Miller et. al. A meta analysis of the past 25 years of weight loss research using diet, exercise or diet plus exercise intervention. International Journal of Obesity, 21:941-947. 1997.

61   Sjodin et. al. The influence of physical activity on BMR. Medicine and Science in Sports and Exercise, 28:85-91. 1996.

62   Ross, D.S., Ardisson, L.J., and Meskell, M.J.: Measurement of thyrotripin clinical and subclinical hyperthyroidism using a new chemiluminescent assay. J. clin, Endocrinol. Metab., 69(3):684-688, 1989.

63   Vanderpump, M.P., Neary, R.H,, Manning, K.,and Clayton, R.N.: Does an increase in the sensitivity of serum thyrotropin assays reduce diagnostic costs for thyroid disease in the community? J. R. Soc. Med., 90(10):547-550, 1997.

64   Weetman, A.P.: Hypothyroidism: screening and subclinical disease. Brit. Med. J., 314:1175, 1997.

65   Vanderpump, M.P.J., Tunbridge, W.M.G., French, J.M., et al.: The development of ischemic heart disease in relation to autoimmune thyroid disease in a 20-year follow-up study of an English community. Thyroid, 6:155-156, 1996.

66   Lowe, J.C.: The Metabolic Treatment of Fibromyalgia. Boulder, McDowell Publishing Co., 2000.

67   Lowe, J.C.: The Metabolic Treatment of Fibromyalgia. Boulder, McDowell Publishing Co., 2000. (pp 813-816).

68   Fraser, W.D., et. al. "Are biochemical tests of thyroid function of any value in monitoring patients receiving thyroxine replacement?" Br. Med. J. 293: 808-810, 1986.

69   Brent, G.A., and Hershman, J.M.: Effects of nonthyroidal illness on thyroid function tests. In The Thyroid Gland: A Practical Clinical Treatise. Edited by Van Middlesworth, Chicago, Year Book Medical Publishers, Inc., 1986.

70   Evans ES, Schooley RA, Evans AB, Jenkins CA, Taurog A. Biological evidence for extrathyroidal thyroxine for-mation. Endocrinology. 1966; 78:983-1001.

71   Wolff J Transport of iodide and other anions in the thy-roid gland. Physiol Rev. 1964; 44:45-90.

72   Venturi, Sebastiano. "Iodine in Evolution." Published in Italian on-line: February 8, 2004, su DIMI-MARCHE NEWS del Dipartimento Interaziendale di Medicina Interna della Regione Marche. Available: www.dimi.marche.it/

73   Imaizumi M, et.al. Risk for ischemic heart disease and all-cause mortality in subclinical hypothyroidism. J Clin Endocrinol Metab. 2004 Jul;89(7):3365-70.

74   Virtanen VK, et.al. Thyroid hormone substitution therapy rapidly enhances left-ventricular diastolic function in hypothyroid patients. Cardiology. 2001;96(2):59-64.

75   Razvi S, et.al. The beneficial effect of L-thyroxine on cardiovascular risk factors, endothelial function, and quality of life in subclinical hypothyroidism: randomized, crossover trial. J Clin Endocrinol Metab. 2007 May;92(5):1715-23. Epub 2007 Feb 13.

76   Hussein WI, et.al. Normalization of hyperhomocysteinemia with L-thyroxine in hypothyroidism. Ann Intern Med. 1999 Sep 7;131(5):348-51.

77   Christ-Crain M, et. al. Elevated C-reactive protein and homocysteine values: cardiovascular risk factors in hypothyroidism? A cross-sectional and a double-blind, placebo-controlled trial. Atherosclerosis. 2003 Feb;166(2):379-86.

78   Barnes, Broda, MD. "Hypothyroidism: The Unsuspected Illness." Thomas Y. Crowell Company, New York. 1976.

79   Ojamaa K, Klemperer JD, Klein I. Acute effects of thyroid hormone on vascular smooth muscle. Thyroid. 1996;85:734–738.

80   Gumieniak O, Perlstein TS, Hopkins PN, Brown NJ, Murphey LJ, Jeunemaitre X, et al. Thyroid function and blood pressure homeostasis in euthyroid subjects. J Clin Endocrinol Metab. 2004;89:3455–3461.

81   Montenegro J, González O, Saracho R, Aguirre R, González O, Martínez I. Changes in renal function in primary hypothyroidism. Am J Kidney Dis. 1996;27:195□ 198.

82   Myrup B, Bregengard C, Faber J. Primary homeostasis in thyroid disease. J Intern Med. 1995;238:59–63.

83   Fommei E, Iervasi G. The role of thyroid hormone in blood pressure homeostasis: evidence from short-term hypothyroidism in humans. J Clin Endocrinol Metab. 2002 May;87(5):1996-2000.

84   Klein I, Danzi S. Thyroid disease and the heart. Circulation 2007; 116: 1725-35.

85   Barnes DJ, O'Connor JD, Bending JJ. Hypothyroidism in the elderly: clinical assessment versus routine screening. Br J Clin Pract 1993; 47: 123-7.

86   Siddiqui AS, D'Costa DF, Moore-Smith B. Covert hypothyroidism with weight loss and atrial fibrillation. Br J Clin Pract 1993; 47 (5): 268.

87   Hypothyroidism. Available: http://www.nlm.nih.gov/medlineplus/ency/article/000353.htm

88   National Fibromyalgia Research Association. Available: http://www.nfra.net/fibromyalgia_definition.php

89   Available: http://www.fibromyalgiaresearch.org/

90   Hershman JM. Hypothalamic and pituitary hypothyroidism. In Progress in the Diagnosis and Treatment of Hypothyroid Conditions. Edited by P.A. Bastenie, M. Bonnyns, and L.VanHaelst, Amsterdam, Excerpta Medica, 1980, pp.40-50.

91   . Tunbridge WMG, Evered DC, and Hall R. The spectrum of thyroid disease in a community survey. Clin. Endocrinol., 1977; 7:481-493.

92   Eisinger J. Hypothyroïdie et fibromyalgie: indications d□ une double hormonothérapie thyroïdienne. Lyon Med. Med., 1999, 35 : 31-36.

93   Lowe JC. Thyroid status of 38 fibromyalgia patients: implications for the etiology of fibromyalgia. Clin. Bull. Myofascial Ther., 1997; 2(1):36-41.

94   Lowe JC, Reichman AJ, Honeyman GS, and Yellin J. Thyroid status of fibromyalgia patients (Abst.). Clin. Bull. Myofascial Ther., 1998; 3(1): 69-70.

95   Biobehavioral Approaches to Pain. Edited by Rhonda J. Moore. 568 pp., illustrated. New York, Springer, 2009.

96   Whybrow PC, et. al. Thyroid function and the response of L-liothyronine in depression. Arch Gen Psychiatry 1972;26:242.

97   Braverman, Lewis E., Utiger, Robert D. Werner and Ingbar's The Thyroid: A Fundamental and Clinical Text. 7th ed. Lippincot-Raven Publishers. 1996. pp 849-51.

98   Hernandez-Rey MD, Armando. "Anovulation." Available: http://emedicine.medscape.com/article/253190-overview

99   Trokoudes, Krinos M, et. al. "Infertility and thyroid disorders." Current Opinion in Obstetrics & Gynecology: August 2006 - Volume 18 - Issue 4 - p 446-451.

100   Wagner MS, Wajner SM, Maia AL. Is there a role for thyroid hormone on spermatogenesis? Microsc Res Tech. 2009 Nov;72(11):796-808.

101   Antonijevic N, et. al. Anemia in hypothyroidism. Med Pregl 1999 Mar-May;52(3-5):136-40.

102   Rochon C, Tauveron I, Dejax C, Benoit P, Capitan P, Fabricio A, Berry C, Champredon C, Thieblot P & Grizard J. Response of glucose disposal to hyperinsulinaemia in human hypothyroidism and hyperthyroidism. Clinical Science 2003 104 7–15.

103   Dimitriadis G, Mitrou P, Lambadiari V, Boutati E, Maratou E, Panagiotakos DB, Koukkou E, Tzanela M, Thalassinos N & Raptis SA. Insulin action in adipose tissue and muscle in hypothyroidism. Journal of Clinical Endocrinology and Metabolism 2006 91 4930–4937.

104   Dimitriadis G, Parry-Billings M, Bevan S, Leighton B, Krause U, Piva T, Tegos K, Challiss RA, Wegener G & Newsholme EA. The effects of insulin on transport and metabolism of glucose in skeletal muscle from hyperthyroid and hypothyroid rats. European Journal of Clinical Investigation 1997 27 475–483.

105   Maratou E, Hadjidakis DJ, Kollias A, Tsegka K, Peppa M, Alevizaki M, Mitrou P, Lambadiari V, Boutati E, Nikzas D, Tountas N, Economopoulos T, Raptis SA, Dimitriadis G. Studies of insulin resistance in patients with clinical and subclinical hypothyroidism. Eur J Endocrinol. 2009 May;160(5):785-90.

106   Roos A, Bakker SJ, Links TP, Gans RO, Wolffenbuttel BH. Thyroid function is associated with components of the metabolic syndrome in euthyroid subjects. J Clin Endocrinol Metab. 2007 Feb;92(2):491-6. Epub 2006 Nov 7.

107   Young T, et al. Epidemiology of obstructive sleep apnea: a population health perspective. Am J Respir Crit Care Med 2002;165:1217-1239.

108   Kryger MH. Management of obstructive sleep apnea: overview. In Principles and Practice of Sleep Medicine. 2nd ed. W.B. Saunders Company, Philadelphia, 1994, p. 738.

109   Smith, TJ, et. al. The effect of thyroid hormone on glycosaminoglycan accumulation in human fibroblasts. Endocrinology, 108(6):2397-99, 1981.

110   Faber, J, et. al. Different effects of thyroid disease on serum levels of procollagen III N-peptide and hyaluronic acid. J. Clin. Endocrinol. Metab., 71(4):1016-21, 1990.

111   Erik D Schraga, MD, Staff Physician, Department of Emergency Medicine, Mills-Peninsula Emergency Medical Associates. Hyperthyroidism, Thyroid Storm, and Graves Disease. Updated: Apr 23, 2010. Available: http://emedicine.medscape.com/article/767130-overview

112   Steven K Dankle, MD, Clinical Associate Professor, Department of Otolaryngology, Medical College of Wisconsin. Thyroid Nodule. Jan 11, 2011. Available: http://emedicine.medscape.com/article/127491-overview

113   Szent-Györgyi, A., Bioenergetics. Academic Press, New York, pg. 112, 1957.

114   Abraham GE. "The Concept of Orthoiodosupplementation and Its Clinical Implications" The Original Internist, 2004.

115   Fenical W. Halogenation in the rhodophyta: A review. J Phycol, 1975; 11:245-259.

116   Abraham GE. "The safe and effective implementation of orthoiodosupplementation in medical practice." The Original Internist, 2004; 11(1):17-36.

117   Hollowell J., Staehling N., Hannon W., Flanders D., Gunter E., Maberly G., Iodine Nutrition in the United States. Trends and Public Health Implications: Iodine Excretion Data from National Health and Nutrition Examination Surveys I and III (1971-1974 and 1988-1994) J. Clinical Endocrinology and Metabolism, 83:3401-3408, 1998.

118   Andersson M, Takkouche B, Egli I, Allen HE, de Benoist B. Bull, World Health Organ. 2005 Jul;83(7):518-25

119   de Luis DA, Aller R, Izaola O. An Med Interna. 2005 Sep;22(9):445-8.

120   Available: http://www.who.int/inf-pr-1999/en/pr99-wha17.htm

121   Available: http://www.cdc/.gov/nchs/products/pubs/pubd/hestats/iodine.htm

122   Hollowell J., Staehling N., Hannon W., Flanders D., Gunter E., Maberly G., Iodine Nutrition in the United States. Trends and Public Health Implications: Iodine Excretion Data from National Health

and Nutrition Examination Surveys I and III (1971-1974 and 1988-1994) J. Clinical Endocrinology and Metabolism, 83:3401-3408, 1998.

123   Editorial: What's Happening to Our Iodine? J. Clinical Endocrinology and Metabolism, 33:3398-3400, 1998.

124   Hollowell JG, et al. J Clin Endocrinol Metab. 1998 Oct;83(10):3401-8.

125   Finley, J.W., Bogardus, G.M., Breast cancer and thyroid disease. Quart. Rev. Surg. Obstet. Gynec. 17:139-147, 1960.

126   Thomas, B.S., Bulbrook, R.D., Russell, M.J., et al, Thyroid function in early breast cancer. Enrop. J. Cancer clin, Oncol, 19:1213-1219, 1983.

127   Thomas, B.S., Bulbrook, R.D., Goodman, M.J., Thyroid Function and the Incidence of Breast Cancer in Hawaiian, British and Japanese Women. Int. J. Cancer, 38:325-329, 1986.

128   Nagataki, S., Shizume, K., Nakao, K., Thyroid Function in Chronic Excess Iodide Ingestion: Comparison of Thyroidal Absolute Iodine Uptake and Degradation of Thyroxine in Euthyroid Japanese Subjects, J. Clin Endo: 27:638-647, 1967.

129   Waterhouse, J., Shanmvgakatnam, K., et al, Cancer incidence in five continents. LARC Scientific Publications, International Agency for Research on Cancer, Lyon, France, 1982.

130   Finley, J.W., Bogardus, G.M., Breast cancer and thyroid disease. Quart. Rev. Surg. Obstet. Gynec. 17:139-147, 1960.

131   Vertianinen E, Puska P, Jousilahti P, Horhonen HJ. Prev Med. 1999 Dec;29(6 Pt 2):S124-9.

132   Lamberg BA. Endocrinol Exp. 1986 Mar;20(1):35-47.

133   Abraham, G.E., The concept of orthoiodosupplementation and its clinical implications. The Original Internist, 11(2):29-38, 2004

134   Pennington JA and Schoen SA., "Total diet study: Estimated dietary intakes of nutritional elements, 1982-1991." Internat J Vit Nutr, 1996; 66:350-362.

135   Brownstein, David. Iodine: Why you need it Why you can't live without it. 2nd Edition. Medical Alternative Press, West Bloomsfield, MI, 2006.

136   Pavelka S. Physiol Res. 2004;53 Suppl 1:S81-90.

137   Vobecky M and Babicky A. "Effect of enhanced bromide intake on the concentration ratio I/Br in the rat thyroid gland." Kio Trace Element Research, 1994; 43:509-513.

138   Velicky J, Titlbach M, Duskova J, et al. "Potassium bromide and the thyroid gland of the rat: morphology and immunohistochemistry, RIA and INNA analysis." Ann Anat, 1997: 179421-431.

139   Van Leeuwen FXR, Hanemaauer R, and Loeber JG. "The effect of sodmide bromide on thyroid function." Arch Toxicol Suppl, 1988; 12:93-97.

140   Levin, M. Brommide psychosis: four varieties. Am. J. Psych. 104:798-804, 1948.

141   Australian Government: Department of the Environment, Water, Heritage, and the Arts. Chlorine Fact Sheet. Available: http://www.npi.gov.au/database/substance-info/profiles/20.html

142   EPA. Perchlorate environmental contamination: toxicological review and risk characterization based on emerging information. 1998.

143   Tonacchera, M. Relative potencies and additivity of perchlorate, thiocyanate, nitrate and iodide on the inhibition of radioactive iodide uptake by the human dosium iodide symporter. Thyroid. 2004. 14. 1012-19.

144   California Environmental Protection Agency, State Water Resources Control Board. 2002. Draft Groundwater Information Sheet. Available at: http://www.waterboards.ca.gov/gama/docs/tcp_jun2003.pdf

145   Brownstein, David. Iodine: Why you need it Why you can't live without it. 2nd Edition. Medical Alternative Press, West Bloomsfield, MI, 2006.

146   Galletti, P. Effect of fluorine on thyroidal iodine metabolism in hyperthyroidism.

147   Available: http://www.zerowasteamerica.org/Fluoride.htm

148   Stubner D, et al. Hypertrophy and hyperplasia during goiter growth and involution in rats - separate bioeffects of TSH and iodine. Acta Endocr, 1967; 116:537-548.

149   Stubner D, et al. Hypertrophy and hyperplasia during goiter growth and involution in rats - separate bioeffects of TSH and iodine. Acta Endocr, 1967; 116:537-548.

150   Zaichick, Vladimir. Et. al. Trace elements and thyroid cancer. Analyst. March 1995, Vol. 120.

151   Zaichick, Vladimir. Et. al. Trace elements and thyroid cancer. Analyst. March 1995, Vol. 120.

152   Abraham GE. "The safe and effective implementation of orthoiodosupplementation in medical practice." The Original Internist, 2004; 11(1):17-36.

153   Brownstein, David. Iodine: Why you need it Why you can't live without it. 2nd Edition. Medical Alternative Press, West Bloomsfield, MI, 2006.

154   Wiseman, R., Breast cancer hypothesis: a single cause for the majority of cases. J Epid Comm Health, 54:851-858, 2000

155   Eskin B., Bartuska D., Dunn M., Jacob G., Dratman M., Mammary Gland Dysplasia in Iodine Deficiency, JAMA, 200:115-119, 1967.

156   Eskin B. Iodine and Mammary Cancer, Adv. Exp. Med. Biol., 91:293-304, 1977.

157   Eskin, B. Iodine Metabolism and Breast Cancer. Trans. New York, Acad. of Sciences, 32:911-947, 1970.

158   Eskin, B. Grotkowski, C.E., Connolly, C.P., et al, Different Tissue Responses for Iodine and Iodide in Rat Thyroid and Mammary Glands. Biological Trace Element Research, 49:9-19, 1995.

159   Ghent, W., Eskin, B., Low, D., Hill, L., Iodine Replacement in Fibrocystic Disease of the Breast, Can. J. Surg., 36:453-460, 1993.

160   Derry, D., Breast Cancer and Iodine, Trafford Publishing, Victoria B.C., 92, 2001.

161   Thomas, B.S., Bulbrook, R.D., Russell, M.J., et al, Thyroid function in early breast cancer. Enrop. J. Cancer clin, Oncol, 19:1213-1219, 1983.

162   Thomas, B.S., Bulbrook, R.D., Goodman, M.J., Thyroid Function and the Incidence of Breast Cancer in Hawaiian, British and Japanese Women. Int. J. Cancer, 38:325-329, 1986.

163   Finley, J.W., Bogardus, G.M., Breast cancer and thyroid disease. Quart. Rev. Surg. Obstet. Gynec. 17:139-147, 1960.

164   Smyth, P. Thyroid Disease and Breast Cancer, J. Endo. Int., 16:396-401, 1993.

165   Delange FM. Iodine deficiency. In: Werner & Ingbar's The Thyroid. Braverman LE and Utiger RD, editors. Lippincott Williams & Wilkins, 2000; 295-329.

166   Eskin, B., Grotkowski, C.E., Connolly, C.P., et al, Different Tissue Responses for Iodine and Iodide in Rat Thyroid and Mammary Glands. Biological Trace Element Research, 49:9-19, 1995.

167   Hypothyroidism. JAMA, 238:1124, 1976Ghent, W., Eskin, B., Low, D., Hill, L., Iodine Replacement in Fibrocystic Disease of the Breast, Can. J. Surg., 36:453-460, 1993.

168   Giani C, Fierabracci P, BonacciR, et al. Relationship between breast cancer and thyroid disease: Relevance of autoimmune thyroid disorders in breast malignancy. J Clin Endocr & Metab, 1996; 81:990-994.

169   Ghandrakant, C., Kapdim MD, Wolfe, J.N., Breast Cancer. Relationship to Thyroid Supplements for hypothyroidism. JAMA, 1976; 238:1124.

170   Eskin, B.A. Thyroid Research. 378:625. 1978.

171   Brownstein, David. Iodine: Why you need it, why you can't live without it. Medical Alternatives Press. West Bloomfield, MI. 2006. pp 83-84.

172   Eskin, BA. Iodine and mammary cancer. Trans. N.Y. Acad. Of Sciences. 1970.

173   Eskin, BA. Mammary gland dysplasia in iodine deficiency. JAMA. 5.22.1967.

174   Gent, W., et al. Iodine Replacement in Fibrocystic Disease of the Breast. Can.J. Surg. 36:453-460, 1993.

175   Gent, W., et al. Iodine Replacement in Fibrocystic Disease of the Breast. Can.J. Surg. 36:453-460, 1993.

176   Stoddard, et al. Int. J. Med. Sci. July 8, 2008.

177   Gent, W., et al. Iodine Replacement in Fibrocystic Disease of the Breast. Can.J. Surg. 36:453-460, 1993.

178   Wang, J,, Effects of tamoxifen on benign breast disease in women at high risk for breast cancer. J. Natl. Cancer Inst., 95 (4):202-207, 2003.

179   Eskin, B., et al. Iodine metabolism and breast cancer. Trans. New York, Acad of Sciences. 32:911-947, 1970.

180   Cummings, et. al. "Prevention of Breast Cancer in Postmenopausal Women: Approaches to Estimating and Reducing Risk." Journal of the National Cancer Institute. Advance Access published online on March 10, 2009. Abstract available: http://jnci.oxfordjournals.org/cgi/content/abstract/djp018

181   Thompson WO, Brailey AG, Thompson PK, et al. "The range of effective iodine dosage in exophthalmic goiter III." Arch Int Med, 1930; 45:430.

182   Thompson Wo, Thompson PK, Brailey AG, et al. "Prolonged treatment of exophthalmic goiter by iodine alone." Arch Int Med, 1930; 45:481-502.

183   Cowell SJ and Mellanby E. The effect of iodine on hyperthyroidism in man. Quart J Med, 1924-1925;18:1-18.

184   DeCourcy JL. The use of Lugol's solution in exophthalmic goiter. Ann Surg, 1927; 86:871-876.

185   Plummer HS and Boothby WM. The Value of iodine in exophthalmic goiter. J Iowa Med Soc, 1924; 14:65.

186   Plummer WA. Iodine in the treatment of goiter. Med Cl North America, 1925; 8:1145-1151.

187   Lahey FH. The use of iodine in goiter. Boston Med & Surg J, 1925; 193:487-490.

188   Starr P, Walcott HP, Segall HN, et al. The effect of iodine in exophthalmic goiter. Arch In Med, 1924; 34:355-364

189   Fraser FR. Iodine in exophthalmic goiter. BMJ, 1925; 1:1.

190   Astwood EB and VanderLaan WP. Thiouracil derivatives of greater activity for the treatment of hyperthyroidism. J Clin Endocr, 1945; 5:424-430.

191   Morton ME, Chaikoff IL, and Rosenfled S. Inhibiting effect of inorganic iodide on the formation in vitro of thyhroine and diiodotyrosine by surviving thyroid tissue. J Biol Chem, 1944; 154:381.

192   Wolff J and Chaikoff IL. Plasma inorganic iodide as a homeostatic regulator of thyroid function. J Biol Chem, 1948;174:555-564.

193   Stanley MM. The direct estimation of the rate of thyroid hormone formation in man. The effect of the idodide ion on thyroid iodine utilization. J Clin Endocr, 1949;9:941-954.

194   Franklin AL, Chaikoff IL, and Lerner SR. The influence of goitrogenic substances on the conversion in vitro of inorganic iodide to thyroixine and diiodotyrosine by thyroid tissue with radioactive iodine as indicator. J Biol Chem, 1944; 153:151-162.

195   Solomon DH, Beck JC, VanderLaan WP, and Astwood EB. Prognosis of hyperthyroidism treated by antithyroid drugs. JAMA, 1953; 152:201-205.

196   Hershman JM, Givens JR, Cassidy CE, and Astwood EB. Long-term outcome of hyperthyroidism treated with antithyroid drugs. J Clin Endocr & Metab, 1966; 26:803-807.

197   Cooper DS. Treatment of Thyrotoxicosis. In: Werner & Ingbar's The Thyroid. Braverman LE and Utiger RD, editors. Lippincott Williams & Wilkins, 2000; 691-715.

198   Abraham, G.E., The safe and effective implementation of orthoiodosupplementation in medical practice. The Original Internist, 11:17-36, 2004.

199   Kelly, Francis C., Iodine in Medicine and Pharmacy Since its Discovery – 1811-1961. Proc R Soc Med 54:831-836, 1961.

200   Bruno R, Ferretti E, et.al. J Clin Endocrinol Metab. 2005 Oct;90(10):5692-7. Epub 2005 Aug 2.

201   Okerlund, M.D., The Clinical Utility of Fluorescent Scanning of the Thyroid. In Medical Applications of Fluorescent Excitation Analysis, Editors Kaufman and Price, CRC Press, Boca Raton Florida, pg 149-160, 1979.

202   Weetman AP. Chronic autoimmune thyroiditis. In: Werner & Ingbar's The Thyroid. Braverman LE and Utiger RD, editors. Lippincott Williams & Wilkins, 2000; 721-732.

203   Follis RH. Further observations on thyroiditis and colloid accumulation in hyperplastic thyroid glands of hamsters receiving excess iodine. Lab Invest, 1964; 13:1590-1599.

204   Belshaw BE and Becker DV. Necrosis of follicular cells and discharge of thyroidal iodine induced by administering iodide to iodine-deficient dogs. J Clin Endocr Metab, 1973; 13:466-474.

205   Mahmoud I, Colin I, et al. Direct toxic effect of iodine in excess on iodine-deficient thyroid gland: epithelial necrosis and inflammation associated with lipofuscin accumulation. Exp Mol Pathol, 1986; 44:259-271.

206   Abraham, G.E., The safe and effective implementation of orthoiodosupplementation in medical practice. The Original Internist, 11:17-36, 2004.

207   Abraham, GE. The Safe and Effective Implementation of Orthoiodosupplementation In Medical Practice. The Original Internist, 11:17-36, 2004.

208   Abraham, Guy E. Iodine supplementation markedly increases urinary excretion of fluoride and bromide - Letters to the Editor. The Townsend Letter. May, 2003. Available: http://findarticles. com/p/articles/mi_m0ISW/is_2003_May/ai_100767875/pg_2?tag=artBody;col1

209   Clinical nutrition: A functional approach, 2nd edition, 2004. Talbel 6.2, p 153-156.

210   Gennaro A.R., Remington: The Science and Practice of Pharmacy, 19th Edition, 1995, Mack Publishing Co., 1267.

211   Abraham GE. The safe and effective implementation of orthoiodosupplementation in medical practice. The Original Internist, 2004; 11(1):17-36.

212   Phillippou G, Koutras DA, Piperingos G, et al. The effect of iodide on serum thyroid hormone levels in normal persons, in hyperthyroid patients, and in hypothyroid patients on thyroxine replacement. Clin Endocr, 1992; 36:573-578.

213   Brownstein, D., Clinical experience with inorganic, non-radioactive iodine/iodide. The Original Internist, 12(3):105-108, 2005.

214   Flechas, J.D., Orthoiodosupplementation in a primary care practice. The Original Internist, 12(2):89-96, 2005.

215   Abraham, Guy E. Iodine: The Universal Nutrient. Townsend Letter. Dec. 2005.

216   Available: http://www.merriam-webster.com/dictionary/stress

217   Available: http://www.merriam-webster.com/dictionary/stress

218   Navy Guidance for Conducting Ecological Risk Assessments http://web.ead.anl.gov/ecorisk/fundamentals/pdf/ecofund.pdf

219   Selye, Hans (1946). The general adaptation syndrome and the diseases of adaptation. Journal of Clinical Endocrinology 6:117-230 Selye, Hans (1952). The Story of the Adaptation Syndrome. Montreal, Quebec, Canada: Acta Inc.

220   Understanding Stress: Characteristics and Caveats Hymie Anisman, Ph.D. and Zul Merali, Ph.D.

221   Holmes, Thomas and Richard Rahe. The Social Readjustment Rating Scale. Journal of Psychosomatic Research. 1967, vol. II p. 214.

222   Positive affect and psychobiological processes relevant to health. Steptoe A, Dockray S, Wardle J. Department of Epidemiology and Public Health, University College London, 1-19 Torrington Place, London WC1E 6BT, UK. a.steptoe@ucl.ac.uk J Pers. 2009 Dec;77(6):1747-76. Epub 2009 Sep 30.

223   Ann N Y Acad Sci. 2005 Dec;1057:466-78. Stress-induced hypocortisolemia diagnosed as psychiatric disorders responsive to hydrocortisone replacement. Schuder SE.

224   Lakartidningen. 2000 Sep 20;97(38):4120-4. [Low cortisol production in chronic stress. The connection stress-somatic disease is a challenge for future research]. Rosmond R, Björntorp P.

225   Clin Sci (Lond). 2001 Dec;101(6):739-47. Cortisol increases gluconeogenesis in humans: its role in the metabolic syndrome. Khani S, Tayek JA.

226   Vicki A. Nejtek, Department of Psychiatry, UT Southwestern Medical Center at Dallas, 5323 Harry Hines Blvd., Dallas, TX 75390-9070, USA. High and low emotion events influence emotional stress perceptions and are associated with salivary cortisol response changes in a consecutive stress paradigm. Darcup, Kathleen, RN, PhD, et. al. Perceived control reduces stress in patients with heart failure. The Journal of Heart and Lung Transplantation. Vol 22, Issue 1, Jan 2008.

227

228   Steptoe A, Dockray S, Wardle J. Positive affect and psychobiological processes relevant to health. J Pers. 2009 Dec;77(6):1747-76. Epub 2009 Sep 30.

229   Nature Reviews Cardiology 7, 468-472 (August 2010) | doi:10.1038/nrcardio.2010.68.

230   Wilson, James. Adrenal Fatigue: the 21st Century Stress Syndrome. Smart Publications, 2001.

231   Garner, Peter R. Adrenal disorders of pregnancy. Chapter 2B. Available: http://www.endotext.org/pregnancy/pregnancy2/pregnancy2b.htm

232   Development of Endocrine Function in the Human Placenta and Fetus, Dorothy B. Villee, M.D., N Engl J Med 1969; 281:473-484, Aug 1969.

233   O'Connell S, Siafarikas A. Addison disease: diagnosis and initial management. Aust Fam Physician. 2010 Nov;39(11):834-7.

234   John F. Kennedy: A Biography; By Michael O'Brien, 2006.

235   Endocrinology: An Integrated Approach. Nussey S, Whitehead S. Oxford: BIOS Scientific Publishers; 2001.

236   Nieman L, Ilias I. Evaluation and treatment of Cushing's syndrome. Amer J of Med. 2005;118:1340–1346.

237   Labeur M, Arzt E, Stalla GK, Páez-Pereda M. New perspectives in the treatment of Cushing's syndrome. Current Drug Targets Immune, Endocrine & Metabolic Disorders. 2004;4:335 342.

238   Klachko, David M. Pseudo-Cushing Syndrome. Available: www.emedicine.com

239   Lin D, Loughlin K. Diagnosis and management of surgical adrenal diseases. Urology. 2005;66:476–483.

240   World Menopause Day. Lancaster, England: International Menopause Society. Available: http://www. imsociety.org/pages/wmday.html.

241   Lokuge S, Frey BN, Foster JA, Soares CN, Steiner M. The rapid effects of estrogen: a mini-review. Behav Pharmacol. 2010;21:465–72.

242   McNair P, Christiansen C, Transbøl I. Effect of menopause and estrogen substitutional therapy on magnesium metabolism. Miner Electrolyte Metab. 1984;10(2):84-7.

243   W.H. Davis and F. Ziady. The Role of Magnesium in Sleep. Montreal Symposium, 1976.

244   Firoz M and Graber M. Bioavailability of U.S. commercial magnesium preparation. Magnes Research 2001;14:257-62.

245   Feigelson HS, Jonas CR, Teras LR, Thun MJ, Calle EE. Weight gain, body mass index, hormone replacement therapy, and postmenopausal breast cancer in a large prospective study. Cancer Epidemiol Biomarkers Prev. 2004;13:220–224.

246   Wade GN, Powers JB. Tamoxifen antagonizes the effects of estradiol on energy balance and estrous behavior in Syrian hamsters. Am J Physiol. 1993;265:R559–562.

247   Rosano GM, Gebara O, Sheiban I, Silvestri A, Wajngarten M, Vitale C, Aldrighi JM, Ramires AF, Fini M, Mercuro G. Acute administration of 17beta-estradiol reduces endothelin-1 release during pacing-induced ischemia. Int J Cardiol. 2007 Mar 2;116(1):34-9. Aldrighi, Jose Epub 2006 Jun 30. Erratum in: Int J Cardiol. 2007 Dec 15;123(1):73.

248   Rosano GM, Leonardo F, Dicandia C, Sheiban I, Pagnotta P, Pappone C, Chierchia SL. Acute electrophysiologic effect of estradiol 17beta in menopausal women. Am J Cardiol. 2000 Dec 15;86(12):1385-7, A5-6.

249   Heitkemper MM, Chang L. Do fluctuations in ovarian hormones affect gastrointestinal symptoms in women with irritable bowel syndrome? Gend Med.2009;6 Suppl 2:152-67. Review.

250   Haggerty CL, Ness RB, Kelsey S, Waterer GW. The impact of estrogen and progesterone on asthma. Ann Allergy Asthma Immunol. 2003 Mar;90(3):284-91; quiz 291-3, 347. Review.

251   Dziedziczko A, Wojtaszek A, Pałgan K. [Bronchial asthma and menopause]. Pol Merkur Lekarski. 2004 Sep;17(99):281-3. Review. Polish.

252   Silberstein SD, Merriam GR. Estrogens, progestins, and headache. Neurology. 1991 Jun;41(6):786-93. Review.

253   Enns DL, Tiidus PM. The influence of estrogen on skeletal muscle: sex matters. Sports Med. 2010 Jan 1;40(1):41-58. Review.

254   Smith RL, Pruthi S, Fitzpatrick LA. Evaluation and management of breast pain. Mayo Clin Proc. 2004 Mar;79(3):353-72. Review.

255   Kumar S, Mansel RE, Scanlon MF, et al. Altered responses of prolactin, luteinizing hormone and follicle stimulating hormone secretion to thyrotropin releasing hormone/gonadotropin releasing hormone stimulation in cyclical mastalgia. Br J Surg. 1984;71: 870-873.

256   Ayers JW, Gidwani GP. The luteal breast: hormonal and sonographic investigation of benign breast disease in patients with cyclic mastalgia. Fertil Steril. 1983;40:779-784.

257   Kumar S, Mansel RE, Hughes LE, et al. Prolactin response to thyrotropin-releasing hormone stimulation and dopaminergic inhibition in benign breast disease. Cancer. 1984;53:1311-1315.

258   Parlati E, Travaglini A, Liberale I, Menini E, Dell'Acqua S. Hormonal profile in benign breast disease: endocrine status of cyclical mastalgia patients. J Endocrinol Invest. 1988;11:679-683.

259   Smith RL, Pruthi S, Fitzpatrick LA. Evaluation and management of breast pain. Mayo Clin Proc. 2004 Mar;79(3):353-72. Review.

260   BeLieu RM. Mastodynia. Obstet Gynecol Clin North Am. 1994; 21:461-477.

261   Gateley CA, Miers M, Mansel RE, Hughes LE. Drug treatments for mastalgia: 17 years experience in the Cardiff Mastalgia Clinic. J R Soc Med. 1992. Jan;85(1):12-5.

262   Genazzani AR, Bernardi F, Pluchino N, Begliuomini S, Lenzi E, Casarosa E, Luisi M. Endocrinology of menopausal transition and its brain implications. CNS Spectr. 2005 Jun;10(6):449-57. Review.

263   Altura BM, Altura BT: Association of alcohol in brain injury, headaches, and stroke with brain-tissue; serum levels of ionized magnesium: review of recent findings and mechanisms of action.Alcohol19 :119 –130,1999.

264   Phillips LS, Langer RD. Postmenopausal hormone therapy: critical reappraisal and a unified hypothesis. Fertil Steril 2005; 83: 558-566.

265   Grodstein F, Manson JE, Stampfer MJ. Hormone therapy and coronary heart disease: the role of time since menopause and age at hormone initiation. J Women's Health (Larchmt) 2006; 15: 35-44.

266   Nabulsi AA, Folsom AR, White A. 1993 Association of hormone-replacement therapy with various cardiovascular risk factors in postmenopausal women. N Engl J Med. 328:1069–1075.

267   Van der Mooren MJ, Demacker PNM, Thomas CMG. 1992 Beneficial effects on serum lipoproteins by 17ß-estradiol-dydrogesterone therapy in postmenopausal women: a prospective study. Eur J Obstet Gynecol Reprod Biol. 47:153☐ 160.

268   Oparil S, Levin RL, Chen YF. 1996 Sex hormones and the vasculature. In: Sowers JR, ed. Endocrinology of the vasculature. Totowa: Humana Press; 225–238.

269   Gisclard V, Miller VM, Vanhoutte PM. 1988 Effect of 17ß-estradiol on endothelium-dependent responses in the rabbit. J Pharmacol Exp Ther. 244:19☐ 22.

270   International Osteoporosis Foundation. Available: http://www.iofbonehealth.org/facts-and-statistics.html

271   NIH Consensus Development Panel on Osteoporosis Prevention, Diagnosis, and Therapy. Osteoporosis prevention, diagnosis, and therapy. JAMA. 2001;285:785–795.

272   Abraham GE, Grewal H: A total dietary program emphasizing magnesium instead of calcium. Effect on the mineral density of calcareous bone in postmenopausal women on hormonal therapy.J Reprod Med35 :503 –507,1990.

273   Sojka JE, Weaver CM: Magnesium supplementation and osteoporosis. Nutr Rev53 :71 –74,1995.

274   Schaafsma A, de Vries PJ, Saris WH: Delay of natural bone loss by higher intakes of specific minerals and vitamins. Crit Rev Food Sci Nutr41 :225 –249,2001.

275   Michaelsson K, Holmberg L, Mallmin H, et al: Diet and hip fracture risk: a case control study. Study Group of the Multiple Risk Survey on Swedish Women for Eating Assessment. Int J Epidemiol24 :771 –782,1995.

276   Volpe SL, Taper LJ, Meacham: The relationship between boron and magnesium status and bone mineral density in the human: a review. Magnes Res6 :291 –296,1993.

277   Schaafsma A, de Vries PJ, Saris WH: Delay of natural bone loss by higher intakes of specific minerals and vitamins. Crit Rev Food Sci Nutr41 :225 –249,2001.

278   Vitamin D Cofactors. Available: http://www.vitamindcouncil.org/newsletter/more-vitamin-d-questions-and-answers.shtml

279   Burger HG. Androgen production in women. Fertil Steril. 2002 Apr;77 Suppl 4:S3-5. Review.

280   Burger HG. Androgen production in women. Fertil Steril. 2002 Apr;77 Suppl 4:S3-5. Review.

281   Speroff L, Glass RH, Kase NG. Clinical gynecologic endocrinology and infertility. 5th ed. Baltimore, MD: Williams and Wilkins, 1994:457–515.

282   Longcope C, Baker RS, Hui SL, Johnston CC Jr. Androgen and estrogen dynamics in women with vertebral crush fractures. Maturitas. 1984;6(4):309-18.

283   Steinberg KK, Freni-Titulaer LW, DePuey EG, Miller DT, Sgoutas DS, Coralli CH, Phillips DL, Rogers TN, Clark RV. Sex steroids and bone density in premenopausal and peri-menopausal women. J Clin Endocrinol Metab. 1989;69(3):533-9.

284   Slemenda C, Longcope C, Peacock M, Hui S, Johnston CC. Sex steroids, bone mass, and bone loss. A prospective study of pre-, peri-, and postmenopausal women. J Clin Invest. 1996;97(1):14-21.

285   Davison SL, Davis SR. Androgenic hormones and aging - The link with female sexual function. Horm Behav. 2011 Jan 5.

286   The North American Menopause Society. The role of testosterone therapy in postmenopausal women: position statement of The North American Menopause Society. Menopause. 2005;12:497–511.

287   Wisniewski AB, Nguyen TT, Dobs AS. Evaluation of high-dose estrogen and high-dose estrogen plus methyltestosterone treatment on cognitive task performance in postmenopausal women. Horm Res. 2002;58(3):150-5.

288   The North American Menopause Society. The role of testosterone therapy in postmenopausal women: position statement of The North American Menopause Society. Menopause. 2005;12:497–511.

289   Traish A, Guay AT, Spark RF; Testosterone Therapy in Women Study Group. Are the Endocrine Society's Clinical Practice Guidelines on Androgen Therapy in Women misguided? A commentary. J Sex Med. 2007 Sep;4(5):1223-34; discussion 1234-5. Review.

290   Cameron DR, Braunstein GD. Androgen replacement therapy in women. Fertil Steril. 2004 Aug;82(2):273-89. Review.

291   Mauvais-Jarvis P, Kuttenn F. [Is progesterone insufficiency carcihogenic]? [Article in French] Nouv Presse Med 1975 Feb 1;4(5):323-326.

292   Lancel M, Faulhaber J, Holsboer F, Rupprecht R. Progesterone induces changes in sleep comparable to those of agonistic GABAA receptor modulators. Am J Physiol 1996 Oct;271(4 Pt 1):E763-E772.

293   Batra SC, Iosif CS. Progesterone receptors in the female lower urinary tract. J Urol 1987 Nov;138(5):1301-4.

294   Miodrag A, Castleden CM, Vallance TR. Sex hormones and the female urinary tract. Drugs 1988 Oct;36(4):491-504.

295   Mauvais-Jarvis P, Kuttenn F. [Is progesterone insufficiency carcihogenic]? [Article in French] Nouv Presse Med 1975 Feb 1;4(5):323-326.

296   Glick ID, Bennett SE. Psychiatric complications of progesterone and oral contraceptives. J Clin Psychopharmacol 1981 Nov;1(6):350-367.

297   Lindheim SR, Presser SC, Ditkoff EC, Vijod MA, Stanczyk FZ, Lobo RA. A possible bimodal effect of estrogen on insulin sensitivity in postmenopausal women and the attenuating effect of added progestin. Fertil Steril 1993 Oct;60(4):664-7.

298   Colacurci N, Zarcone R, Mollo A, Russo G, Passaro M, de Seta L, de Franciscis P. Effects of hormone replacement therapy on glucose metabolism. Panminerva Med 1998 Mar;40(1):18-21.

299   Kumagai S, Holmang A, Bjorntorp P. The effects of estrogen and progesterone on insulin sensitivity in female rats. Acta Physiol Scand 1993 Sep;149(1):91-7.

300   Lindheim SR, Presser SC, Ditkoff EC, Vijod MA, Stanczyk FZ, Lobo RA. A possible bimodal effect of estrogen on insulin sensitivity in postmenopausal women and the attenuating effect of added progestin. Fertil Steril 1993 Oct;60(4):664-7.

301   Tsibris JC, Raynor LO, Buhi WC, Buggie J, Spellacy WN. Insulin receptors in circulating erythrocytes and monocytes from women on oral contraceptives or pregnant women near term. J Clin Endocrinol Metab 1980 Oct;51(4):711-7.

302   Verhaar HJ, Damen CA, Duursma SA, Scheven BA. A comparison of the action of progestins and estrogen on the growth and differentiation of normal adult human osteoblast-like cells in vitro. Bone 1994 May;15(3):307-311.

303   Heersche JN, Bellows CG, Ishida Y. The decrease in bone mass associated with aging and menopause. J Prosthet Dent 1998 Jan;79(1):14-16.

304   Tremollieres FA, Strong DD, Baylink DJ, Mohan S. Progesterone and promegestone stimulate human bone cell proliferation and insulin-like growth factor-2 production. Acta Endocrinol -Copenh 1992 Apr;126(4):329-337.

305   Barengolts EI, Kouznetsova T, Segalene A, Lathon P, Odvina C, Kukreja SC, Unterman TG. Effects of progesterone on serum levels of IGF-1 and on femur IGF-1 mRNA in ovariectomized rats. J Bone Miner Res 1996 Oct;11(10):1406-1412.

306   Arner P. Effects of testosterone on fat cell lipolysis. Species differences and possible role in polycystic ovarian syndrome. Biochimie. 2005. Jan;87(1):39-43.

307   Dicker A, Rydén M, Näslund E, Muehlen IE, Wirén M, Lafontan M, Arner P. Effect of testosterone on lipolysis in human pre-adiposities from different fat depots. Diabetologia. 2004 Mar;47(3):420-8. Epub 2004 Jan 30.

308   Toth MJ, Tchernof A, Sites CK, Poehlman ET 2000 Effect of menopausal status on body composition and abdominal fat distribution. Int J Obes Relat Metab Disord 24:226–231.

309   Ramirez ME, McMurry MP, Wiebke GA, Felten KJ, Ren K, Meikle AW, Iverius PH. Evidence for sex steroid inhibition of lipoprotein lipase in men: comparison of abdominal and femoral adipose tissue. Metabolism. 1997 Feb;46(2):179-85.

310   Price TM, O'Brien SN, Welter BH, George R, Anandjiwala J, Kilgore M 1998 Estrogen regulation of adipose tissue lipoprotein lipase—possible mechanism of body fat distribution. Am J Obstet Gynecol 178:101–107.

311   Mystkowski P, Seeley RJ, Hahn TM, Baskin DG, Havel PJ, Matsumoto AM, Wilkinson CW, Peacock-Kinzig K, Blake KA, Schwartz MW. Hypothalamic melanin-concentrating hormone and estrogen-induced weight loss. J Neurosci. 2000 Nov 15;20(22):8637-42.

312   Gray A, Feldman HA, McKinlay JB, Longcope C. 1991 Age, disease, and changing sex hormone levels in middle-aged men: results of the Massachusetts male aging study. J Clin Endocrinol Metab. 73:1016–1025.

313   Njolstad I., et. al. Smoking, serum lipids, blood pressure, and sex differences in myocardial infarction. A 12-year follow-up of the Finnmark Study. Circulation 1996;93:450–6.

314   Jones RD, et. al. Testosterone and atherosclerosis in aging men: purported association and clinical implications. Am J Cardiovasc Drugs. 2005;5:141–54.

315   Scragg JL, et. al. Testosterone is a potent inhibitor of L-type Ca(2+) channels. Biochem Biophys Res Commun 2004;318:503–6.

316   Malkin CJ. Testosterone replacement in hypogonadal men with angina improves ischemic threshold and quality of life. Heart 2004;90:871–6.

317   Bagatell CJ, et. al. Androgens in men – uses and abuses. N Engl J Med 1996;334:707–14.

318   Mainous AG, III, Baker R, Koopman RJ, et al. Impact of the population at risk of diabetes on projections of diabetes burden in the United States: an epidemic on the way. Diabetologia. 2007;50:934–40.

319   Kapoor D. Testosterone replacement therapy improves insulin resistance, glycaemic control, visceral adiposity and hypercholesterolaemia in hypogonadal men with type II diabetes. Eur J Endocrinol 2006;154:899–906.

320　Heufelder AE, et. al. 52-Week treatment with diet and exercise plus transdermal testosterone reverses the metabolic syndrome and improves glycaemic control in men with newly diagnosed type II diabetes and subnormal plasma testosterone. J Androl 2009;30:726–33.

321　Selvin E, Feinleib M, Zhang L, et al. Androgens and diabetes in men: results from the Third National Health and Nutrition Examination Survey (NHANES III) Diabetes Care. 2007;30:234–8.

322　Araujo AB, Travison TG, Leder BZ, McKinlay JB. Correlations between serum testosterone, estradiol, and sex hormone-binding globulin and bone mineral density in a diverse sample of men. J Clin Endocrinol Metab. 2008;93:2135–41.

323　Ebeling PR. Clinical practice. Osteoporosis in men. N Engl J Med. 2008;358:1474–82.

324　Shores MM. Low testosterone is associated with decreased function and increased mortality risk: a preliminary study of men in a geriatric rehabilitation unit. J Am Geriatr Soc 2004;52:2077–81.

325　Shores MM, et.al. Low serum testosterone and mortality in male veterans. Arch Intern Med 2006;166:1660–5.

326　Laughlin GA. Low serum testosterone and mortality in older men. J Clin Endocrinol Metab 2008;93:68–75.

327　Khaw KT, et. al. Endogenous testosterone and mortality due to all causes, cardiovascular disease, and cancer in men: European prospective investigation into cancer in Norfolk (EPIC-Norfolk) Prospective Population Study. Circulation 2007;116:2694–701.

328　Isidori AM, Giannetta E, Gianfrilli D, Greco EA, Bonifacio V, Aversa A, Isidori A, Fabbri A, Lenzi A. Effect of testosterone on sexual function in men: results of meta-analysis. Clin Endocrinol.(Oxf). 2005;63: 239 –243.

329　Schiavi RC, Rehman J. Sexuality and aging. Urol Clin North Am. 1995 Nov;22(4):711-26. Review.

330　Kaufman JM, Vermeulen A. The decline of androgen levels in elderly men and its clinical and therapeutic implications. Endocrinol Rev. 2005;26: 833 –876.

331　Cho NH, Ahn CW, Park JY, Ahn TY, Lee HW, Park TS, Kim IJ, Pomerantz K, Park C, Kimm KC, Choi DS. Elevated homocysteine as a risk factor for the development of diabetes in women with a previous history of gestational diabetes mellitus: a 4-year prospective study. Diabetes Care. 2005;28: 2750 –2755.

332　Morley JE, Kaiser F, Raum WJ, Perry HM 3rd, Flood JF, Jensen J, Silver AJ, Roberts E. Potentially predictive and manipulable blood serum correlates of aging in the healthy human male: progressive decreases in bioavailable testosterone, dehydroepiandrosterone sulfate, and the ratio of insulin-like growth factor 1 to growth hormone. Proc Natl Acad Sci U S A. 1997 Jul 8;94(14):7537-42.

333　McKeever WF, Deyo A. Testosterone, dihydrotestosterone and spatial task performance of males. Bull Psychonomic Soc. 1990;28:305–308.

334　Moffat SD, Zonderman AB, Metter EJ, Kawas C, Blackman MR, Harman SM, et al. Free testosterone and risk for Alzheimer disease in older men. Neurology. 2004;62:188–193.

335　Wang C, Alexander G, Berman N, Salehian B, Davidson T, McDonald V, Steiner B, Hull L, Callegari C, Swerdloff RS. Testosterone replacement therapy improves mood in hypogonadal men--a clinical research center study. J Clin Endocrinol Metab.
1996 Oct;81(10):3578-83.

336　Ferrando AA, Sheffield-Moore M, Paddon-Jones D, Wolfe RR, Urban RJ. Differential anabolic effects of testosterone and amino acid feeding in older men. J Clin Endocrinol Metab. 2003;88:358–362.

337　Longcope C, Feldman HA, McKinlay JB, Araujo AB. Diet and sex hormone-binding globulin. J Clin Endocrinol Metab. 2000 Jan;85(1):293-6.

338   Carruba Estrogens and Mechanisms of Prostate Cancer Progression. Ann N Y Acad Sci. 2006;1089:201–7. doi: 10.1196/annals.1386.027.

339   Degroot, et. al. The Thyroid & Its Diseases. 6th ed. 1996.

340   Available: http://en.wikipedia.org/wiki/Reductionism

341   Lowe, J.C.: The Metabolic Treatment of Fibromyalgia. Boulder, McDowell Publishing Co., 2000.

342   BMA (1992) The BMA guide to pesticides, chemicals and health, Report of the Board of Science and Education, British Medical Association.

343   Robbins C. Poisoned harvest: A consumer's guide to pesticide use and abuse. Victor Gollancz Ltd, p. 300 – 313. 1991.

344   Balch JF and Balch PA, 1997, Prescriptions for nutritional healing, 2nd edition, Avery publishers, USA p. 176-183.

345   Soil Association (2001) Organic Farming, food quality and human health: a review of the evidence.

346   Worthington V (2001) Nutritional quality of organic versus conventional fruits, vegetables, and grains. The Journal of Complimentary Medicine, vol. 7, No. 2, p. 161 - 173.

347   Hemminki K, Zhang H, Czene K. Incidence trends and familial risks in invasive and in situ cutaneous melanoma by sun-exposed body sites. Int J Cancer. 2003 May 10;104(6):764–71.

348   Journal of the National Cancer Institute, Vol. 97, No. 3, February 2, 2005.

349   Heaney RP. Long-latency deficiency disease: insights from calcium and vitamin D. Am J Clin Nutr 2003;78:912-9.

350   Griffin MD, Xing N, Kumar R. Vitamin D and its analogs as regulators of immune activation and antigen presentation. Annu Rev Nutr. 2003;23:117-145.

351   Zeitz U, Weber K, Soegiarto DW, Wolf E, Balling R, Erben RG. Impaired insulin secretory capacity in mice lacking a functional vitamin D receptor. FASEB J. 2003;17(3):509-511.

352   Sigmund CD. Regulation of renin expression and blood pressure by vitamin D(3). J Clin Invest. 2002;110(2):155-156.

353   Available: www.vitamindcouncil.org

354   Holick MF. Environmental factors that influence the cutaneous production of vitamin D. Am J Clin Nutr. 1995 Mar;61(3 Suppl):638S–645S.

355   Vitamin D Cofactors. Available: http://www.vitamindcouncil.org/

356   Wood, Daren. National Park Visitation Statistics. Available: http://usparks.about.com/od/natlparkbasics/a/Natlparkvisitor.htm

357   Stone, B. Sleep and low doses of alcohol. Electroencephalography and Clinical Neurophysiology. 1980; 48: 706-709.

358   Newsweek, 6 Nov. 1995, 60-63.

359   Wilber, Ken, et. al. "Integral Life Practice." Shambhala Press. Boston, MA. 2008. pp 50-51. Excerpt Available: http://integrallife.com/awaken/shadow/practice-3-2-1-shadow-process

360   van Praag HM, Lemus C. Monoamine precursors in the treatment of psychiatric disorders. In: Wurtman RJ, Wurtman JJ, eds. Nutrition and the Brain. New York: Raven Press; 1986:89-139.

361   den Boer JA, Westenberg HG. Behavioral, neuroendocrine, and biochemical effects of 5-hydroxytryptophan administration in panic disorder. Psychiatry Res 1990;31:267-278.

362   Goodwin GM, Cowen PJ, Fairburn CG, et al. Plasma concentrations of tryptophan and dieting. BMJ 1990;300:1499-1500.

363   Cangiano C, Ceci F, Cascino A, et al. Eating behavior and adherence to dietary prescriptions in obese adult subjects treated with 5-hydroxytryptophan. Am J Clin Nutr 1992;56:863-867.

364   Cangiano C, Ceci F, Cairella M, et al. Effects of 5-hydroxytryptophan on eating behavior and adherence to dietary prescriptions in obese adult subjects. Adv Exp Med Biol 1991;294:591-593.

365   McCarty MF: Does bitter melon contain an activator of AMP-activated kinase? Med Hypotheses 2004 , 63(2):340-343.

366   Krawinkel MB, Keding GB: Bitter gourd (Momordica Charantia): A dietary approach to hyperglycemia. Nutr Rev 2006 , 64:331-337.

367   Shetty AK, Kumar GS, Sambaiah K, Salimath PV: Effect of bitter gourd (Momordica charantia) on glycaemic status in streptozotocin induced diabetic rats. Plant Foods Hum Nutr 2005 , 60(3):109-112.

368   Chao CY, Huang C: Bitter Gourd (Momordica charantia) Extract Activates Peroxisome Proliferator-Activated Receptors and Upregulates the Expression of the Acyl CoA Oxidase Gene in H4IIEC3 Hepatoma Cells. J Biomed Sci 2003 , 10:782-791.

369   Cefalu WT, Ye J, Wang ZQ: Efficacy of dietary supplementation with botanicals on carbohydrate metabolism in humans.   Endocr Metab Immune Disord Drug Targets. 2008 , 8(2):76-81.

370   Basch E, Gabardi S, Ulbricht C: Bitter melon (Momordica charantia): a review of efficacy and safety. Am J Health Syst Pharm 2003 , 60(4):356-359.

371   Available: http://www.nutratechinc.com/advz/advz.php?p=2

372   Stanko RT, Tietze DL, Arch JE. Body composition, energy utilization, and nitrogen metabolism with a 4.25-MJ/d low-energy diet supplemented with pyruvate. Am J Clin Nutr 1992;56:630–5.

373   Stanko RT, Reynolds HR, Hoyson R, et al. Pyruvate supplementation of a low-cholesterol, low-fat diet: Effects on plasma lipid concentration and body composition in hyperlipidemic patients. Am J Clin Nutr 1994;59:423–7.

374   Kalman D, Colker CM, Wilets I, et al. The effects of pyruvate supplementation on body composition in overweight individuals. Nutrition 1999;15:337–40.

375   Kalman D, Colker CM, Stark S, et al. Effect of pyruvate supplementation on body composition and mood. Curr Ther Res 1998;59:793–802.

376   Shindea UA, Sharma G, Xu YJ, Dhalla NS, Goyal RK. Insulin sensitizing action of chromium picolinate in various experimental models of diabetes mellitus. J Trace Elem Med Biol. 2004;18(1):23-32.

377   Pittler MH, Stevinson C, Ernst E. Chromium picolinate for reducing body weight: meta-analysis of randomized trials. Int J Obes Relat Metab Disord. Apr;27(4):522-9. 2003.

378   Kaats GR, Blum K, Fisher JA and Adelman JA. Effects of chromium picolinate supplementation on body composition: A randomized, double-masked, placebo-controlled study. Current Therapeutic Research, 57(10):747-765, Oct. 1996.

379   Cefalu, W. T., Bell-Farrow, A. D., Stegner, J., Wang, Z. Q., King, T., Morgan, T. and Terry, J. G. (1999), Effect of chromium picolinate on insulin sensitivity in vivo. The Journal of Trace Elements in Experimental Medicine, 12: 71□ 83.

380   Broadhurst CL, Domenico P. Clinical studies on chromium picolinate supplementation in diabetes mellitus--a review. Diabetes Technol Ther. 2006. Dec;8(6):677-87. Review.

381   Oknin VIu, Fedotova AV, Veĭn AM. [Use of citrulline malate (stimol) in patients with autonomic dystonia associated with arterial hypotension]. Zh Nevrol Psikhiatr Im S S Korsakova. 1999;99(1):30-3. Russian.

382   Fedorova VI. [Autonomic disorders in persons with asthenic syndrome and their correction with citrulline malate]. Zh Nevrol Psikhiatr Im S S Korsakova. 2000;100(4):32-6. Russian.

383   Pérez-Guisado J, Jakeman PM. Citrulline malate enhances athletic anaerobic performance and relieves muscle soreness. J Strength Cond Res. 2010 May;24(5):1215-22.

384   Sureda A, Córdova A, Ferrer MD, Pérez G, Tur JA, Pons A. L-citrulline-malate influence over branched chain amino acid utilization during exercise. Eur J Appl Physiol. 2010 Sep;110(2):341-51. Epub 2010 May 25.

385   Schwedhelm E, Maas R, Freese R, Jung D, Lukacs Z, Jambrecina A, Spickler W, Schulze F, Böger RH. Pharmacokinetic and pharmacodynamic properties of oral L-citrulline and L-arginine: impact on nitric oxide metabolism. Br J Clin Pharmacol. 2008 Jan;65(1):51-9. Epub 2007 Jul 27.

386   Cormio L, De Siati M, Lorusso F, Selvaggio O, Mirabella L, Sanguedolce F, Carrieri G. Oral L-citrulline supplementation improves erection hardness in men with mild erectile dysfunction. Urology. 2011 Jan;77(1):119-22.

387   Schwedhelm E, Maas R, Freese R, Jung D, Lukacs Z, Jambrecina A, Spickler W, Schulze F, Böger RH. Pharmacokinetic and pharmacodynamic properties of oral L-citrulline and L-arginine: impact on nitric oxide metabolism. Br J Clin Pharmacol. 2008 Jan;65(1):51-9. Epub 2007 Jul 27.

388   Rougé C, Des Robert C, Robins A, Le Bacquer O, Volteau C, De La Cochetière MF, Darmaun D. Manipulation of citrulline availability in humans. Am J Physiol Gastrointest Liver Physiol. 2007 Nov;293(5):G1061-7. Epub 2007 Sep 27.

389   Br J Clin Pharmacol. 1986 Aug;22(2):177-82. Comparative pharmacokinetics of caffeine and its primary demethylated metabolites paraxanthine, theobromine and theophylline in man. Lelo A, Birkett DJ, Robson RA, Miners JO.

390   Food Chem Toxicol. 1984 May;22(5):365-9. Comparative toxicities of dietary caffeine and theobromine in the rat. Gans JH.

391   Okuda H, Morimoto C, Tsujita T. Relationship between cyclic AMP production and lipolysis induced by forskolin in rat fat cells. J Lipid Res 1992;33:225-231.

392   Allen DO, Ahmed B, Naseer K. Relationships between cyclic AMP levels and lipolysis in fat cells after isoproterenol and forskolin stimulation. J Pharmacol Exp Ther 1986;238:659-664.

393   Han LK, Morimoto C, Yu RH, Okuda H. Effects of Coleus forskohlii on fat storage in ovariectomized rats. Yakugaku Zasshi 2005; 125:449-453.

394   Haye B, Aublin JL, Champion S, et al. Chronic and acute effects of forskolin on isolated thyroid cell metabolism. Mol Cell Endocrinol 1985;43:41-50.

395   Roger PP, Servais P, Dumont JE. Regulation of dog thyroid epithelial cell cycle by forskolin, and adenylate cyclase activator. Exp Cell Res 1987;172:282-292.

396   Lindner, E., Dohadwalla, A.N., and Bhattacharya, B.K.: Positive inotropic and blood pressure lowering activity of a diterpene derivative isolated from Coleus forskohli: Forskolin. Arzneimittelforschung, 28(2):284-9, 1978.

397   Dubey, M.P., Srimal, R.C., Nityanand, S., et al.: Pharmacological studies on coleonol, a hypotensive diterpene from Coleus forskohlii. J. Ethnopharmacol., 3(1):1-13, 1981.

398   Kreider RB, et al. Effects of Coleus forskohlii supplementation on body composition and markers of health in sedentary overweight females. Experimental Biology 2002 Late Breaking Abstracts. LB305: 2002.

399   Hedin L, Rosberg S. Forskolin effects on the cAMP system and steroidogenesis in the immature rat ovary. Mol Cell Endocrinol. 1983 Nov;33(1):69-80.

400   Yoshizumi WM, Tsourounis C. Effects of creatine supplementation on renal function. J Herb Pharmacother. 2004;4(1):1-7. Review. PubMed PMID: 15273072.

401   Persky AM, Rawson ES. Safety of creatine supplementation. Subcell Biochem. 2007;46:275-89. Review.

402   Haeri MR, Izaddoost M, Ardekani MR, Nobar MR, White KN. The effect of fenugreek
        4-hydroxyisoleucine on liver function biomarkers and glucose in diabetic and fructose-fed rats.
        Phytother Res. 2009 Jan;23(1):61-4.

403   Jetté L, Harvey L, Eugeni K, Levens N. 4-Hydroxyisoleucine: a plant-derived treatment for metabolic
        syndrome. Curr Opin Investig Drugs. 2009 Apr;10(4):353-8. Review.

404   Narender T, Puri A, Shweta, Khaliq T, Saxena R, Bhatia G, Chandra R. 4-hydroxyisoleucine an
        unusual amino acid as antidyslipidemic and antihyperglycemic agent. Bioorg Med Chem Lett. 2006
        Jan 15;16(2):293-6. Epub 2005 Oct 21.

405   Broca C, Gross R, Petit P, Sauvaire Y, Manteghetti M, Tournier M, Masiello P, Gomis R, Ribes G.
        4-Hydroxyisoleucine: experimental evidence of its insulinotropic and antidiabetic properties. Am J
        Physiol. 1999 Oct;277(4 Pt 1):E617-23.

406   Gupta A, Gupta R, Lal B. Effect of Trigonella foenum-graecum (fenugreek) seeds on glycaemic
        control and insulin resistance in type II diabetes mellitus: a double blind placebo controlled study. J
        Assoc Physicians India 2001;49:1057–61.

407   Raghuram TC, Sharma RD, Sivakumar B, Sahay BK. Effect of fenugreek seeds on intravenous glucose
        disposition in non-insulin dependent diabetic patients. Phytother Res 1994;8(2):83–6.

408   Madar A, et. al. Glucose-lowering effect of fenugreek in non-insulin dependent diabetics. Eur J Clin
        Nutr 1988;42:51-54.

409   Sharma RD, Raghuram TC. Hypoglycemic effect of fenugreek seeds in non-insulin dependent
        diabetics subjects. Nutr Res 1990;10(7):731–9.

410   Gupta A et al., J Assoc Physicians India 2001: 49: pp 1057-1061.

411   Vuksan V, et.al. Reduction in postprandial glucose excursion and prolongation of satiety: possible
        explanation of the long-term effects of whole grain Salba (Salvia Hispanica L.). Eur J Clin Nutr. 2010
        Apr;64(4):436-8. Epub 2010 Jan 20.

412   Vuksan V, et.al. Supplementation of conventional therapy with the novel grain Salba (Salvia hispanica
        L.) improves major and emerging cardiovascular risk factors in type II diabetes: results of a randomized
        controlled trial. Diabetes Care. 2007 Nov;30(11):2804-10. Epub 2007 Aug 8.

413   Cusi, K, Defronzo, RA. Metformin: a review of its metabolic effects. Diabetes Reviews 1998. 6:89-
        131.

414   Bailey, CJ, Turner, RC. Metformin. N Engl J Med 1996. 334:574-579.

415   UKPDS GroupEffects of intensive blood-glucose control with metformin on complications in
        overweight patients with type II diabetes Lancet 1998. 352:854-865.

416   Cusi, K, Defronzo, RA. Metformin: a review of its metabolic effects. Diabetes Reviews 1998. 6:89-
        131.

417   Vitamin Research News 2001, 15(3): 4-5.

418   Palit P, Furman BL, Gray AI Novel weight-reducing activity of Galega officinalis in mice. J Pharm
        Pharmacol 1999, 51(11):1313-1319.

419   Changhong Li, Aron Allen, Jae Kwagh, Nicolai M. Doliba, Wei Qin, Habiba Najafi, Heather W. Collins,
        Franz M. Matschinsky, Charles A. Stanley, and Thomas J. Smith (2006). Green Tea Polyphenols
        Modulate Insulin Secretion by Inhibiting Glutamate Dehydrogenase. J. Biol. Chem., Vol. 281, Issue
        15, 10214-10221, April 14, 2006

420   W. Rumpler, J. Seale, B. Clevidence, et al (2001). Oolong tea increases metabolic rate and fat oxidation
        in men. Journal of Nutrition; 131: 2848-2852.

421   Duloo AG, Duret C, Rohrer D, Girardier L, Mensi N, Fathi M, Chantre P, Vandermander (1999).
        Efficacy of a green tea extract rich in catechin polyphenols and caffeine in increasing 24-h

energy expenditure and fat oxidation in humans. The American journal of clinical nutrition. 1999 Dec;70(6):1040-5.

422   Hursel, R. et. al. The effects of green tea on weight loss and weight maintenance: a meta-analysis. Int J Obes (Lond). 2009 Sep;33(9):956-61. Epub 2009 Jul 14.

423   Hill AM, et. al. Can EGCG reduce abdominal fat in obese subjects? J. Am. Col. Nutr. 2007 Aug;26(4):396S-402S.

424   Sasazuki S et all (2000). A relation between green tea consumption and severity of coronary atherosclerosis among Japanese men and women. Ann Epidemiol 10:401-408.

425   Chemical Research in Toxicology, vol 20, p 583.

426   Mead, Nathaniel. Diet and Nutrition: Temperance in Green Tea. Environ Health Perspect. 2007 September; 115(9): A445

427   R.A. Isbrucker, et. al. Safety Studies on EGCG preparations. Food and Chemical Toxicology. Vol 44, Issue 5, May 2006, Pages 636-650.

428   Kinghorn, A. Douglas; Compadre, César M. (2001). Less Common High Potency Sweeteners. In Nabors, Lyn O'Brien. Alternative Sweeteners. CRC Press. pp. 209⃞ 33.

429   Shanmugasundaram ER, Rajeswari G, Baskaran K, et al. Use of Gymnema sylvestre leaf in the control of blood glucose in insulin-dependent diabetes mellitus. J Ethnopharmacol 1990;30:281-294.

430   Baskaran K, Ahamath BK, Shanmugasundaram KR, Shanmugasundaram ER. Antidiabetic effect of a leaf extract from Gymnema sylvestre in non-insulin-dependent diabetes mellitus patients. J Ethnopharmacol 1990;30:295-305.

431   Sahu N., Mahato S.B., Sarkar S.K., Poddar G. Triterpenoid Saponins from Gymnema sylvestre. Phytochem. 1996;41:1181–1185.

432   Yoshikawa K., Kondo Y., Arihara S., Matsuura K. Antisweet natural products IX structures of gymnemic acids XV-XVIII from Gymnema sylvestre R. Br. Chem. Pharm. Bull. 1993;41:1730–1732.

433   Boigk G, Stroedter L, Herbst H, Waldschmidt J, Riecken EO, Schuppan D. Silymarin retards collagen accumulation in early and advanced biliary fibrosis secondary to complete bile duct obliteration in rats. Hepatology. 1997 Sep;26(3):643-9.

434   Deák G, Müzes G, Láng I, Niederland V, Nékám K, Gonzalez-Cabello R, Gergely P, Fehér J. [Immunomodulator effect of silymarin therapy in chronic alcoholic liver diseases]. Orv Hetil. 1990 Jun 17;131(24):1291-2, 1295-6. Review. Hungarian.

435   Muriel P, Mourelle M. Prevention by silymarin of membrane alterations in acute CCl4 liver damage. J Appl Toxicol. 1990 Aug;10(4):275-9.

436   Available: http://www.thorne.com/altmedrev/.fulltext/4/4/272.pdf

437   Bracesco N, et.al. "Antioxidant activity of a botanical extract preparation of Ilex paraguariensis: Prevention of DNA double-strand breaks in saccharomyces cerevisiae and human low-density lipoprotein oxidation." J Alt Com Med. 2003 Jun;9(3):379-87.

438   Filip, R. Antioxidant activity of Ilex paraguariensis and related species. Nutrition Research, Volume 20, Issue 10, Pages 1437-1446.

439   Kabat GC, O'Leary ES, Gammon MD, Sepkovic DW, Teitelbaum SL, Britton JA, Terry MB, Neugut AI, Bradlow HL. Estrogen metabolism and breast cancer. Epidemiology.2006 Jan;17(1):80-8.

440   Im A, Vogel VG, Ahrendt G, Lloyd S, Ragin C, Garte S, Taioli E. Urinary estrogen metabolites in women at high risk for breast cancer. Carcinogenesis. 2009 Sep;30(9):1532-5. Epub 2009 Jun 5.

441   Chan EK, Sepkovic DW, Yoo Bowne HJ, Yu GP, Schantz SP. A hormonal association between estrogen metabolism and proliferative thyroid disease. Otolaryngol Head Neck Surg. 2006 Jun;134(6):893-900

442   Bradlow, HL, et. al. 2-hydroyxgestone, The "good" estrogen. J Endocrinol 1996. Sep;150 Suppl 5259-65.

443   Bentz AT, Schneider CM, Westerlind KC. The relationship between physical activity and 2-hydroxyestrone, 16alpha-hydroxyestrone, and the 2/16 ratio in premenopausal women (United States). Cancer Causes Control. 2005 May;16(4):455-61.

444   Fowke, JH, et. al. Brassica vegetable consumption shifts healthy estrogen metabolism in postmenopausal women. Cancer Epidemiol Biomarkers Prev. 2000 Aug;9(8):773-9.

445   Vivar OI, Saunier EF, Leitman DC, Firestone GL, Bjeldanes LF. Selective activation of estrogen receptor-beta target genes by 3,3'-diindolylmethane. Endocrinology. 2010 Apr;151(4):1662-7. Epub 2010 Feb 16.

446   Mildred S. Seelig, MD, Burton M. Altura, PhD and Bella T. Altura, PhD. Benefits and Risks of Sex Hormone Replacement in Postmenopausal Women. Journal of the American College of Nutrition, Vol. 23, No. 5, 482S-496S (2004).

447   Kanadys WM, Leszczyńska-Gorzelak B, Oleszczuk J. [Efficacy and safety of Black cohosh (Actaea/Cimicifuga racemosa) in the treatment of vasomotor symptoms--review of clinical trials]. Ginekol Pol. 2008 Apr;79(4):287-96. Review. Polish.

448   Mahady GB, Fabricant D, Chadwick LR, Dietz B. Black cohosh: an alternative therapy for menopause? Nutr Clin Care. 2002 Nov-Dec;5(6):283-9. Review.

449   Mahady GB. Black cohosh (Actaea/Cimicifuga racemosa): review of the clinical data for safety and efficacy in menopausal symptoms. Treat Endocrinol. 2005;4(3):177-84. Review.

450   Wuttke W, Seidlova-Wuttke D, Gorkow C. The Cimicifuga preparation BNO 1055 vs. conjugated estrogens in a double-blind placebo-controlled study: effects on menopause symptoms and bone markers. Maturitas. 2003;44 (Suppl 1):S67–77.

451   Low Dog T, Powell KL, Weisman SM. Critical evaluation of the safety of Cimicifuga racemosa in menopause symptom relief. Menopause. 2003. Jul-Aug;10(4):299-313. Review.

452   Einer-Jensen N, Zhao J, Andersen KP, Kristoffersen K. Cimicifuga and Melbrosia lack oestrogenic effects in mice and rats. Maturitas. 1996;25:149–53.

453   Freudenstein J, Dasenbrock C, Nisslein T. Lack of promotion of estrogen-dependent mammary gland tumors in vivo by an isopropanolic Cimicifuga racemosa extract. Cancer Res. 2002;62:3448–52.

454   Seidlova-Wuttke D, Jarry H, Becker T, Christoffel V, Wuttke W. Pharmacology of Cimicifuga racemosa extract BNO 1055 in rats: bone, fat and uterus. Maturitas. 2003;44 (Suppl 1):S39–50.

455   Burdette JE, Liu J, Chen SN, et al. Black cohosh acts as a mixed competitive ligand and partial agonist of the serotonin receptor. J Agric Food Chem. 2003;51:5661–70.

456   Mahady GB. Is black cohosh estrogenic? Nutr Rev. 2003;61:183–6.

457   Tharakan B, Manyam BV. Botanical therapies in sexual dysfunction. Phytotherapy Research. 2005;19(6):457–463.

458   Hudson T. Maca: new insights on an ancient plant. Integrative Medicine: A Clinician's Journal. 2008;7(6):54–57.

459   McKay D. Nutrients and botanicals for erectile dysfunction: examining the evidence. Altern Med Rev. 2004 Mar;9(1):4-16.

460   Gonzales GF, Cordova A, Vega K, Chung A, Villena A, Gonez C, Castillo S. Effect of Lepidium meyenii (MACA) on sexual desire and its absent relationship with serum testosterone levels in adult healthy men. Andrologia. 2002;34(6):367–372.

461   Brooks NA, Wilcox G, Walker KZ, Ashton JF, Cox MB, Stojanovska L. Beneficial effects of Lepidium meyenii (Maca) on psychological symptoms and measures of sexual dysfunction in postmenopausal women are not related to estrogen or androgen content. Menopause. 2008;15(6):1157–1162.

462   Dording CM, Fisher L, Papakostas G, Farabaugh A, Sonawalla S, Fava M, Mischoulon D. A double-blind, randomized, pilot dose-finding study of maca root (L. meyenii) for the management of SSRI-induced sexual dysfunction. CNS Neurosci Ther. 2008;14(3):182–191.

463   Gonzales GF, Cordova A, Gonzales C, Chung A, Vega K, Villena A. Lepidium meyenii (Maca) improved semen parameters in adult men. Asian J Androl. 2001;3(4):301–303.

464   Gonzales GF, Cordova A, Vega K, Chung A, Villena A, Gonez C. Effect of Lepidium meyenii (Maca), a root with aphrodisiac and fertility-enhancing properties, on serum reproductive hormone levels in adult healthy men. J Endocrinol. 2003;176(1):163–168.

465   Brooks NA, Wilcox G, Walker KZ, Ashton JF, Cox MB, Stojanovska L. Beneficial effects of Lepidium meyenii (Maca) on psychological symptoms and measures of sexual dysfunction in postmenopausal women are not related to estrogen or androgen content. Menopause. 2008;15(6):1157–1162.

466   Zenico T, Cicero AF, Valmorri L, Mercuriali M, Bercovich E. Subjective effects of Lepidium meyenii (Maca) extract on well-being and sexual performances in patients with mild erectile dysfunction: a randomised, double-blind clinical trial. Andrologia. 2009;41(2):95–99.

467   MacConnie SE, Barkan A, Lampman RM, Schork MA, Beitins IZ, 1986 Decreased hypothalamic gonadotropin-releasing hormone secretion in male marathon runners. N Engl J Med 315: 411-417.

468   Luger A, Deuster PA, Kyle SB, et al, 1987 Acute hypothalamic-pituitary-adrenal responses to the stress of treadmill exercise. Physiologic adaptations to physical training. N Engl J Med 316: 1309-1315.

469   Tsigos C, Papanicolaou DA, Kyrou I, Raptis SA, Chrousos GP, 1999 Dose-dependent effects of recombinant human interleukin-6 on the pituitary-testicular axis. J Interferon Cytokine Res 19: 1271-1276.

470   Rabin DS, Schmidt PJ, Campbell G, Gold PW, Jensvold M, Rubinow DR, et al, 1990 Hypothalamic-pituitary-adrenal function in patients with the premenstrual syndrome. J Clin Endocrinol Metab 71: 1158-1162.

471   Rivier C, Rivier J, Vale W, 1986 Stress-induced inhibition of reproductive functions: role of endogenous corticotropin-releasing factor. Science 231: 607-609.

472   Adaikan PG, Srilatha B. Oestrogen-mediated hormonal imbalance precipitates erectile dysfunction. Int J Impot Res. 2003 Feb;15(1):38-43.

473   Rozati R, Reddy PP, Reddanna P, Mujtaba R. Role of environmental estrogens in the deterioration of male factor fertility. Fertil Steril. 2002 Dec;78(6):1187-94.

474   Ritchie JM, Vial SL, Fuortes LJ, Guo H, Reedy VE, Smith EM. Organochlorines and risk of prostate cancer. J Occup Environ Med. 2003 Jul;45(7):692-702.

475   Sharpe RM. The 'oestrogen hypothesis'- where do we stand now? Int J Androl. 2003 Feb;26(1):2-15. Review.

476   Schultheiss OC, Campbell KL, McClelland DC. Implicit power motivation moderates men's testosterone responses to imagined and real dominance success. Horm Behav. 1999 Dec;36(3):234-41.

477   Veldhuis JD, Iranmanesh A, Godschalk M, Mulligan T. 2000 Older men manifest multifold synchrony disruption of reproductive neurohormone outflow. J Clin Endocrinol Metab 85:1477–1486.

478   Schiavi RC, White D, Mandeli J 1992 Pituitary-gonadal function during sleep in healthy aging men. Psychoneuroendocrinology 17:599–609.

479   Hishkowitz M, Moore CA, O'Connor S, Beallamy M, Cunningham GR 1997 Androgen and sleep related erections. J Psychosomat Res 42:541–546.

480   Vingren JL, Kraemer WJ, Ratamess NA, Anderson JM, Volek JS, Maresh CM. Testosterone physiology in resistance exercise and training: the up-stream regulatory elements. Sports Med. 2010 Dec 1;40(12):1037-53.

481   Kraemer WJ, Ratamess NA. Hormonal responses and adaptations to resistance exercise and training. Sports Med. 2005;35(4):339-61. Review.

482   Gordon GG, Altman K, Southren AL, Rubin E, Lieber CS. Effect of alcohol (ethanol) administration on sex-hormone metabolism in normal men. N Engl J Med. 1976 Oct 7;295(15):793-7.

483   Rubin E, Lieber CS, Altman K, Gordon GG, Southren AL. Prolonged ethanol consumption increases testosterone metabolism in the liver. Science. 1976 Feb 13;191(4227):563-4.

484   Välimäki MJ, Härkönen M, Eriksson CJ, Ylikahri RH. Sex hormones and adrenocortical steroids in men acutely intoxicated with ethanol. Alcohol. 1984 Jan-Feb;1(1):89-93.

485   Iturriaga H, Lioi X, Valladares L. Sex hormone-binding globulin in non-cirrhotic alcoholic patients during early withdrawal and after longer abstinence. Alcohol. 1999 Nov-Dec;34(6):903-9.

486   O'Donnell AB, Araujo AB, McKinlay JB. The health of normally aging men: The Massachusetts Male Aging Study (1987-2004). Exp Gerontol. 2004 Jul;39(7):975-84. Review.

487   Infertility in the modern world: present and future prospects, Gillian R. Bentley,C. G. N. Mascie-Taylor, Cambridge University Press, p.99-100.

488   Assinder S, Davis R, Fenwick M, Glover A. Adult-only exposure of male rats to a diet of high phytoestrogen content increases apoptosis of meiotic and post-meiotic germ cells. Reproduction. 2007;133:11–9.

489   Sliwa L. [The influence of soybean riches of phytoestrogens diet in mouse testis histological structure] Folia Med Cracov. 2005;46:121–31.

490   Hamilton-Reeves JM, Vazquez G, Duval SJ, Phipps WR, Kurzer MS, Messina MJ (2010). "Clinical studies show no effects of soy protein or isoflavones on reproductive hormones in men: results of a meta-analysis". Fertil Steril. 94 (3): 997–1007.

491   Costello LC, Franklin RB. Zinc is decreased in prostate cancer: an established relationship of prostate cancer! J Biol Inorg Chem. 2011 Jan;16(1):3-8. Epub 2010 Dec 8. Review.

492   Bedwal RS, Bahuguna A. Zinc, copper and selenium in reproduction. Experientia. 1994 Jul 15;50(7):626-40. Review.

493   Om AS, Chung KW. Dietary zinc deficiency alters 5 alpha-reduction and aromatization of testosterone and androgen and estrogen receptors in rat liver. J Nutr. 1996 Apr;126(4):842-8.

494   Available: http://nutritiondata.self.com/facts/finfish-and-shellfish-products/4192/2

495   Sandstead HH. Requirements and toxicity of essential trace elements, illustrated by zinc and copper. Am J Clin Nutr. 1995;61(suppl 3):621S-624S.

496   Available: http://www.merckmanuals.com/professional/sec01/ch005/ch005j.html

497   Golik A, Zaidenstein R, Dishi V, et al. Effects of captopril and enalapril on zinc metabolism in hypertensive patients. J Am Coll Nutr. 1998;17:75-78.

498   Webb JL. Nutritional effects of oral contraceptive use: a review. J Reprod Med. 1980;25:150-156.

499   Reyes AJ, Olhaberry JV, Leary WP, et al. Urinary zinc excretion, diuretics, zinc deficiency and some side-effects of diuretics. S Afr Med J. 1983;64:936-941.

500   Sturniolo GC, Montino MC, Rossetto L, et al. Inhibition of gastric acid secretion reduces zinc absorption in man. J Am Coll Nutr. 1991;10:372-375.

501 Dawson-Hughes B, Seligson FH, Hughes VA. Effects of calcium carbonate and hydroxyapatite on zinc and iron retention in postmenopausal women. Am J Clin Nutr. 1986;44:83-88.

502 Spencer H, Kramer L, Norris C, et al. Effect of calcium and phosphorus on zinc metabolism in man. Am J Clin Nutr. 1984;40:1213-1218.

503 Tee TT, Cheah YH, Hawariah LP. F16, a fraction from Eurycoma longifolia jack extract, induces apoptosis via a caspase-9-independent manner in MCF-7 cells. Anticancer Res. 2007;27:3425–30.

504 Farouk AE, Benafri A. Antibacterial activity of Eurycoma longifolia Jack. A Malaysian medicinal plant. Saudi Med J. 2007;28:1422–4.

505 Chan KL, Choo CY, Abdullah NR, Ismail Z. Antiplasmodial studies of Eurycoma longifolia Jack using the lactate dehydrogenase assay of Plasmodium falciparum. J Ethnopharmacol. 2004;92:223–7.

506 Sholikhah EN, Wijayanti MA, Nurani LH, Mustofa Stage specificity of pasak bumi root (Eurycoma longifolia Jack) isolate on Plasmodium falciparum cycles. Med J Malaysia. 2008;63(Suppl A):98–9.

507 Chan KL, Low BS, Teh CH, Das PK. The effect of Eurycoma longifolia on sperm quality of male rats. Nat Prod Commun. 2009 Oct;4(10):1331-6.

508 Zanoli P, Zavatti M, Montanari C, Baraldi M. Influence of Eurycoma longifolia on the copulatory activity of sexually sluggish and impotent male rats. J Ethnopharmacol. 2009 Nov 12;126(2):308-13.

509 Wahab NA, Mokhtar NM, Halim WN, Das S. The effect of eurycoma longifolia Jack on spermatogenesis in estrogen-treated rats. Clinics (Sao Paulo). 2010;65(1):93-8.

510 Lie-Chwen Lin, et. al. Reinvestigation of the Chemical Constituents of Eurycoma longifolia. National Research Institute of Chinese Medicine, Shih-Pai, Taipei 112, Taiwan, R.O.C. Department of Physiology, National Yang-Ming University, Shih-Pai, Taipei 112, Taiwan, R.O.C. Received in March 2, 2001; Accepted in March 31, 2001. Available: http://jwc1.mc.ntu.edu.tw/cpj/Material/53-2/532097abs.htm

511 Hamzah S, Yusof A. The Ergogenic Effects of Eurycoma Longifolia Jack: A Pilot Study. Br J Sports Med. 2003;37:464–70.

512 Mullen JO, Juchau MR, Fouts JR. Studies of 3,4-benzpyrene, 3-methylcholanthrene, chlordane, and methyltestosterone as stimulators of hepatic microsomal enzyme systems in the rat. Biochem Pharmacol 1966; 15: 137–144.

513 Bird DR, Vowles KD. Liver damage from long-term methyltestosterone. Lancet 1977; 2: 400–401.

514 Bagheri SA, Boyer JL. Peliosis hepatis associated with androgenic-anabolic steroid therapy: a severe form of hepatic injury. Ann Intern Med 1974; 81: 610–618.

515 Stanczyk FZ, Paulson RJ, Roy S. Percutaneous administration of progesterone: blood levels and endometrial protection. Menopause. 2005 Mar;12(2):232-7. Review.

516 Lewis JG, McGill H, Patton VM, Elder PA. Caution on the use of saliva measurements to monitor absorption of progesterone from transdermal creams in postmenopausal women. Maturitas. 2002 Jan 30;41(1):1-6.

517 Benster B, Carey A, Wadsworth F, Vashisht A, Domoney C, Studd J. A double-blind placebo-controlled study to evaluate the effect of progestelle progesterone cream on postmenopausal women. Menopause Int. 2009 Jun;15(2):63-9.

518 Wren BG, Champion SM, Willetts K, Manga RZ, Eden JA. Transdermal progesterone and its effect on vasomotor symptoms, blood lipid levels, bone metabolic markers, moods, and quality of life for postmenopausal women. Menopause. 2003 Jan-Feb;10(1):13-8.

519 Lobo RA. Estrogen replacement: the evolving role of alternative delivery systems. Am J Obstet Gynecol 1995; 173:981

520 Christiansen C, Alexandersen P. Future management of HRT for the prevention and treatment of osteoporosis, state of the art. Presented at the IV European Congress on Menopause, Vienna, October 1997.

521 Stevenson JC, Cust MP, Gangar KF, et al. Effects of transdermal versus oral hormone replacement therapy on bone density in spine and proximal femur in postmenopausal women. Lancet 1990; 335:265–9.

522 Holtorf, Ken. "The Safety and Effectiveness of Bioidentical Hormone Replacement Therapy." Available: http://www.holtorfmed.com/nss-folder/pdf/BHRT-PGM-2009.pdf

523 Chlebowski RT, Anderson GL, Gass M, Lane DS, Aragaki AK, Kuller LH, Manson JE, Stefanick ML, Ockene J, Sarto GE, Johnson KC, Wactawski-Wende J, Ravdin PM, Schenken R, Hendrix SL, Rajkovic A, Rohan TE, Yasmeen S, Prentice RL; WHI Investigators. Estrogen plus progestin and breast cancer incidence and mortality in postmenopausal women. JAMA. 2010 Oct 20;304(15):1684-92.

524 Jose-Manuel Fernández-Real, et. al. Thyroid Function Is Intrinsically Linked to Insulin Sensitivity and Endothelium-Dependent Vasodilation in Healthy Euthyroid Subjects. The Journal of Clinical Endocrinology & Metabolism Vol. 91, No. 9 3337-3343.

525 Werner and Ingbar's The Thyroid. 7th ed. p 859.

526 Kazutosi, Nisizawa. 2002. Seaweeds Kaiso: Bountiful Harvest From the Seas. Sustenance for Health and Wellbeing.

527 Kazutosi, Nisizawa.2002. Seaweeds Kaiso: Bountiful Harvest from the Seas. Sustenance for Health and Wellbeing.

528 A Lanni, M Moreno, A Lombardi, and F Goglia. Calorigenic effect of diiodothyronines in the rat. J Physiol. 1996 August 1; 494(Pt 3): 831–837.

529 Moreno M, et. al. Metabolic effects of thyroid hormone derivatives. Thyroid. 2008 Feb;18(2):239-53.

530 The Effect Of Virgin Coconut Oil Supplementation For Community-Acquired Pneumonia In Children Aged 3 To 60 Months Admitted At The Philippine Children's Medical Center: A Single Blinded Randomized Controlled Trial, CHEST, October 29, 2008

531 In vitro antimicrobial properties of coconut oil on Candida species in Ibadan, Nigeria. J Med Food. 2007 Jun 10(2):384-7.

532 In vitro killing of Candida albicans by fatty acids and monoglycerides. Antimicrob Agents Chemother. 2001 Nov 45(11):3209-12.

533 Antimicrobial Activity of Saturated Fatty Acids and Fatty Amines against Methicillin-Resistant Staphylococcus aureus. Biological & Pharmaceutical Bulletin, Vol. 27 (2004) , No. 9 1321.

534 Inactivation of enveloped viruses and killing of cells by fatty acids and monoglycerides. Antimicrob Agents Chemother. 1987 Jan 31(1):27-31.

535 The role of coconut and coconut oil in coronary heart disease in Kerala, south India. Trop Doct. 1997 Oct 27(4):215-7.

536 Cholesterol, coconuts, and diet on Polynesian atolls: a natural experiment: the Pukapuka and Tokelau island studies. Am J Clin Nutr. 1981 Aug;34(8): 1552-61.

537 The Tokelau Island Migrant Study: serum lipid concentration in two environments. J Chronic Dis. 1981; 34(2-3):45-55.

538 Absorption of individual fatty acids from long chain or medium chain triglycerides in very small infants. Am J Clin Nutr. 1986 May;43(5): 745-51.

539 Medium-chain triglyceride feeding in premature infants: effects on calcium and magnesium absorption. Pediatrics. 1978 Apr;61(4): 537-45.

540   Menhaden, coconut, and corn oils and mammary tumor incidence in BALB/c virgin female mice treated with DMBA. Nutr Cancer. 1993; 20(2):99-106.

541   The influence of dietary medium chain triglycerides on rat mammary tumor development. Lipids 1987 Jun;22(6):455-61.

542   St-Onge MP, Jones PJ. Greater rise in fat oxidation with medium-chain triglyceride consumption relative to long-chain triglyceride is associated with lower initial body weight and greater loss of subcutaneous adipose tissue. Int J Obes Relat Metab Disord. 2003 Dec 27(12):1565-71.

543   Physiological effects of medium-chain triglycerides: potential agents in the prevention of obesity. J Nutr. 2002 Mar;132(3):329-32.

544   Medium- versus long-chain triglycerides for 27 days increases fat oxidation and energy expenditure without resulting in changes in body composition in overweight women. Int J Obes Relat Metab Disord. 2003 Jan;27(1):95-102.

545   Thermogenesis in humans during overfeeding with medium-chain triglycerides. Metabolism. 1989 Jul;38(7):641-8.

546   St-Onge, M.P., and Jones, P.J.H., 2002. Physiological effects of medium-chain triglycerides: potential agents in the prevention of obesity. Journal of Nutrition 132(3):329-332.

547   Fife, B., 2002. Eat Fat, Look Thin: A Safe and Natural Way to Lose Weight Permanently, Piccadilly Books, Ltd., Colorado Springs, CO.

548   Medical diagnostic x rays and thyroid cancer. J. Natl Cancer Inst.1995 Nov 1;87(21):1613-21.

549   R Gartner, et. al. Selenium supplementation in patients with autoimmune thyroiditis decrease thyroid peroxidase antibody concentrations. The Jour of Clin Endo & Metab, vol. 87; No, 4, 1687-1691.

550   Zimmermann MB, Köhrle J. The impact of iron and selenium deficiencies on iodine and thyroid metabolism: biochemistry and relevance to public health. Thyroid. 2002 Oct;12(10):867-78.

551   Kelly Barranger. Anemias. In: Arcangelo V, Peterson A, eds. Pharmacotherapeutics for Advanced Practice, A Practical Approach. Second Edition. Philadelphia, PA: Lippincott Williams and Wilkins; 2006:800.

552   Centers for Disease Control and Prevention. Recommendations to Prevent and Control Iron Deficiency in the United States. MWR 1998; 47(No. RR-3):1-29.

553   Tripathy, Y.B., et. al. Thyroid stimulating actions of guggulsterone obtained from Comiphora mukul. Planta medica. 1985, 78-80.

554   Panda S, Kar A. Guggul induces T3 production. Life Sci 1999;65 (12):137-41.

555   Tripathy, Y.B., Tripathy, P., Malhotra, O.P.and Tripathy, S.N. (1988) Thyroid stimulating action of (Z) guggulsterone. Mechanism of action. Planta Medica 271-276.

556   Owsley and Chiang. Guggulsterone antagonizes farnesoid X receptor induction of bile salt export pump but activates pregnane X receptor to inhibit cholesterol 7a-hydroxylase gene. Biochem.Biophys. Res.Comm. 2003. 304 191.

557   Burris, et al. The hypolipidemic natural product guggulsterone is a promiscuous steroid receptor ligand. Mol.Pharmacol. 2005. 67, 948.

558   Antonio J., Colker CM, Torina GC, et al. Effects of a Standardized Guggulsterone Phosphate Supplement on Body Composition in Overweight Adults: A Pilot Study. Current Therapeutic Research 1999; 60(4):220-227.

559   Lowe, J.C.: Comparative effects of Cynomel and Hypo Support Formula. Thyroid Science, 4(10):CR1-8, 2009.

560   Lowe, J.C.: Comparison of Cynomel and Hypo Support Formula: Their physiological effects. Thyroid Science, 4(3):CLS1-11, 2009.

561   FDA: Recalls and Field Corrections: Drugs—Class II, May 11, 2005. www.fda.gov/bbs/topics/ enforce/2005/ENF00899.html

562   Johnson, S.B.: Endogenous substance bioavailability and bioequivalence: levothyroxine sodium tablets, March 13, 2003. http://www.fda.gov/ohrms/dockets/ac/03/slides/3926S2_07_Johnson.ppt

563   Braverman and Utiger. Werner and Ingbar's The Thyroid: A Fundamental and Clinical Text. 7th Ed. 1996.

564   Kimball, O.O.: Clinical Hypothyroidism. Kentucky Med.. J., 31:488-495, 1933.

565   Wharton, G.B.: Unrecognized hypothyroidism. Canadian Med. Assoc. J., 40:371-376, 1939.

566   Barnes, B.: Basal temperature versus basal metabolism. J.A.M.A., 119:1072-1074, 1942.

567   Goglia et al. FEBS Letters. 452, 115-120 (1999).

568   Lombardi et al. Biochem J. 330, 521-526 (1998).

569   Moreno et al. Life Sciences. 62(26), 2369-2377 (1998).

570   Cimmino et al. J of Endocrinology. 149, 319-325 (1996).

571   Chung-Yau Lo, et. al. High prevalence of cyclooxygenase 2 expression in papillary thyroid carcinoma. European Journal of Endocrinology, Vol. 152, Issue 4, 545-550.

572   Kurylowicz A, et. al. The role of nuclear factor-kappa B in the development of autoimmune diseases: a link between genes and environment. Acta Biochem Pol 2008; 55(4): 629-47.

573   Manna SK, et. al. Resveratrol suppresses TNF-induced activation of nuclear transcription factors NF-kappa B, activator protein-1, and apoptosis: potential role of reactive oxygen intermediates and lipid peroxidation. J Immunol. 2000 Jun 15;164(12):6509-19.

574   Yumi Yamamoto and Richard B. Gaynor. Therapeutic potential of inhibition of the NF-ϰB pathway in the treatment of inflammation and cancer. J. Clin. Invest. 107(2): 135-142 (2001). doi:10.1172/ JCI11914.

575   Martínez-Flórez S, et. al. Quercetin attenuates nuclear factor-kappaB activation and nitric oxide production in interleukin-1beta-activated rat hepatocytes. J Nutr. 2005 Jun;135(6):1359-65.

576   Available: http://www.boswellin.com/research5.html

577   Szeto FL, Sun J, Kong J, Duan Y, Liao A, Madara JL, et al. Involvement of the vitamin D receptor in the regulation of NF-kappaB activity in fibroblasts. The Journal of steroid biochemistry and molecular biology 2007;103(3-5):563-6.

578   Harvey, R. Lycopus europaeus L. and Lycopus virginicus L.: A review of Scientific research. British Journal of Phytotherapy 4(20, 55-65) 1995.

579   Auf'mkolk M, Ingbar JC, Kubota K, et al. Extracts and auto-oxidized constituents of certain plants inhibit the receptor-binding and biological activity of Graves' immunoglobulins. Endocrin 1985;116:1687-93.

580   Auf'mkolk M, Ingbar JC, Kubota K, et al. Extracts and auto-oxidized constituents of certain plants inhibit the receptor-binding and the biological activity of Graves' immunoglobulins. Endocrinol 1985;116:1687-93.

581   Marcelle Pick, RNC, MDN, OB/GYN, NP. Are you wired and tired? Your Proven 30-day Program for overcoming adrenal fatigue and feeling fantastic again. Hay House, 2011.

582   Arroyo, CF, Med. Jou. and Rac., Jan 2, 1924. Cxix, pg. 25

583   Galbois A, Rudler M, Massard J, Fulla Y, Bennani A. Assessment of adrenal function in cirrhotic patients: salivary Cortisol should be preferred. J Hepatol. 2010 Jun;52(6):839-45. Epub 2010 Mar 15.

584   Thevenot T, Borot S, Remy-Martin A. Assessment of adrenal function in cirrhotic patients using concentration of serum-free and salivary Cortisol. Liver Int. 2011 Mar;31(3):425-433. Epub 2011 Jan 13.

585   Michael T Murray MD Joseph L Pizzorno ND. Encyclopedia Of Natural Medicine. Prima Publishing. 1998. Page 368.

586   Available: http://www.merriam-webster.com/dictionary/diet

587   Available: http://en.wikipedia.org/wiki/Immunoglobulin_G

588   Available: http://www.takemeaway.com/our-story

589   Mastorakos G, Pavlatou M, Diamanti-Kandarakis E, Chrousos GP. Exercise and the stress system. Hormones (Athens). 2005 Apr-Jun;4(2):73-89.

590   The Practice of Chinese Medicine: The Treatment of Diseases with Acupuncture and Chinese Herb, Giovanni Maciocia CAc(Nanjing).

591   Transcendental Meditation, mindfulness, and longevity: An experimental study with the elderly. Alexander, Charles N.; Langer, Ellen J.; Newman, Ronnie I.; Chandler, Howard M.; Davies, John L. Journal of Personality and Social Psychology, Vol 57(6), Dec 1989, 950-96

592   Chacko SA, Sul J, Song Y, Li X, LeBlanc J, You Y, Butch A, Liu S. Magnesium supplementation, metabolic and inflammatory markers, and global genomic and proteomic profiling: a randomized, double-blind, controlled, crossover trial in overweight individuals. J Clin Nutr. 2011 Feb;93(2):463-73. Epub 2010 Dec 15.

593   Siener R, Jahnen A, Hesse A. Bioavailability of magnesium from different pharmaceutical formulations. Urol Res. 2011 Apr;39(2):123-7. Epub 2010 Sep 23.

594   Ullmann Y, Klein Y, Savulescu D, Borovoi I, Egozi D, Gavish M, Nagler R. Salivary monitoring related to major surgery. Eur J Clin Invest. 2010 Dec;40(12):1074-80.

595   Padayatty SJ, Doppman JL, Chang R, Wang Y, Gill J, Papanicolaou DA, Levine M. Human adrenal glands secrete vitamin C in response to adrenocorticotrophic hormone. Am J Clin Nutr. 2007 Jul;86(1):145-9.

596   Available: http://en.wikipedia.org/wiki/Pantothenic_acid

597   Available: http://www.biochem.arizona.edu/classes/bioc460/summer/460web/lecture/metabolism/pdh-tca.pdf

598   Susan M. Webb, Manuel Puig-Domingo. Clinical Endocrinology Role of melatonin in health and disease. Volume 42, Issue 3, pages 221–234, March 1995.

599   Robert L Sack, et. al. Annals of Medicine Use of melatonin for sleep and circadian rhythm disorders 1998, Vol. 30, No. 1 , Pages 115-121.

600   I S Young, J V Woodside. Antioxidants in health and disease. J Clin Pathol 2001;54:176–186.

601   Schrauzer GN. J Am Coll Nutr. 2001 Feb;20(1):1-4. Nutritional selenium supplements: product types, quality, and safety.

602   RA Potmis, VK Nonavinakere, HR Rasekh, II. Effect of selenium (Se) on plasma ACTH,[beta]-endorphin, corticosterone and glucose in rat: influence of adrenal enucleation and metyrapone pretreatment. Early Toxicology, 1993.

603   Miao-Lin Hua, Hee Poh Nga. Dietary selenium and vitamin E affect adrenal and brain dehydroepiandrosterone levels in young rats. J. of Nutritional Biochemistry 1998.

604   Souci SW, Fachmann E, Kraut H (2008). Food Composition and Nutrition Tables. Medpharm Scientific Publishers Stuttgart.

605   Hirayama S, Masuda Y, Rabeler R (). Effect of phosphatidylserine administration on symptoms of attention-deficit/hyperactivity disorder in children. Agro Food 17 (5): 32–36. September/October 2006. Available: http://www.lipamin-ps.com/ftp/agro_16_20.pdf.

606   Available: http://www.nal.usda.gov/fnic/foodcomp/search

607   Merck Index, 14th Edition, p.1327. Published by Merck & Co. Inc.

608   Meikle AW, Tyler FH. Potency and duration of action of glucocorticoids. Effects of hydrocortisone, prednisone and dexamethasone on human pituitary-adrenal function. Am J Med. 1977 Aug;63(2):200-7.

609   William McK. Jeffries. Safe Uses of Cortisol. Charles C. Thomas Publishing Ltd. 2004. 3rd Edition.

610   Roberts AD, Charler ML, Papadopoulos A, Wessely S, Chalder T, Cleare AJ. Does hypocortisolism predict a poor response to cognitive behavioural therapy in chronic fatigue syndrome? Psychol Med. 2010 Mar;40(3):515-22.

611   Cleare A et al. Hypothalamo-Pituitary-Adrenal Axis Dysfunction in Chronic Fatigue Syndrome, and the Effects of Low-Dose Hydrocortisone Therapy. The Journal of Clinical Endocrinology & Metabolism 2001. 86(8):3545–3554.

612   Cleare AJ et al. Low-dose hydrocortisone in chronic fatigue syndrome: a randomized crossover trial. Lancet 1999 Feb 6;353(9151):455.

613   Gaab J, Huster D, Peisen R, Engert V, Schad T, Schurmeyer TH, Ehlert U. Low-dose dexamethasone suppression test in chronic fatigue syndrome and health. Psychosom Med. 2002 Mar-Apr;64(2):311-8.

614   Cleare AJ; Bearn J; Allain T; McGregor A; Wessely S; Murray RM; O'Keane V. Contrasting neuroendocrine responses in depression and chronic fatigue syndrome, J Affect Disord, 1995 Aug 18, Issue: 4 Volume: 34 Page: 283-9.

615   Jefferies W. Cortisol and Immunity. Medical Hypotheses 1991;34:198-208.

616   Teitelbaum J, Bird B, Greenfield R, Weiss A, Muenz L, Gould L. Effective Treatment of Chronic Fatigue Syndrome (CFIDS) & Fibromyalgia (FMS) - A Randomized, Double-Blind, Placebo-Controlled, Intent To Treat Study. Journal of Chronic Fatigue Syndrome Volume 8, Issue 2 – 2001.

617   Available: http://cms.herbalgram.org/herbclip/077/review41425.html

618   Chen R , Yuan C . China Journal of Chinese Materia Medica . 1991 ; 16 (10): 617-619.

619   Yasue H , Itoh T , Mizuno Y , Harada E . Severe hypokalemia, rhabdomyolysis, muscle paralysis, and respiratory impairment in a hypertensive patient taking herbal medicines containing licorice . Intern Med . 2007 ; 46 (9): 575-578.

620   Quinkler M , Stewart PM . Hypertension and the cortisol-cortisone shuttle . J Clin Endocrinol Metab . 2003 ; 88 (6): 2384-2392

621   Journal of Ethnopharmacology Volume 71, Issues 1-2, July 2000, Pages 193-200 Immunomodulatory activity of Withania somniferaLeemol Davisa and Girija Kuttan.

622   Available: http://www.drugs.com/npp/ashwaganda.html#ref5

623   Available: http://bearmedicineherbals.com/nettle-seed-as-adrenal-trophorestorative-adaptogen.html

624   Zhao J, Nakamura N, Hattori M, Kuboyama T, Tohda C, Komatsu K. Withanolide derivatives from the roots of Withania somnifera and their neurite outgrowth activities. Chem Pharm Bull (Tokyo) . 2002;50(6):760-765.

625   Cooley K, Szczurko O, Perri D, et al. (2009). Naturopathic care for anxiety: a randomized controlled trial ISRCTN78958974. PLoS ONE 4 (8): e6628.

626   Available: http://www.herbaltransitions.com/materiamedica/Withania.htm

627   Available: http://www.statehealthfacts.org/profileind.jsp?cat=5&rgn=4&sub=66

628   Prometrium Description. Available: http://www.rxlist.com/cgi/generic/progesterone.htm

629   Gardner, Amanda. HRT Debate Not Over Yet: Experts say treatment still has value despite latest finding on link to breast cancer. Available: http://health.msn.com/centers/breastcancer/ArticlePage. aspx?cp-documentid=100150987

630   Kenyon AT, et al. Endocrinology (1938) 23 135.

631   Breast Cancer Action. Newsletter #20 October 2003. Available: http://www.bcaction.org/Pages/ SearchablePages/1993Newsletters/Newsletter020B.html

632   Salmon U, et. al.: Use of estradiol subcutaneous pellet in humans. Scienc 1939, 90:162.

633   Women's Health Initiative Participant Website. Available: http://www.whi.org/

634   Tutera, Gino. Marked Reduction of Breast, Endometrial, and Ovarian Cancer in Users of Bio-Identical Estradiol and Testosterone Subcutaneous Pellets.

635   Veurink M, Koster M, Berg LT. The history of DES, lessons to be learned. Pharm World Sci. 2005 Jun;27(3):139-43. Review.

636   National Cancer Institute. DES Research Update 1999: Current Knowledge, Future Directions. National Cancer Institute, 1999. (30% incr br ca risk in women using des during preg).

637   Smith, R NJ; Studd, J. WW. British Journal of Hospital Medicine. "Recent Advances in Hormone Replacement Therapy. 1993.

638   The United States Pharmacopeia: The National Formulary. 2007 edition. Volume 1: 511-14.

639   Pharmacy Compounding Subject to Pharmacy Approval: The facts don't fit. Available: http://www. iacprx.org/site/PageServer?pagename=P2C2_FactsDontFit

640   Compounding in the News: Midland Ruling. Available: http://www.iacprx.org/site/ PageServer?pagename=Comp_News_P2C2

641   Available: http://compoundingtoday.com/FDA/FDAPre1938Drugs.cfm

642   Lazarou J, Pomeranz BH, Corey PN. Incidence of adverse drug reactions in hospitalized patients: a meta-analysis of prospective studies. JAMA. 1998 Apr 15;279(15):1200-5.

643   Suh DC , Woodall BS, Shin SK , Hermes-De Santis ER. Clinical and economic impact of adverse drug reactions in hospitalized patients. Ann Pharmacother. 2000 Dec;34(12):1373-9.